Nurses' Guide to Teaching Diabetes Self-Management

Second Edition

Rita Girouard Mertig, MS, RNC, CNS, DE

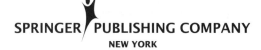

SPRINGER PUBLISHING COMPANY
NEW YORK

Springer Publishing Company, LLC
11 West 42nd Street
New York, NY 10036
www.springerpub.com

Acquisitions Editor: Margaret Zuccarini
Composition: S4Carlisle Publishing Services

ISBN: 978-0-8261-0827-2
E-book ISBN: 978-0-8261-0828-9

11 12 13/ 5 4 3 2 1

The author and the publisher of this Work have made every effort to use sources believed to be reliable to provide information that is accurate and compatible with the standards generally accepted at the time of publication. Because medical science is continually advancing, our knowledge base continues to expand. Therefore, as new information becomes available, changes in procedures become necessary. We recommend that the reader always consult current research and specific institutional policies before performing any clinical procedure. The author and publisher shall not be liable for any special, consequential, or exemplary damages resulting, in whole or in part, from the readers' use of, or reliance on, the information contained in this book. The publisher has no responsibility for the persistence or accuracy of URLs for external or third-party Internet websites referred to in this publication and does not guarantee that any content on such websites is, or will remain, accurate or appropriate.

Library of Congress Cataloging-in-Publication Data
Mertig, Rita G.
    Nurses' guide to teaching diabetes self-management/Rita Girouard Mertig. —2nd ed.
        p. ; cm.
    Includes bibliographical references and index.
    ISBN-13: 978-0-8261-0827-2
    ISBN-10: 0-8261-0827-X
    ISBN-13: 978-0-8261-0828-9 (E-book)
    I. Title.
    [DNLM: 1. Diabetes Mellitus—therapy—Nurses' Instruction.   2. Patient Education as Topic—Nurses' Instruction.   3. Diabetes Mellitus—psychology—Nurses' Instruction.   4. Nurse-Patient Relations—Nurses' Instruction.   5. Self Care—psychology—Nurses' Instruction. WK 850]
    616.4′620231—dc23
                                                                                    2011036750

Printed in the United States of America by Hamilton Printing

Nurses' Guide to Teaching Diabetes Self-Management

Rita Girouard Mertig, MS, RNC, CNS, DE, received her BSN from Georgetown University (1966), an MS from the University of California San Francisco (1969), and an MS from the Adult Nurse Practitioner Program at Virginia Commonwealth University, Medical College of Virginia. She received certification in RNC Maternal-Newborn Nursing in 1997 and as a Clinical Nurse Specialist in 1998. She taught nursing for more than 22 years, most recently at John Tyler Community College in Chester, Virginia, where she taught maternity nursing, pediatric nursing, and psychiatric mental health nursing along with nutrition and test-taking skills. Since 1986 she has given seminars on diabetes to various groups, ranging from the lay public to students and professional nurses (in 1989 she won the ADA, Virginia Affiliate "Diabetes Educator of the Year"). Ms. Mertig is a Certified Childbirth Educator and a member of the American Association of Diabetes Educators, the Association of Women's Health, Obstetric and Neonatal Nurses, and Sigma Theta Tau. In addition to writing chapters in nursing fundamentals textbooks, she is the author of *Teaching Nursing in an Associate Degree Program* (published by Springer Publishing Company in 2003).

This book is dedicated to my husband, Bob, and our adult children, Karen and Kelley, and also to the many former nursing students, now registered nurses, who gave me the inspiration to write the first edition of this book. This second edition is also dedicated to you.

Contents

Preface

When life hands you a lemon, make lemonade.

When I was in nursing school learning about diabetes mellitus and all of its complications, I decided that if I had diabetes I would never have children. I thought it was a horrible legacy to pass on to future generations. When I was diagnosed with diabetes in my late 30s, I already had children and the guilt I experienced was enormous. I also went through all of Dr. Elisabeth Kübler-Ross's "stages of grief" (denial, anger, bargaining, depression, and acceptance). They are as pertinent to loss of perceived health as they are to loss of a body part or of life itself when a terminal diagnosis is given. The plans I had made for my life, my family, and my career would never be realized. Not me! I wasted 3 months of my life in denial, eating very few carbohydrates, exercising after every meal, and seeing another physician for an alternative diagnosis, all to no avail. I was also angry at everyone I knew who smoked, was overweight, or who did not exercise, and I was very angry with God. Why me? I took care of my body and look at the thanks I got.

When I finally decided that "yes, it is me, but … ," the bargaining began. OK, as long as I don't have to take insulin, I can manage life with diabetes. Meanwhile, I was reading everything I could get my hands on and asking my physician a million questions. This was back in the days before widespread use of glucose monitors. Human insulin had just come on the market, and the only oral hypoglycemic drugs were first-generation sulfonylureas, such as Orinase, Tolinase, and Diabinese, drugs that are rarely used today. When two tablets of Diabinese, a maximum dose, failed to decrease my blood sugar, I was put on insulin. I gave myself my first shot of insulin in the examination room under the supervision of a nurse. I did it perfectly, having given many injections to others during my nursing career. I had also taught and supervised many student nurses giving injections for several years. However, after this first injection, I cried for 20 to 30 minutes. It didn't hurt, but my denial was over. I could no longer pretend my diabetes pills were vitamins. My bargaining had failed. I did have diabetes and would be giving myself insulin injections for the rest of my probably shortened life. It might also mean I'd be on dialysis, perhaps blind and missing a few toes, or worse, before I finally died. To put it mildly, I was very depressed.

I don't know what helped me to turn my attitude around, to finally accept my fate and work at making the best of what I considered to be a dismal future. Maybe it was the hope I received from all of my research about diabetes management. Maybe it was my husband's faith in my ability to overcome adversity. Another factor that helped me to come to grips with this diagnosis was that I had to be a positive role model for my children just in case I had passed on this hereditary disease. I had to demonstrate that there was "life after diagnosis."

I have detailed my coming to terms with this disease to help nurses and other healthcare professionals who read this book to understand how the grieving process applies to a diagnosis of a chronic illness such as diabetes, the emotional and physical impact of such a turn of events, and the enormous energy it takes to achieve acceptance so as to work toward the best possible outcome. Please remember my story when you read Chapter 12 on client noncompliance.

To those readers who share my diagnosis, I hope you recognize some of your own struggles in my tale and know that you are not alone. The more you share your own feeling and fears, the faster you will move toward acceptance and the better you will be able to work toward achieving the most positive state of wellness possible.

I have been attempting to write this book for years. My first draft started out as a chronological account of my life with diabetes. Such chapters as "Life after Diagnosis" and "Six Months and Counting" helped me to deal with what I was experiencing and how I was evolving as a person. This was more of a journal than the book that you now have in your hands. Several years ago, as I was becoming an "expert" on the subject, I started to write about the new research in diabetes management: new medication and insulins, new dietary guidelines, and therapies on the horizons. I gave these handouts to my students so that they could be aware of and look forward to the implementation of cutting-edge technology for diabetes management. Each year I added more and more to the list as research on diabetes escalated. My original 2-page handout grew to 10 pages, even though I moved some of the items into my lecture because they were now standards of care. That project alone was very empowering to me and to my students, who were in the process of becoming tomorrow's nurses. As I shared this handout with those who attended my support group for diabetics, I hoped they, too, were encouraged by the giant leaps forward in the management of their condition.

The second edition of this book is written for all of the healthcare professionals who interact with clients who have diabetes and not just for nurses. I realize that as a dietician, a physical or occupational therapist, a social worker, or a pharmacist, you want to help people with diabetes to control their disease. You may or may not know a lot of information that might help you to do that. In Part I of this book I have included many specifics about diabetes that might help you see the big picture and get a better understanding of all of the ins and outs of living with this condition. But it is the information in Part II that will help you to put it all together with regard to a particular individual. Giving canned "speeches" probably will only serve to anger people and convince them that you really do not understand their particular situation. Experimenting with the many teaching and motivating techniques used in the various chapters will expand your repertoire. "Same old, same old" speeches about diabetes will become "assessment and implementation" of an individualized approach to helping each person with diabetes apply self-management skills. This should be very empowering for both of you.

The other new aspect of this second edition is the addition of a chapter on chronic complications. This is a chapter I could not have written five years ago because I feared these complications. After living with type 1 diabetes for 25 years, I am now experiencing some of these complications. My attitude toward them has changed. Instead of viewing them as a failure of blood sugar control or, worse, as a punishment for not being perfect, I see them as another challenge to overcome. No one should think of chronic complications as inevitable. However, there are so many treatments for each that if any should arise, it is not the end of the world. As with diabetes, early detection and treatment are what matters. On the other hand, chronic complications should never be used as a threat to force a client to be "compliant." This strategy does not work.

Other additions to this edition include greatly expanded nutrition and exercise chapters, as well as updates in all of the other chapters. Teaching and motivating clients to want to control blood sugars by monitoring what they eat and include exercise in their daily life is a hard sell if you don't make it real for them. That means you have to figure out what is important to them and "make them an offer they can't refuse."

Acknowledgment

I would like to thank in a special way Dr. James Combs of the Virginia Eye Institute, my ophthalmologist and retinal specialist, for all of his encouragement in writing this second edition. His help in editing the part about visual complications related to diabetes is also greatly appreciated.

Thanks also to Dr. Scott Vantre of Virginia Foot and Ankle Center, my podiatrist, who also has been very supportive and helpful in the material concerning diabetic foot and ankle complications.

To Rosanne Ostrowski, my massage therapist, thanks for being my go-to person when I need to vent and talk about what diabetes means in my life. I always feel so much better physically and mentally after my appointment.

To the clients who come to my diabetes and weight management class at CrossOver Ministries Clinic, thanks for letting me be a part of your life and for sharing your stories with me.

Thanks also to Margaret Zuccarini, Nursing Publisher at Springer Publishing Company, for all your encouragement and understanding of my request for delays due to problems with my vision.

Rita Girouard Mertig

PART I

The Diabetes Conundrum

What is in a name? Well, as it turns out, quite a bit. The American Diabetes Association has been reclassifying and renaming the types of diabetes over the years as more is understood about the pathology and etiology of each. A major effort was made in 1997 to get rid of old and misleading nomenclature. *Type 1 diabetes* is no longer called *juvenile onset diabetes* because people like me are being diagnosed in their 40s and older. Likewise, *type 2 diabetes* is not thought of as just *adult onset diabetes* because obese children as young as 4 years old meet the criteria. Also, treatment with insulin is not the deciding factor between type 1 and type 2 diabetes, because insulin is but one of the many medications appropriately used to treat persons with type 2 diabetes. In this second edition I include more about prediabetes and have added LADA (latent autoimmune diabetes in adults) to expand on what used to be called type 1.5 diabetes.

What we all must focus on is the very distinct pathology differentiating the two main forms of diabetes, type 1 and type 2. We must continually remain as updated and current as possible. Why is this important? Knowing what kind of diabetes a person has will help a healthcare professional to anticipate problems, use strategies to prevent these complications, troubleshoot to decide what is going on, and apply correct interventions. For instance, a person with type 1 diabetes is more prone to rapid changes in blood sugar than someone with type 2 diabetes. A client with type 2 who is taking insulin or an oral medication that increases production of insulin is more likely to experience a low blood sugar than someone who is controlled by diet and exercise or by an oral agent that increases tissue sensitivity to the insulin.

Chapters 1 through 5 of this book explore the ins and outs of diabetes so that healthcare practitioners and clients will understand, in more depth, what is currently known about this mystifying disease. Before nurses and other healthcare professionals can teach clients how to live with diabetes, they must first understand the ramifications of each type of diabetes diagnosed.

Chapter 6 covers chronic complications that may not ever happen. Effective blood sugar control over the years can postpone or prevent their occurrence, but knowing the symptoms can catch them early if they do occur. Asking a client with diabetes about some of these symptoms should be part of the care given by any healthcare professional and will increase the likelihood that they will be diagnosed and treated early.

ONE

Diabetes: The Basics

Forewarned, forearmed; to be prepared is half the victory.
—Miguel de Cervantes

Diabetes mellitus is a group of metabolic diseases characterized by hyperglycemia resulting from defects in insulin secretion, insulin action, or both. The chronic hyperglycemia of diabetes is associated with long-term damage, dysfunction, and failure of different organs, especially the eyes, kidneys, nerves, heart, and blood vessels (American Diabetes Association [ADA], 2011, p. S62).

In fall 2010, the Centers for Disease Control and Prevention (CDC) estimated that 25.8 million, up from 20.8 million in 2005, adults over 20 years of age in the United States, or 8.3% of the population, have *diabetes mellitus*. Of this number, 18.8 million are diagnosed, thus leaving 7.0 million, or 27% of the total, as yet undiagnosed. If current trends continue, the CDC estimates that as many as one in three adults in the United States could have diabetes by 2050. This is because the population as a whole is aging, an increase in minority groups with a high risk for type 2 diabetes is expected, and people with diabetes are living longer (National Diabetes Information Clearinghouse [NDIC], 2011). Therefore, it is imperative that all healthcare professionals be prepared to help this population by learning as much as possible about all of the aspects of this disease and how to teach diabetes self-management.

Prior to the 1997 changes made in the diagnostic criteria, it was once estimated that half of all persons with diabetes did not know they had the disease. The 1997 ADA diagnostic and classification criteria lowered the fasting blood sugar requirement from 140 mg/dl (milligrams per deciliter) to 126 mg/dl, resulting in many more people being diagnosed and treated. The goal was to identify and treat as many persons as possible to prevent long-term complications; what one does not know can and will hurt a person. Healthcare professionals should apply this concept to their own lives and impart it to clients who have or are at risk for diabetes.

HOW INSULIN WORKS

Diabetes was first recognized 2,000 years ago in ancient Greece, but it was not until 1909 that insulin was identified as the bodily substance that controlled blood glucose levels. It took another decade before this substance was distilled from the pancreas of a dog and purified for injection into humans.

Insulin is a protein and a hormone secreted by the beta cells found throughout the pancreas. When blood sugar rises after a meal, insulin is secreted to help glucose (blood sugar) move into the cells of the body to be used as fuel. If there is more glucose than needed for cellular energy, insulin helps sugar to fill storage places in the liver and skeletal muscles for later use. Glucose is stored there as *glycogen*. When the amount of glucose in the blood exceeds these two needs, the rest is stored in fat cells, causing weight gain. Another role for insulin is to prevent inappropriate release of glycogen from the liver when it is not needed. In other words, blood glucose levels are not dropping. However, if blood sugar levels drop due to, for example, prolonged exercise or a skipped meal, another pancreatic hormone, *glucagon*, is secreted to allow the stored glycogen to be released from the liver (Figure 1.1) to maintain normal blood glucose levels. This is very important because the cells of the brain and nervous system only burn glucose for energy. The rest of the body can function by burning fat and protein for energy in the absence of blood glucose, but the brain cannot.

The beta cells that produce insulin and the alpha cells that produce glucagon are part of the islets of Langerhans that are scattered throughout the pancreas. This fact is important to remember as you read at the end of this chapter about the new islet cell transplantation procedure being used to reverse type 1 diabetes. Another important fact to remember is that in

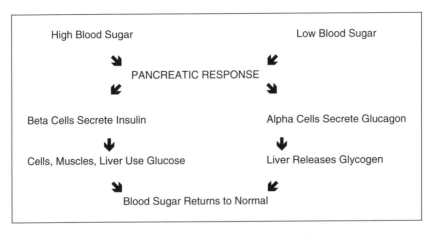

FIGURE 1.1 How the Pancreas Regulates Blood Sugar

a normal pancreas, only approximately one-fourth of the beta cells are needed to keep blood sugar levels within normal range. The other three-fourths of the cells may be called upon when more insulin is needed—for example, when blood glucose load is high, when excessive weight makes cells insulin resistant, when stress and other hormones increase the release of stored glycogen, or when the body is fighting an infection or other physical condition such as an injury or pregnancy. Only when the need for insulin outstrips the supply does blood sugar level rise.

CLASSIFICATION OF DIABETES

The pathology that causes each type of diabetes is very different, which should explain why a person with type 2 diabetes cannot become a person with type 1 simply because insulin is prescribed to control blood sugar. (See Table 1.1 for differences.)

Type 1 diabetes is an autoimmune disease in which the body's own immune system attacks and destroys the beta cells of the pancreas. Thus, in a short span of time, from weeks to a few months, the body does not even have the one-fourth of beta cells functioning to prevent a rise in blood sugar. These are not the clients who live for years with undiagnosed diabetes. Clients with type 1 diabetes are diagnosed relatively quickly due to the symptoms of a potentially life-threatening *ketoacidosis*. When the body ceases to produce sufficient insulin, the cells are starved of their preferred fuel, glucose. The body then begins to burn fat and then protein for energy. The breakdown of fat produces fatty acids and ketones that begin to poison the body. Burning fat and protein reduces fat and lean muscle mass, causing life-threatening weight loss. The body is literally wasting away because the cells have no way of getting to the ever-rising sugar in the blood without insulin to transport it past the cell wall. And as if that was not bad enough, the high blood glucose level increases the concentration of the blood so water is pulled from cells and *interstitial fluid* (fluid around the cells) to dilute the sugar concentration in the blood. Kidneys then excrete some of the excess sugar and water as very sweet urine (*glycosuria*). Without injections of insulin, the body and its cells become very dehydrated, to the point of multiorgan failure. Prior to the discovery of insulin in the 1920s, all children with this disease died. Today, persons with type 1 diabetes account for only 5% to 10% of those with diabetes, and with lifestyle modifications, blood sugar control, and insulin injections, they can live long, productive lives.

Type 2 diabetes, on the other hand, stems from cellular insulin resistance, an insufficient amount of insulin to overcome this resistance, or a production of insulin that the body cannot use efficiently. For many it is a combination of all three factors. Insulin resistance is often found in persons who are overweight or obese. Those obese persons who have not inherited the genes for type 2 diabetes simply produce a large amount

TABLE 1.1
Diabetes Classifications

	CAUSE	FASTING BLOOD SUGAR/A1C	HEREDITY AGE AT DIAGNOSIS	INSULIN PRODUCTION
Normal		70–99 mg/dl/4%–5.6%		Normal
Prediabetes	Decreased insulin sensitivity	100–125 mg/dl/5.7%–6.4%	Very strong Adult	Increased production
Type 1	Autoimmune destruction of beta cells	≥126 mg/dl ≥6.5%	Not common Youth/adult	Very little to none
LADA	Autoimmune destruction of beta cells	≥126 mg/dl ≥6.5%	Not common Adult >25 yr	Decreasing to none within a few years
MODY	Insulin resistance	≥126 mg/dl ≥6.5%	Very strong Youth <25 yr	Insufficient
Type 2	Insulin resistance, inadequate amount of insulin	≥126 mg/dl ≥6.5%	Very strong Adult	Increased then decreased
Gestational diabetes	Pancreatic hormones cause insulin resistance, insufficient insulin	Abnormal 2-hr OGTT @ 24–28 wk	Very strong	Increased but insufficient
Other: pancreatitis, pancreatic and other cancers, drugs (steroids, diuretics, antirejection medications, HIV/AIDS medications)	Abnormal production of hormones causing insulin resistance	≥126 mg/dl ≥6.5%	Sometimes	Decreased to none if pancreas is removed

of insulin to overcome this resistance and maintain normal blood sugar levels. When type 2 diabetes "runs in the family," weight gain often results in a diagnosis. According to Christopher Saudek and Simeon Margolis, "About 80% of people with type 2 diabetes are overweight or obese, and the risk of type 2 diabetes rises as a person's weight increases" (Saudek & Margolis, 2011, p. 7). Because this form of diabetes has a strong genetic component, the population at risk for developing type 2 diabetes includes members of the following ethnic groups:

- African Americans
- Asian Americans
- Pacific Islanders, such as Hawaiians and Filipinos
- Native Americans (American Indians)
- Mexican Americans

In addition, all overweight and obese individuals have an increased risk of developing the metabolic syndrome, the components of which include obesity, dyslipidemia (low high-density lipoprotein [HDL] levels and high triglyceride levels), hypertension, and insulin resistance. This syndrome affects at least one of every five overweight people and increases their risk of being diagnosed with type 2 diabetes (Saudek & Margolis, 2011). If those who are experiencing any of these components and are concerned that they might be developing type 2 diabetes, they can check to see what their risk is of developing type 2 in the next 5 years. The *PreDx Diabetes Risk Score test*, developed by Tethys Bioscience, measures seven biomarkers (chemical measurements of biological processes underlying type 2 diabetes) and calculates a prediagnosis risk score. It must be ordered by a healthcare professional. To learn more about this test, go to http://predxdiabetes.com.

CLINICAL EXAMPLE: Anyone with type 2 diabetes is at high risk for developing heart disease, hypertension, stroke, blood vessel problems leading to amputation, vision problems, kidney disease, and nervous system difficulties. Type 2 diabetes is much more than just a "touch of sugar." It is as serious a disease as type 1 diabetes, and individuals with type 2 diabetes need to make the same concerted effort to eat healthy foods and lose weight, increase activity level, and control blood sugar with medication, if needed.

In Table 1.1, LADA is listed after type 1 diabetes. Type 1 is most often diagnosed in children, adolescents, and young adults after some kind of environmental factor, such as a virus or other illness triggers the immune system to attack and destroy the insulin-producing beta cells of the pancreas. This destruction is rapid and the resulting symptomatic hyperglycemia occurs within weeks to months. The person affected with LADA is usually over 25 years of age and experiences this beta cell destruction much more gradually over a period of a few years. This group of people are usually thin or of normal weight, do not have a family history of diabetes, and are not insulin resistant. They are often misdiagnosed as having type 2 diabetes and are prescribed oral hypoglycemic agents. These agents may work for a short time but soon fail to control blood sugar levels. There is some evidence that if these individuals are given insulin at diagnosis, the beta cell destruction may be halted (Gebel, 2010b). Because this is an autoimmune phenomenon like type 1 diabetes, they need insulin injections for life as well. Because of my history of periodic hyperglycemia over a 5-year period, this is probably what I have experienced.

Maturity-onset diabetes of the young (MODY), on the other hand, is a rare form of diabetes caused by a single aberrant gene, a group of which regulates the flow of insulin. This decreases the pancreas' ability to make sufficient insulin. Most forms of MODY are inheritable dominant (only one affected parent is needed to pass on the disease) genetic defects, which affect those under 25 years of age. Persons diagnosed with MODY are usually not overweight and do not exhibit other risk factors for type 2 diabetes, such as hypertension and dyslipidemia (Gebel, 2010a). This condition is often controlled with oral agents and sometimes insulin. These clients still produce insulin but often may need insulin injections to normalize blood glucose as do some clients with type 2 diabetes. It is important and now possible to conduct DNA tests on saliva for this mutant gene so that the most appropriate treatment can be used to control blood sugar for these individuals. Genetic testing should also be performed with family members and can be performed prenatally to detect this condition in the fetus.

Another more common type of diabetes is *gestational diabetes mellitus* (GDM), which only occurs during pregnancy. It occurs in about 2% to 10% of all pregnancies in the United States, resulting in about 135,000 cases diagnosed each year. Ninety percent of all women who have pregnancies complicated by diabetes have GDM (CDC, 2011). Women who are overweight or obese, have a family history of type 2 diabetes, and/or are from the high-risk populations listed earlier have a much greater risk of developing GDM than does the general population.

CLINICAL EXAMPLE: Pregnancy and the resulting placental hormones cause some degree of insulin resistance in all women. However, a healthy pancreas is able to produce more and more insulin to keep blood sugars within normal range as the pregnancy advances. Today it is recommended that all women be given a 75-g, 2-hour oral glucose tolerance test (OGTT) as a screening tool between 24 and 28 weeks of gestation. If any of the glucose levels are at or above the norm, GDM is diagnosed (ADA, 2011). In the past it took two abnormal results for a diagnosis. This new diagnostic criterion will increase the number of women with GDM by 18% according to an international, multicenter study using only one abnormal value. Because the health of both mother and fetus depends on tight glucose control during pregnancy, this should improve pregnancy outcomes. Immediately after pregnancy, 5% to 10% of women with GDM are found to have diabetes, usually type 2, and so should be screened for diabetes 6 to 12 weeks postpartum. The rest of these women have a 40% to 60% risk of developing type 2 diabetes later in life, often within 10 to 20 years of the pregnancy (ADA, 2011). You can read more about diabetes during pregnancy in Chapter 10.

There is a fourth classification of diabetes termed "other," which encompasses those who have a diseased pancreas caused by cancer or infection and those with drug-induced hyperglycemia, as is often the case with chronic use of prednisone or other corticosteroid medications, some diuretics, antirejection medications, and HIV/AIDS drugs. A list of drugs that increase blood sugar is provided in Chapter 5.

In recent years we have heard a lot about *prediabetes,* a term that has replaced *impaired glucose tolerance (IGT)* and *impaired fasting glucose (IFG)* to increase the attention of both healthcare providers and clients to the fact that time is running out to prevent future cases of diabetes, *cardiovascular disease (CVD),* and stroke (Saudek & Margolis, 2011). Prior to developing type 2 diabetes, most clients have had difficulty with glucose tolerance, perhaps for years. This includes a number of people who have the metabolic syndrome. Research has shown that organ damage often begins during the prediabetes years. Normal fasting blood sugar once was 70 to 109 mg/dl, and IFG was 110 to 125 mg/dl. In 2003, these criteria were lowered to help motivate those with prediabetes to follow guidelines and prevent or delay the diagnosis of type 2 diabetes and long-term complications. These guidelines include weight loss, exercise, and lifestyle modifications. Currently, prediabetes is diagnosed when a fasting blood sugar is between 100 and 125 mg/dl or an A1c level is 5.7% to 6.4%. There are about 57 million Americans diagnosed with prediabetes today. This is an increase from 40 million in the 2005 statistics. As stated in the *Johns Hopkins White Papers* on diabetes, "Without lifestyle changes or medication, many of [individuals with prediabetes] will develop type 2 diabetes in the next 10 years" (Saudek & Margolis, 2011, p. 10). The hope is that, if forewarned, clients will make the changes in their life to lower fasting blood sugar levels to less than 100 mg/dl and that you, as a healthcare practitioner, will be more concerned about the health consequences to your patients in the years prior to their official diagnosis of type 2 diabetes.

DIAGNOSTIC CRITERIA

Most people with diabetes are diagnosed with a fasting blood glucose of 126 mg/dl or higher or a random blood glucose of 200 mg/dl or higher. In 2010, the ADA added an A1c of 6.5% or more to the diagnostic criteria. *Hemoglobin A1c*, or simply *A1c*, is a blood test that measures one's average blood sugar level over 2 to 3 months. To put this in perspective, a person without diabetes would have an A1c of 4% to 5.6% (ADA, 2011). Common symptoms of diabetes that might initiate a blood glucose test include excessive urination, excessive thirst, weight loss despite cravings for sweets (type 1), fatigue, skin lesions that do not heal, repeat infection, and any end organ damage associated with chronic diabetic complication, particularly cardiovascular and neuropathic problems (type 2). Current ADA recommendations for screening people without symptoms include a fasting blood sugar, an A1c, or a 2-hour 75-g OGTT for all individuals 45 years of age and older and, if the results are normal, repeating this test at least every 3 years. Screening should be done earlier than age 45 years and/or be done more frequently for those who have any of the following risk factors:

- Overweight body mass index (BMI $\geq$25 kg/m^2)
- Habitually physically inactive
- First-degree relative with diabetes (parent, sibling, child)
- Member of a high-risk race/ethnic population (e.g., African American, Asian American, Pacific Islander, Native American, Mexican American)
- Women who delivered a baby weighing $\geq$9 pounds or diagnosed with GDM
- Hypertension ($\geq$140/90 mm Hg) or on medication for hypertension
- HDL cholesterol $\geq$35 mg/dl and/or triglyceride level $\geq$250 mg/dl
- Women with polycystic ovarian syndrome (PCOS)
- A1c $\geq$5.7%, IGT, or IFG on a previous testing
- Any other clinical condition associated with insulin resistance (e.g., severe obesity, acanthosis nigricans)
- History of CVD
  (Modified from Table 4 from Standards of Medical Care in Diabetes—2011 in *Diabetes Care, 34,* S11-S61 [2011] used with permission from the American Diabetes Association.)

Because the incidence of type 2 diabetes in adolescents and children has increased dramatically in the past 10 years, those who meet the criteria listed below are thus at increased risk for developing type 2 diabetes in childhood and should be tested at puberty or age 10, whichever comes first, and retested at least every 3 years using a fasting blood sugar or an A1c blood test.

- Overweight (BMI >85th percentile for age and sex, weight for height >85th percentile, or weight >120% of ideal for height)

Plus any two of the following risk factors:

- Family history of type 2 diabetes in first- or second-degree relative
- Race/ethnicity (African American, Asian American, Pacific Islander, Native American, Mexican American)

- Signs of insulin resistance or conditions associated with insulin resistance (acanthosis nigricans, hypertension, dyslipidemia, or PCOS, or small-for-gestational-age birth weight)
- Maternal history of diabetes or GDM during the pregnancy with this child. (Modified from Table 5 from Standards of Medical Care in Diabetes—2011 in *Diabetes Care, 34,* S11-S61 [2011] used with permission from the American Diabetes Association.)

Children who present with signs and symptoms of diabetes, such as excessive urination, constant thirst, excessive craving for sweets, and rapid, unintentional weight loss, probably have type 1 diabetes and are in immediate danger of developing diabetic ketoacidosis, which can be life threatening.

CLINICAL EXAMPLE: Testing for islet cell antibodies may identify children and adults at risk for developing type 1 diabetes, such as those with a previous brief period of hyperglycemia or who have relatives with type 1 diabetes. Those who screen positive for antibodies should be counseled concerning their risk for developing diabetes and can be directed to clinical studies' testing method to prevent or reverse type 1 diabetes.

Genetics of Diabetes

If your clients are concerned about the potential of passing on this hereditary disease, as I was, consider the following information from the ADA:

1. For both type 1 and type 2 diabetes, a person must inherit a predisposition to the disease.
2. As stated earlier, something in their environment must trigger the onset of diabetes. With type 1, it is probably a virus. Type 2 is generally precipitated by obesity and too little exercise, and it has a much greater genetic basis than type 1.
3. Women who develop GDM are more likely to have a family history of diabetes, especially on their mother's side, and to be overweight prior to the pregnancy. Women who have had GDM have an increased risk of developing type 2 diabetes within 10 years of the pregnancy.
4. With identical twins, if one has type 1 diabetes, the other has a 1-in-2 risk of developing type 1. However, if one twin has type 2 diabetes, the other has a 3-in-4 risk of developing type 2.

The child's risk for developing type 1 diabetes is as follows:

- The child of a man with type 1 has a 1-in-17 risk.
- The child of a woman with type 1 who gave birth to this child before age 25 has a 1-in-25 risk, but if the child was born after the mother turned 25, his or her risk decreases to 1 in 100.

- The child's risk doubles if the parent's diabetes was diagnosed before age 11.
- If both parents have type 1 diabetes, the child's risk jumps to between 1 in 10 and 1 in 4.
- Siblings of someone with type 1 diabetes have a 1-in-17 risk of developing it.
- In addition, most Caucasians with type 1 have an *HLA-DR3* or *HLA-DR4* gene. If the parent and child are White and share these genes, the child is at higher risk for developing type 1. Similarly, the *HLA-DR7* gene increases the risk of African Americans, and the *HLA-BR9* gene increases the risk of Japanese.
- Type 1 diabetes is less common if the child has been breastfeed and solid foods were delayed until later in the first year of life.
- High levels of antibodies against insulin, against the islet cells in the pancreas, or to an enzyme called *glutamic acid decarboxylase* indicate that a child has a higher risk of developing type 1 diabetes.

What about the child's risk of developing type 2 diabetes?

- Type 2 tends to "run in families" partly because children are taught poor eating habits and nonexercising behaviors from parents.
- A child's risk for type 2 is 1 in 7 if the parent was diagnosed with type 2 before the age of 50. It drops to 1 in 13 if the parent was diagnosed after age 50.
- A child's risk is greater if the mother has type 2 diabetes. If both mother and father have type 2, the risk for the child is 1 in 2.
- Children of people with MODY, a rare form of type 2 diabetes discussed earlier in this chapter, have a 1-in-2 risk of developing MODY as well (ADA, n.d.).

A risk factor does not mean a certainty. Clients need to remember that environmental factors must also exist. Parents need to encourage their children to eat a healthy diet and move more by playing active games. For more on the genetics of diabetes, see the National Institutes of Health (NIH)'s *The Genetic Landscape of Diabetes* by Laura Dean, MD, and Jo McEntyre, PhD, at http://www.ncbi.nlm.nih.gov/bookshelf/br.fcgi?book=diabetes, a free online book for people interested in learning more.

WHAT IS ON THE HORIZON FOR PREVENTION AND CURE?

The following are some types of research that may provide answers to better control, prevention, and perhaps a cure. Most of these research studies listed next are preclinical and must meet with success in mice or other animals before being used on human subjects, so there is a long way to go. Research in the treatment and cure of diabetes is funded by grants from the ADA, the Juvenile Diabetes Research Foundation (JDRF), and the NIH. As you read the following, consider the facts that donations are down for all charities and the federal government has recently cut funds for research in all areas. This will greatly impact future diabetes research.

Type 1 Diabetes

Here are some of the ongoing research studies to prevent and cure type 1 diabetes.

Stopping the Immune Destruction of the Beta Cell of the Pancreas

1. A vaccine to prevent type 1 diabetes.
   Stage of development: The vaccine, named Diamyd (rhGAD65) and produced by Diamyd Medical, is in Phase III trials with an estimated completion date of October 2011. The vaccine is given to newly diagnosed type 1 diabetics in an attempt to permanently preserve remaining beta cells from ongoing destruction. Anything that can halt the immune destruction in type 1 diabetes may be also useful in any autoimmune disease.

2. Several groups of researchers are studying rare variations in a single gene that can lead to a wide variety of autoimmune disorders. The gene encodes an enzyme protein called *sialic acid acetylesterase* (SIAE). This enzyme regulates the activity of the immune system's antibody-producing B cells. About 2% to 3% of people with autoimmune disorders have defects in the enzyme that allow these B cells to run amok and make antibodies that attack specific body cells. Individuals manifesting susceptibility to autoimmune disease type 6 can have juvenile idiopathic arthritis, rheumatoid arthritis, multiple sclerosis, Sjögren syndrome, systemic lupus erythematosus, ulcerative colitis, or Crohn disease, as well as type 1 diabetes. The hope is that a treatment can be developed to stop this from happening.

3. Alba Therapeutics is conducting trials of an oral medication called AT-1001, a zonulin inhibitor, that may prevent intestinal permeability caused by excessive amounts of the human protein zonulin. Increased permeability of the intestinal wall "allows undigested foodstuff, toxins, and other bacterial and viral particles access to the immune system . . . which leads to the production of antibodies that can destroy the insulin-producing islet cells of the pancreas among people genetically predisposed to developing type 1 diabetes" (Fasano, 2005). If this medication is given to patients in the earliest stages of type 1, it might halt the process and preserve beta cell function.

4. Another potential drug to halt autoimmune destruction is a CD3 monoclonal antibody infused over several days in clients with recent-onset type 1 diabetes. In a 2005 clinical trial, this short-term treatment preserved

residual beta cell function for at least 2 years (Herold, 2005). A more recent NIH Type 1 Diabetes Trial Net clinical study, tested whether teplizumab, an anti-CD3 monoclonal antibody, which is thought to stop that part of the immune system that attacks the beta cells of the pancreas, will halt this process in newly diagnosed type 1 diabetics. These studies are Phase II trials and are estimated to have results in late 2011 to mid-2012.

5. The researchers at the JDRF Center working on immunological tolerance in type 1 diabetes at Harvard Medical School have found the genetic region that usually stops errant T cells of the immune system from attacking the body's tissue, such as the beta cell. The immune system, which protects the body from "non-self" invaders such as bacteria and viruses, also sometimes releases "misguided" T cells, which have the potential to attack the body's own cells. There is a safeguard mechanism that should find and destroy such errant T cells, a process called tolerance. However, in people with autoimmune diseases, such as type 1 diabetes, rheumatoid arthritis, multiple sclerosis, types of hypothyroidism and hyperthyroidism, and others, the immune system's safeguard mechanism is defective. Thus, these errant T cells seek the body's tissue genetically marked for destruction, such as the pancreas' beta cells, and kill them. The JDRF researchers are now looking for the precise genes that control this safeguard mechanism. Once the genes are identified, procedures to "fix" the defect can be developed to prevent or halt this process of destruction (Keymeulen, 2005). The number of people with the genetic predisposition for autoimmune diseases could benefit enormously from this discovery.

6. The journal *Immunity*, in July 2004, published a series of experiments conducted by scientists from various research centers around the world that worked in a different way to prevent the immune system from attacking its own cells. During their research, they discovered a transcription factor, PPAR-gamma, in the dendritic cells, the immature immune cells. When rosiglitazone (Avandia), a drug already used with type 2 diabetes to increase insulin sensitivity, was added to these dendritic cells, PPAR-gamma activity was increased, which activated natural killer T (NKT) cells. The researchers working on this project believe that this drug used in this manner can increase the immune system's recognition and tolerance of "self," thus preventing autoimmune destruction of cells such as the insulin-producing beta cells. PPAR-gamma also regulates "the expression of a gene called CD1d, which encodes a glycoprotein responsible for the presentation of self and foreign lipids to T cells" (Howard Hughes Medical Institute, 2004). Current studies are using pioglitazone (Actos) instead of Avandia due to the U.S. Food and Drug Administration warning in February 2011 that Avandia put patients at risk for heart failure. By continuing to study the PPAR-gamma pathway in nonobese diabetic mice and its effects on the *CD1d* gene and NKT cells, the hope is that the autoimmune process can be prevented or at least halted.

Replacing Beta Cells

1. Pancreas and kidney transplantations have been done successfully for several years. The down side to any transplantation is the potential complications of immunologic suppression to prevent rejection of the transplanted organs. This is currently a lifelong suppression, which results in the recipient being very susceptible to infections, illnesses, and cancers. It, therefore, is only done as a last resort in selected individuals in renal failure. Moreover, there is always the possibility of rejection despite the potent, daily, and expensive immunosuppressive drug cocktails. Unlike kidney transplantation, live donors of part of their pancreas are no longer used because this often leads to the donor developing diabetes. This procedure does not represent the great hope for type 1 diabetics because the cure may be worse than the disease.

2. What about islet cells transplantation? In 1974 the first human islet cell transplantations were performed. This therapy has had minimal success for years because some of the immunosuppressant drugs, namely corticosteroids, actually destroyed the islets. To understand the process of islet cell transplantation, it may be useful to point out some insulin physiology. Insulin produced by the pancreatic beta cells is not in a form that the body can use. It is sometimes called "pro-insulin" and must be sent to the liver where the C-peptide amino acid chain is cleaved off, leaving the A and B chains. This insulin is now ready for distribution to the body via the blood vessels. Proof that the body is producing insulin can be found by testing the blood for C-peptide amino acid chains. Because insulin produced by islet cells must first go to the liver, it makes sense to inject islet cell transplants directly into the liver instead of the pancreas. Islet cell transplantation using the Edmonton Protocol (Edmonton, Canada) has been at least 50% successful since its inception in 2000. What makes this procedure work has to do with the drugs used to prevent rejection. By omitting any corticosteroids, which destroy islet cells and raise blood pressure and cholesterol levels, islet cells are preserved and continue to function for years. The immunosuppressant drugs used with the Edmonton Protocol include sirolimus, which negates the need for steroids and decreases the dose of the second drug, tacrolimus. Tacrolimus can raise blood pressure and ultimately be toxic to kidneys. It is also toxic to islet cells (Dinsmoor, 2005). The third drug, daclizumab, is used only for a short period of time to prevent initial rejection of the islet cells. Because type 1 diabetes is an autoimmune disease, immunosuppression is needed to protect the implanted islet cells as well as prevent rejection. Insulin is usually produced for 1 year and in some cases up to 5 years after the transplantation, but most patients need insulin injections after 1 year. Islet cell transplantation remains a research procedure (Saudek & Margolis, 2011).

3. Transplantation of a patient's own islet cells (autologous) has been performed at several medical centers across the country and worldwide where a pancreas had to be removed due to chronic pancreatitis. This removal would have cause "surgical diabetes" and the patient would have required insulin as well as pancreatic enzyme replacement for life. By isolating the patient's own islet cells from his or her removed pancreas and reinjecting them into the liver, the client's insulin production was resumed. This could potentially also be done in the early stages of type 1 diabetes prior to significant beta cell destruction.

4. To increase the viability and continued function of transplanted beta cells, the ADA is sponsoring a research project to test whether embedding these islet cells in a biomimetic gel-like nanomatrix omental pouch will protect them so they will last longer.

Beta Cell Regeneration

This new field, beta cell regeneration, is based on getting beta cells of the pancreas to reproduce themselves in order to replace those cells lost through aging or disease. This would provide no limit to the number of beta cells an individual could produce, which would eliminate two of the most troublesome difficulties with islet cell transplantation: shortages of islet cell donors and immunosuppressive drugs. If the beta cells in mice replicate themselves, why cannot human beta cells do it?

1. In November 2004, researchers at the NIH caused human pancreatic cells to revert to a more primitive form so they could multiply and produce islet cells that produced insulin. The drawback was that these cells produced far less insulin than the original beta cells. The fact that this replication could happen at all ensures continued research on this topic. Would it not be wonderful if type 1 diabetics could grow their own beta cells to replace those destroyed by their errant immune system? Another interesting fact discovered early in 2005 was that the majority of type 1 diabetics continue to form insulin-producing beta cells, even those diabetics with long-standing diabetes (Juvenile Diabetes Research Foundation, 2005). Now all we have to do is stop the autoimmune destruction and find ways to increase beta cell replication to return the insulin production back to normal.

2. Stem cell research is actively involved in finding ways to grow beta cells. One such study conducted at Georgetown University Medical Center in Washington, DC, by G. Ian Gallicano has demonstrated that spermatogonial stem cells (SSCs) can be transformed into beta-islet cells that produce insulin. SSCs are precursors of human sperm. By extracting these SSCs from the testes of dead organ donors, they can be directed to form a kind of cell in the body just like embryonic stem cells.

Gallicano states that the same may be true of the precursor stem cells of female egg cells (Jha, 2010).

3. Liver cells using the *PDX-1* gene can be converted into beta cells producing insulin. *PDX-1*–transdifferentiated adult liver cells not only produced, stored, and secreted insulin in a glucose-regulated manner but also ameliorated diabetes when implanted in diabetic mice.

4. Scientists report in the *Journal of Dental Research* (JDR) that stem cells from teeth can be transformed into cells that produce insulin in a glucose-dependent manner. In 2000, scientists from the NIH first reported isolating stem cells from dental pulp. In 2009, it was shown that stem cells from periodontal ligaments could produce insulin. Now scientists are able to change dental pulp stem cells into islet-like cells that could produce insulin in response to elevated glucose levels (Govindasamy, 2011).

Type 2 Diabetes

The following are some of the ongoing research studies being conducted to better understand and treat type 2 diabetes.

- Type 2 diabetes may also be triggered by an autoimmune process. NIH-funded research study identified immune system antibodies in people who are obese and insulin-resistant that are not present in people who are obese without insulin resistance. The researchers also tested a drug that modifies the immune system in mice fed a fatty diet and found that the medication could help maintain normal blood sugar levels. More research on human subjects is needed to see if this premise holds true in humans.
- A Johns Hopkins University team of researchers are working on a way to stimulate the body to make more brown fat (the fat that babies burn to keep warm) instead of white fat, which is unhealthy. By suppressing the appetite-stimulating protein NPY in the brain of rats, the rodents decreased their food intake and weight even when feed a high-fat diet. The rats also developed more brown fat and lost some white fat. Brown fat is more biologically active (like in babies) and can burn more calories. As we age, we lose brown fat and replace it with white fat, which can cause CVD and cancer. Researchers are trying to affect this change by injecting brown fat stem cells under the skin in humans so they will burn white fat and cause weight loss.
- The search for the genes responsible for type 2 diabetes is ongoing. In the future, gene therapy may help to target better diabetes medication to control blood sugar levels in people with particular genes or even alter these genes to cure this form of diabetes.

■ Harvard University scientists have discovered that reducing the function of a transmembrane protein, klotho, in obese mice with high blood glucose levels made them lean and decreased blood sugar levels. Because humans also have klotho, targeting this protein with a new class of medication might reduce obesity and blood sugar, thereby preventing type 2 diabetes in the process (Ohnishi, Kato, Akiyoshi, Atfi, & Razzaque, 2011).

■ An NIH study showed that the protein osteocalcin, which stimulates bone-forming cells osteoblasts in mice, also stimulates insulin production and decreases insulin resistance in body cells when activated by osteoclasts, which break down old bone. This research may be promising in controlling type 2 diabetes (Clemens & Karsenty, 2011).

Because what we do not know about our health can and does cause damage to glucose-sensitive organs, diagnosis of anyone at risk for diabetes and treatment at the earliest possible opportunity are critical. A diagnosis of diabetes can be very overwhelming and frightening for anyone. I hope that, with the information on various treatment options available today, living within the guidelines of a healthy lifestyle as outlined in the following chapters will be as doable for you and your clients as it has become for me. No one is perfect, but the goal of being healthy and living a healthy life should be important for everyone, not just those of us with diabetes.

REFERENCES

American Diabetes Association. (n.d.). *Genetics of diabetes*. Retrieved March 18, 2011, from http://www.diabetes.org/diabetes-basics/genetics-of-diabetes.html

American Diabetes Association. (2011). Standards of medical care in diabetes—2011. *Diabetes Care, 34*, S11–S61.

Centers for Disease Control and Prevention (CDC). (2011). *National Diabetes Fact Sheet, 2011*. Atlanta, GA: US Department of Health and Human Services.

Clemens, T. L., & Karsenty, G. (2011). The osteoblast: An insulin target cell controlling glucose homeostasis. *Journal of Bone and Mineral Research, 26*(4), 677–680.

Dinsmoor, R. S. (2005, Spring). Rebooting the immune system. *JDRF Countdown*, 8–17.

Fasano, A. (2005). Potential method for preventing type 1 diabetes. *Proceedings of the National Academy of Science, 102*:2916–2921.

Gebel, E. (2010a, May). *Another kind of diabetes: MODY*. Retrieved March 14, 2011, from http://forecast.diabetes.org/magazine/features/another-kind-diabetes-mody

Gebel, E. (2010b, May). *The other diabetes: LADA, or 1.5*. Retrieved March 14, 2011, from http://forecast.diabetes.org/magazine/features/other-diabetes-lada-or-type-1.5

Gordan, S. (2011). *Do immune system ills help drive type 2 diabetes?* Retrieved April 5, 2011, from http://health.usnews.com/health-news/diet-fitness/diabetes/articles/2011/04/17/do-immune-system-ills-help-drive-type-2-diabetes

Govindasamy, V., Ronald, V. S., Abdullah, A. N., Nathan, K. R., Ab Aziz, Z. A., Abdullah, M. H., . . . Bhonde, R. R. (2011). Differentiation of dental pulp stem cells into islet like aggregates. *Journal of Dental Research, 90*(5), 646–652.

Herold, K. C. (2005). Anti-CD3 antibodies stabilizes insulin secretion in diabetes. *Diabetes, 54,* 1763–1769.

Howard Hughes Medical Institute. (2005, July 21). A pathway to blocking autoimmunity. *ScienceDaily.* Retrieved March 4, 2011, from http://www.sciencedaily.com/releases/2004/07/040721091234.htm

Jha, A. (2010). Sperm stem cells can be turned into insulin-making cells to treat diabetes. *The Guardian.* Retrieved March 4, 2011, from http://www.guardian.co.uk/science/2010/dec/12/sperm-stem-cells-insulin-diabetes

Juvenile Diabetes Research Foundation. (2005, Spring). Researchers make strides in understanding beta cell regeneration. *Discoveries,* p. 5.

Keymeulen, B. (2005). CD3 antibodies may be helpful in recent-onset type 1 diabetes. *New England Journal of Medicine, 352,* 2598–2608, 2642–2644.

National Diabetes Information Clearinghouse. (2011). Total prevalence of diabetes in the United States, all ages, 2011. *National Diabetes Statistics.* Retrieved March 1, 2011, from http://www.diabetes.niddk.nih.gov/dm/pubs/statistics/index.aspx

Ohnishi, M., Kato, S., Akiyoshi, J., Atfi, A., & Razzaque, M.S. (2011, March 7). Dietary and genetic evidence for enhancing glucose metabolism and reducing obesity by inhibiting klotho functions. *FASEB Journal, 25,* 2031–2039.

Saudek, C. D., & Margolis, S. (2011). *Johns Hopkins White Papers: Diabetes.* Baltimore, MD: Johns Hopkins University School of Medicine.

TWO

Treatment:
Medical Nutritional Therapy

Diabetics have *to do what everyone else* ought *to do.*

The ADA states that the goals of treatment for diabetes are to prevent or delay long-term complications while minimizing acute manifestations such as hypoglycemia. Nutrition, exercise, and medication, when needed, are the cornerstones of successfully treating all classifications of diabetes. In addition to diet and physical activity, there are lifestyle modifications, which include smoking cessation and normalization of blood pressure and blood cholesterol (ADA, 2011). Nurses and other healthcare professionals need to remind their clients that these are goals of a healthy lifestyle for all people, not just those diagnosed with diabetes.

Early on in my career as a diabetic, a very wise physician said to me that which I have quoted above. It changed my life and my attitude toward myself and this disease. As I attempted to control my blood sugars by eating nutritiously, exercising, and giving multiple injections of insulin, I felt superior to my peers instead of feeling sorry for myself. I then felt I was choosing to live a healthy lifestyle instead of being forced into it. Sometimes bad things can have good consequences.

NUTRITION

Diet is simply what we eat: good, bad, or indifferent. We can have a healthy or unhealthy diet. The word, *diet* by itself, has no negative connotations except what we choose to give it. It can be high fat, high carbohydrate, high fast food, high junk food, high calorie, or restrictive in terms of all of the above, or it can be so low in calories as to deprive our body of the nutrients to sustain life. Therefore, focusing on nutrition and avoiding the negative images, the word diet has come to evoke, may improve attitudes and motivation to make healthier food choices. Medical nutritional therapy to achieve and maintain appropriate weight for age, gender, and height must begin with a thorough evaluation of a client's dietary history. Culture lifestyle, finances, and a person's readiness to learn and change must be considered. Many people with diabetes need the help of a registered dietitian to make the changes required to stay healthy and normalize blood sugars; however, all healthcare practitioners should become more familiar with nutrition for their own well-being as well as for client teaching. For that reason, look at the rest of this chapter as an exploration into an adventure in healthy eating.

CLINICAL EXAMPLE: The basic elements of a diet include carbohydrates, protein, fats, vitamins, minerals, and water. Of these six nutrients, the only ones that provide calories are carbohydrates and protein, which have 4 calories per gram, and fat, which yields a whopping 9 calories per gram. Anyone who wants to lose weight must definitely be concerned about how much fat he or she consumes.

Carbohydrates

Blood sugar is influenced by the amount and type of carbohydrates consumed and whether protein and fat are eaten along with it.

CLINICAL EXAMPLE: An orange is metabolized more slowly than orange juice and takes longer to increase blood sugar. An orange eaten after cereal and milk or eggs and sausage takes even longer to metabolize. Protein and fat eaten with carbohydrate-containing foods slow down its absorption and, thus, the resulting blood sugar rise.

Dietary carbohydrate is the major contributor to blood glucose concentration after a meal. According to Warshaw and Boderman (2001, p. 1), "Carbohydrates begin to raise blood glucose within 15 minutes after initiation of food intake and are converted to nearly 100% glucose within 2 hours . . . The ADA nutrition recommendations encourage a focus on total carbohydrate intake rather than differentiating between types of carbohydrates."

Carbohydrates are an important source of energy, fiber, minerals, and water-soluble vitamins such as the B complex and vitamin C. Because almost all carbohydrates one eats (except for fiber) are absorbed into the blood as glucose, the recommended range of carbohydrate intake is 45% to 65% of the total calories. In addition, because the brain and central nervous system, as opposed to other tissues of the body, can only use glucose as an energy source, restricting one's total carbohydrate intake to <130 g/day is a bad idea. Carbohydrates come from fruit (fructose), milk (lactose), grains such as bread and cereal, starches such as pasta and rice, starchy vegetables (corn, peas, and all kinds of beans), and table sugar (sucrose). Yes, people with diabetes can eat sugar. The body metabolizes sugar as a carbohydrate. However, not all carbs are created equal. The empty carbohydrate calories in regular sodas and sugary desserts and snacks contain no nutritive value and should be limited. Desserts and snacks with sugar or high-fructose corn syrup also usually have a high fat content, contributing to increased calories and weight gain. Clients who administer insulin for glucose control should try to match the number of carbohydrates in a meal or snack with the appropriate amount of insulin (see Chapter 4).

Fiber is a complex carbohydrate that does not get absorbed in the body, so technically it should be subtracted from the total carb grams. For most people, the recommended amount of fiber per day should equal 20 to 35 grams (g), depending on total caloric intake, age, and sex.

CLINICAL EXAMPLE: If a client eats 2,000 calories, his/her diet should contain 28 g of fiber or 14 g per 1,000 calories for men older than 50 years and 31 g/day for men younger than 50 years. For women younger than 50 years or older than 50 years, the amount of fiber per day should be 25 or 22 g, respectively (Cheskin, Roberts, & Margolis, 2011).

Fiber decreases the speed with which food travels through the digestive system, helps to retain bulk and water in the stool as it enters the rectum, and stimulates the urge to defecate, thus preventing constipation. This slowed movement also increases satiety, so a person eats less. Fiber-rich foods are usually low in calories and fat, which also helps weight loss. In addition, soluble fiber is a magnet for cholesterol and carries it out of the body, lowering low-density lipoproteins (LDL, the "bad" cholesterol). Soluble fiber is included in oats, oatmeal, barley, dry beans and peas, citrus fruits, and apples and pears with their skins. Wheat bran in any whole grain cereals, breads, crackers and pasta, brown rice, bulgur, or wheat berries are examples of foods containing insoluble fiber, as are most vegetables, including potatoes if eaten with skins, fresh fruit with edible skin, and fresh vegetables consumed separately or in a salad.

CLINICAL EXAMPLE: When buying cereal or bread, a person should look for those labeled *whole wheat*, not just *wheat* or *100% wheat*, and *whole multigrain*, not just *twelve-grain*, *fifteen-grain*, or *multigrain*. If a client is not used to eating fiber-rich foods, he or she should be advised to start slowly or he or she may feel gassy and bloated. The client also needs six to eight glasses of noncarbonated liquid to help flush the fiber out of the body. Too much fiber without sufficient increase in fluid volume can cause a bowel obstruction.

Natural Versus Artificial Sweeteners

Table sugar (sucrose) is a natural sweetener. So are fructose, honey, molasses, maple sugar, high-fructose corn syrup, and agave nectar. Agave nectar comes from the agave plant, a Mexican fruit. Its sweetness is derived from fructose, which has carbohydrate grams and calories. Because it is much sweeter than sugar, much less is needed. Sugars have empty calories, but carbs can be moderately consumed by persons with diabetes. Another natural sweetener comes from the *Stevia* plant. In December 2008, the Food and Drug Administration (FDA) gave a "generally recognized as safe" status to Truvia and PureVia, both of which are wholly derived from the *Stevia* plant and have no calories. Since then, combinations have come on the market, such as Only Sweet, a combination of maltodextrine and *Stevia*, also with zero calories, and Sun Crystals, a combination of Truvia and pure cane sugar that has 5 calories per packet. With obesity and diabetes on the rise, other products are sure to follow. All of these preparations can be found in regular grocery stores and are safe in moderation for nonpregnant adults.

What about artificial sweeteners? The newest one that I am aware of has been on the market since its FDA approval in 1998. It is the yellow packet, sucralose, with the trade name Splenda (and many chain store equivalents). It has been deemed safe by many studies and by the FDA. It is 600 times sweeter than sugar, and it can be used in baking and at high heat levels. Although it is made from chemically altered sugar, it is not absorbed by the body and thus has no calories. To increase fiber in the diet, 1 g of fiber is added to specially marked packets of Splenda, which increases the carbs to 2 g per packet but still zero calories. Splenda is also marketed as a sugar blend and a brown sugar blend for baking. These blends decrease the sugar needed in baked goods by half but still have 10 calories and two carbs per half-teaspoon. To eat something made with these Splenda blends, clients need the carbohydrate gram information to decide on an insulin dose, or they can ask how much of this blend was used and divide by the number of servings per cake, pie, or cookie. If it is more than half a teaspoon per serving, they should be advised to cut their serving to this amount. They could also multiply the number of half-teaspoons of the serving size by 10 calories and two carbs, or use the nutrition facts listed in the recipe. Even though the sugar is decreased, these baked goods provide calories and carbs that must be counted.

Two other commonly used artificial sweeteners include saccharin (Sweet & Low and other store brands), in the pink packets, and aspartame (Equal, NutraSweet, and other store brand names), in the blue packets. Both are unstable at high temperatures and are safe in moderate amounts. However, many object to the taste or bitter aftertaste with saccharin or fear the old studies in animals that linked saccharin in large amounts with cancer. Some people react with headaches when they use aspartame. Those who have the rare inherited disorder phenylketonuria (PKU) diagnosed during the newborn period should avoid anything sweetened with aspartame because they cannot metabolize the phenylalanine it contains. Anything sweetened with aspartame has a warning label to this effect. A less commonly available sweetener is acesulfame K (Sunett and Sweet One). Another artificial sweetener is sodium cyclamate, which was banned in the United States in 1969 but can still be found in other countries.

I need to say a word about sugar-free candy, gum, chocolate, and other products. They are often sweetened with a *sugar alcohol*, which is listed on the nutrition facts label under "total carbohydrates" if present. The list includes mannitol, sorbitol, xylitol, maltitol, lactitol, isomalt, erythritol, and hydrogenated starch hydrolysates. They do contribute to blood sugar but are slowly absorbed and only half of the sugar alcohol grams need be counted. They also stimulate the bowels, and even a listed serving size may cause cramps and diarrhea in some people. I discuss sugar-free chocolate further in the section labeled "Fats."

CLINICAL EXAMPLE: Until I was diagnosed with diabetes, I used to hate the words "in moderation." What does it really mean? The meaning becomes clear when people monitor their blood sugar and weight to see how consuming these products affect their body, from no effect to greatly increasing blood glucose levels and weight gain. When considering whether a sweetener is safe, remember that if sugar, or any other carbohydrate source, raises blood glucose to an unhealthy level, glucose-sensitive organs, such as the eyes, kidneys, heart, blood vessels, and nerve endings, can be affected. The bottom line is that sugar or its substitutes can be used in small amounts to enhance the enjoyment of foods. However, your client may want to consider choosing more nutrient-dense foods, such as fresh or frozen unsweetened fruit and nonfat yogurt, to satisfy their sweet tooth, with a small serving of low-caloric sweet treats on occasion. Nutrient-dense foods provide a high dose of vitamins and minerals for a low-calorie count.

Protein

Protein is needed to build and repair cells and body tissue as well as to enhance the immune system's response to germs, to maintain fluid and electrolyte and acid–base balance, to produce hemoglobin in red cells, and to build or maintain muscle mass. The ADA recommends that low-fat protein comprise 10% to 35% of the calories consumed. Items such as lean meat, chicken, turkey, ham, or fish, as well as low-fat or nonfat dairy products, should be eaten every day.

If your client is a vegetarian, he or she should be substituting vegetable protein from a variety of sources, such as whole grains, legumes (e.g., beans and lentils), vegetables, and starches, as well as eggs and low-fat dairy products, to meet protein needs. Most of these foods will also increase carbohydrate intake, so they need to be counted carefully, especially if the client is taking insulin or taking a medication that increases his or her own insulin production.

For vegans, who eat no animal products, meeting calcium, iron, and vitamin B_{12} needs can be difficult, and they may need to supplement their diets with a multivitamin and mineral source. Calcium, which is needed for strong teeth and bones, is found not only in dairy products such as milk, cheese, and yogurt but also in soy products, such as soy milk, soy yogurt, and tofu, as well as in green leafy vegetables and in legumes such as beans and peas in lesser amounts. Iron is part of the hemoglobin molecule in red cells and thus is needed for the transport of oxygen to all of the cells of the body. The iron in vegetables and legumes is much harder to digest and absorb than that in egg yolks and red meat, so eating more vegetables containing iron or taking an iron supplement may be necessary. Vitamin B_{12}, which is needed for red blood cell production, is found naturally only in animal products. There are pastas and other vegan foods fortified with this essential nutrient, which makes reading package labels important.

There are so many good, low-calorie protein choices that, unless a person is sick or unable to consume them, artificial or supplemental protein sources are unnecessary, expensive, and probably unwise.

Fats

Fats are a very important part of our diet. They help the absorption of fat-soluble vitamins and provide essential fatty acids (which the body needs but cannot manufacture). They provide concentrated stored energy and fuel muscle movement. Fat cells pad internal organs and insulate the body against temperature extremes. They also form the major component of cell walls and are the raw material from which hormones, enzymes, bile, and vitamin D are made. Fats also stimulate appetite, make meats tender, and contribute to the feeling of fullness. The problem is that they provide 9 calories per gram and contribute to weight gain more than any other nutrient. But let's look at the good, the bad, and the ugly fats. The American Heart Association and the American Cancer Society, as well as the ADA, recommend that fat should be limited to 25% to 35% of calories per day and that no more than 7% should come from the saturated fat of animal products, such as meat, poultry, and full-fat dairy products. *trans*-Fatty acids in any oils that are hydrogenated or partially hydrogenated should be limited as much as possible (ADA, 2010). Saturated (the bad) fats and *trans* (the ugly) fats contribute to total cholesterol and triglycerides in the body and eventually to heart disease, atherosclerosis, high blood pressure, and stroke, as well as some cancers, such as breast and colon cancers.

Most fat should come from polyunsaturated (the good) sources, such as vegetable oil and fish oil, and monounsaturated (better) sources, such as canola oil, olive oil, nuts, and avocadoes. Ten percent or more of calories should come from monounsaturated sources. In 2006, guidelines for nutritional labels were revised to state that manufacturers must list the kinds of fats in each product; however, if the amount of anything, including *trans*-fats, is 0.5 mg or less per serving, the manufacturer is allowed to list it as zero. If a person chooses to have more than one serving of the product, the *trans*-fats and other ingredients could add up. If the words *hydrogenated* or *partially hydrogenated* are included anywhere in the list of ingredients, *trans*-fat is present.

Elsewhere in this chapter, I recommend fresh vegetable salads as a way to lose weight, fill up, and take advantage of their high fiber and nutrient content. However, anyone can turn a wonderful salad into a high-calorie, high-fat meal or side dish by dousing it with a high-fat creamy or oily dressing. Advise clients to look for light, fat-free, low-calorie bottled dressing at the grocery store and ask for the same at restaurants, then request that it come on the side. They will use much less dressing than the server will put on the salad if the dressing comes separately. Another source of high saturated fat is butter, made from the cream of cow's milk and thus 100% saturated fat. Stick margarine is no better because it is hydrogenated oil and so contains a lot of *trans*-fats and has the same number of calories per serving as butter. Better choices include spreads in tubs (read labels for the lowest amount of saturated and *trans*-fats) and butter sprays. Also, a lot less of the product will be used than with a spread in stick form.

Natural Versus Artificial Fat Products

Natural fats come from animal products, such as butter, margarine, mayonnaise, cream, and cheese, as well as vegetable sources, such as nuts, nut butters (e.g., peanut butter), and chocolate. Butter and margarine contain 100 calories per 1-tablespoon serving size, mostly from the 11 g of fat they contain, of which 7 g are saturated. In addition, most brands of stick margarine contain hydrogenated oil, which contains *trans*-fats, so margarine is actually not healthier than butter. One tablespoon of full-fat mayonnaise, which is made from egg yolks, contains 80 calories and 9 g of fat; the same serving size of light mayonnaise has half the calories and half the fat, most of which is unsaturated and is a rich source of omega-3 fatty acids. If clients use mayonnaise, encourage them to try the light version. Full-fat dairy products, including cream, cheese, whole milk, and yogurt, contain saturated fat and thus should be limited, especially if they are trying to lose weight or are at high risk for heart disease. Fortunately, they all come in lighter versions that greatly reduce, or eliminate, the fat content.

CLINICAL EXAMPLE: The only differences among whole milk, 2% milk, and nonfat (skim) milk are the amounts of fat and thus calories. All milk has the same carbohydrate, calcium, and protein content. Mixing 2% and skim milk or looking for 1% milk is a good alternative if a client chooses not to drink skim milk. The same goes for yogurt, but fat-free yogurt with more than 100 calories and 20 g of carbs per 6-ounce cup probably has a syrupy fruit mixture that will increase the carb content and raise blood sugar. Clients can make their own by adding cut-up ripe fresh fruit to plain fat-free yogurt and adding artificial sweetener if needed. Reduced-fat cheese will decrease the calories but not the protein, calcium, or the taste. Fat-free cheese, however, may taste like plastic to some people.

Nuts and nut butters such as peanut butter or almond butter contain 190 to 200 calories, 6 to 7 g of carbs, 7 to 9 g of protein per serving, and 16 to 17 g of fat, most unsaturated. They comprise some of the good fats because they are unsaturated and are a good source of omega-3 fatty acids. They are also a good source of protein. However, clients should stick to the serving size (¼ cup of nuts and 2 tablespoons of nut butters), or weight gain due to their high-calorie count is a distinct possibility.

Oils are another source of fat calories, so a little goes a long way. Frying foods should be avoided, because even canola or olive oil will be absorbed by the chicken, fish, or vegetable being fried and increase the calorie content of foods no matter what the oil label states. Clients can choose to "oven fry," bake, or stir-fry foods using aerosolized oil (like Pam) or olive oil or canola oil in a spritzer to decrease the amount.

Now we come to my favorite indulgence: chocolate. I was once told I could not have chocolate any more. I said I would find a way to keep it in my diet, and I did. Current research has proved that a small amount of dark chocolate, my personal favorite, eaten every day, is heart healthy because it is rich in flavonoids and antioxidants. It relaxes blood vessels, thus decreasing blood pressure, improves mood, and puts a smile on your face. Pure, unsweetened cocoa powder has almost no fat or carbohydrates. Unsweetened baking chocolate does have cocoa butter and thus fat calories. According to the FDA, semisweet or dark chocolate must have at least 35% chocolate liquor (nonalcoholic) as well as cocoa butter and sugar. Dark chocolate can have as much as 90% chocolate liquor, which replaces most of the cocoa butter and sugar. If it contains over 60% to 70% chocolate liquor, it may taste pasty and bitter. Milk chocolate, however, only has 10% to 15% chocolate liquor and more cocoa butter, sugar, and milk or cream. White chocolate has no chocolate liquor (Hershey Company, n.d.). None of the chocolate preparations, including the sugar-free variety, are a low-calorie food because they contain a lot of fat grams. But a 1-ounce serving size of dark chocolate may be well worth the calories.

The only artificial fat or fat substitute is olestra, brand name Olean. It is a synthetic oil that is not absorbed by the gut, so there are no fat calories. Snacks made with this substance do taste like the full-fat variety; however, this compound takes fat-soluble vitamins, such as A, D, E, and K, as well as carotinoids (precursors to vitamin A) out of the body as well. Because this fat substitute exits the body in the stool, many people experience cramps, diarrhea, or oily brown staining on underpants, especially if the serving size is exceeded. Procter & Gamble received FDA approval to use olestra as a food additive in 1996. Clients may remember the controversy surrounding olestra-containing WOW! potato chips, manufactured a few years ago by the Frito-Lay corporation, which was required to note on the product label the fact that it contained olestra as well as a list of possible side effects. The FDA-mandated list of the preceding side effects was removed in 2003, but the negative publicity remained. WOW! chips were taken off the market, but Frito-Lay continues to use olestra in their "light" potato chips, Ruffles, Doritos, Tostitos, and other snack foods. Pringles "light" potato chips, all flavors, also contain olestra. They all state "made with olestra" on the front of the package, and Olean or olestra is the second listed ingredient after potatoes. Olestra is *not* in the reduced-fat or baked chips of any manufacturer. Olean may also be found in other "light" or fat-free baked goods, frozen desserts, and snack foods (Center for Science in the Public Interest, 2004). For more facts about olestra, visit *www.cspinet .org/olestra*. If a client chooses to eat these products, he or she should be warned to stick to the serving size at the top of the nutrition facts label. Clients can check the ingredients label for Olean or olestra, and they can avoid these products if they experience gastrointestinal repercussions. If it sounds and tastes too good to be true, it just might be. As another alternative to full-fat snacks, they can try "baked" products and pretzels, but they should compare the carb content with the real thing. When manufacturers take out fat, which has 9 calories per gram, they may replace it with carbohydrates or protein, which only have 4 calories per gram. The extra protein will not increase blood sugar, but the increased carbs will. Snacking on fresh fruit and veggies is a healthier plan.

In Table 2.1 and the information that follows, I have listed the recommended percentages and what they mean in terms of the range of grams for each nutrient based on the number of calories per day. You or your client can crunch the numbers and individualize this table by following the formula underneath.

NUTRITION LABELS

To figure out the percentage of carbohydrates, protein, and fat a client consumes, the client needs to know how to read a nutrition label. If he or she is not familiar with nutrition labels, he or she can get a package, can, or bread wrapper and follow along while you explain what it contains.

TABLE 2.1
Grams of Carbs, Protein, and Fat

CALORIES (CAL)/DAY	CARBS (4 CAL) 45%–65% OF CAL	PROTEIN (4 CAL) 10%–35% OF CAL	FAT (9 CAL) 25%–35% OF CAL
1,200	135–195 g	30–105 g	33–47 g
1,500	169–244 g	37.5–131 g	42–58 g
1,800	202.5–292.5 g	45–157.5 g	50–70 g
2,000	225–325 g	50–175 g	55.5–78 g
2,200	247.5–357.5 g	55–192.5 g	61–85.5 g
2,500	281–406 g	62.5–219 g	69.5–97 g
3,000	337.5–487.5 g	75–262.5 g	83–117 g

Calories × percent changed to decimal = calories from nutrient
Calories from nutrient ÷ 4 or 9 = Number of grams
for this nutrient

Examples:

1,200 cal × 45% (0.45) = 540 calories from carbohydrates
540 calories ÷ 4 cal/g = 135 g of carbohydrates

1,200 cal × 65% (0.65) = 780 calories from carbohydrates
780 calories ÷ 4 cal/g = 195 g of carbohydrates

Example Breakdown of a 1,200 Calorie Weight Loss Diet

Meal	Carbs: 45%	Protein: 30%	Fat: 25%
Breakfast	40 g	15 g	10 g
Snack	10 g	10 g	0 g
Lunch	30 g	20 g	10 g
Snack	15 g	0 g	0 g
Dinner	30 g	30 g	10 g
Snack	15 g	15 g	3 g
Dietary total	135 g	90 g	33 g

Source: Reprinted with permission from Mertig, R. G. (2011). *What nurses know . . . Diabetes.* New York, NY: Demos Health.

The client can also visit the FDA website *www.fda.gov/food/labelingnutrition/ consumerinformation/ucm078889.htm* (US Food and Drug Administration, n.d.). The most important thing to look at is the serving size, which is right under the words *Nutrition Facts* at the top. It can be listed as the number of slices, the size of the slice in ounces, the number of cups, from ¼ cup or more, or some other measurable amount (e.g., number of crackers). In the beginning, and periodically throughout an adventure in healthy eating, a person needs to use measuring cups and spoons to get accurate serving sizes and then put what is measured (the serving size) onto a plate typically used for this food. Clients should be directed to notice how much of the plate it covers. After awhile, they may be able to estimate the proper serving size. I still measure cereal and milk because I am tempted to pour more than the correct serving size, and they both contain carbs. It is also helpful to note how many servings a package contains.

CLINICAL EXAMPLE: Clients might be shocked to learn that most macaroni and cheese boxes contain four servings, especially if they have been splitting it with one other person (or eating all of it themselves). Once the concept of the serving size is understood, they need to realize that every number or percentage listed below it refers to that exact amount. That means if they are eating twice the serving size, they must multiply all the numbers on the nutrition facts label by 2, and so on.

A client should also look at calories per serving and the number of calories from fat. Divide this number by the total calories to get the percentage of fat per serving. Everyone who wants to lose weight should aim for 30% (0.3) or less. The FDA considers a food that contains fewer than 100 total calories as a low-caloric food, 100 to 399 calories as having a moderate amount of calories, and more than 400 calories or more as a high-calorie food (US FDA, n. d.). Next, look at fat and protein grams. Unless a person is trying to gain weight, the lower the fat grams and the higher the protein grams, the better. If a client is counting carbs, the total carbohydrate grams is important, not just the grams of sugar, which is included in that total. I have already discussed the importance of fiber; clients should look for at least 5 g of fiber per serving of cereal and 2½ to 3 g per slice of bread. Comparing labels and buying the better source of fiber that tastes good to that person and his or her family represent an investment in health.

The last items of note on the label are sodium and potassium. Both relate to blood pressure, which can be a problem with anyone who has diabetes. Sodium contributes to raising blood pressure, and potassium helps lower it. It is estimated that the average American consumes about 3,000 mg of sodium per day (Consumer Reports, 2010). We all need sodium in our body to maintain the appropriate concentration of blood and for electrolyte balance; however, the daily sodium intake for healthy people should be about the equivalent of a teaspoon of table salt, or 2,300 mg. If a client is already concerned about hypertension or is on medication to lower it, a low-sodium diet (≤2,300 mg) is a must. Advise clients to stick to fresh or frozen fruit (no sugar added) and fresh or frozen vegetables (not in butter sauce) and to limit canned products, deli meats, or processed foods. If they use canned vegetables, they should rinse the contents thoroughly and not use the liquid, to reduce the sodium. Rinsing canned beans also reduces the potential for intestinal gas.

According to *Consumer Reports Health.org* last reviewed August 2010, 75% of salt intake in the United States comes from packaged and restaurant foods. For example, if clients do not prepare their own spaghetti sauce, they should check and compare commercial preparations to find the lowest sodium content per serving size. A person can easily consume half or more of their 2,300 mg of sodium per day with just a ½ cup serving size of this product. Just like getting used to a low-fat diet, a low-sodium diet takes time. Sodium should be reduced gradually. This can be accomplished by putting the salt shaker in a cabinet to make it inconvenient to use; replacing salt with pepper, the available blends of herbs and spices (e.g., Mrs. Dash), and/or Morton's Lite Salt (a mixture of sodium and potassium chloride); and limiting salty snacks such as potato chips and pretzels and, when they are consumed, sticking to the serving size.

CLINICAL EXAMPLE: Besides reducing blood pressure, potassium also helps with fluid and electrolyte balance as well as nerve stimulation of muscles, including the heart muscle. Most potassium is found in cells, but the small amount in blood is critical in maintaining heart rhythm and kidney function. When potassium levels are too low, a person may experience leg and arm muscle cramps, nausea, vomiting, weakness, fatigue, heart palpitations, and abdominal cramps, bloating, or constipation.

Increasing potassium in the diet is as simple as eating more fresh fruits, such as bananas, cantaloupe, and citrus fruit, and vegetables, such as carrots, tomatoes, winter squash, and potatoes. Visit *www.dashdiet.org* for more information on the dietary alternative to stop hypertension (DASH) diet, which is low in sodium and high in potassium. It includes fresh fruits, vegetables, and whole-grain products. Box 2.1 lists examples of foods that lower blood pressure.

Because reading labels can be time consuming at first, suggest that clients start by looking at the products they already have in their refrigerators and/or pantries. On the next grocery shopping excursion, clients can start with bread or cereal if they find the products they have been buying are high in calories and fat and low in fiber. Next, they can look at milk and other dairy products for low-calorie, low-fat milk, and yogurt choices. Reduced-fat cheese adds calories, protein, and calcium to meals without adding carbohydrate grams.

WEIGHT LOSS

Weight loss is recommended for anyone whose BMI indicates that she or he is overweight or obese (see Box 2.2). Even a small weight loss of 7% of current weight or 10 to 20 pounds can reverse insulin resistance and improve blood sugar. This might be a selling point to use with clients. Weight loss should be achieved over a period of time with a loss of 1 to 2 pounds per week. This can

---

BOX 2.1
Foods That Lower Blood Pressure

FIBER-RICH FOODS
Whole-grain foods
    Brown rice
    Whole wheat bread
    High-fiber cereals
Fruit with edible peel or seeds
    Pears
    Apples
    Berries
    Figs, prunes
Vegetables
    Artichokes
    Celery
    Legumes
    Broccoli
    Peas

POTASSIUM-RICH FOODS
Salt substitutes (100% potassium chloride)
Light salt (half potassium chloride, half sodium chloride)
Fresh fruits and vegetables

Source: Reprinted with permission from Mertig, R. G. (2011). *What nurses know . . . Diabetes*. New York, NY: Demos Health.

---

be achieved by portion control, decreasing intake of high-calorie foods and foods with empty calories, and increasing physical activity. Calories ingested must not exceed calories burned or weight gain will result. Calorie intake for most adults should not be less than 1,000 to 1,200 Kcal/day for women or 1,200 to 1,600 Kcal/day for men. Anything less will result in a reprogramming of the rate at which calories are burned (Collazo-Clavell, 2009).

CLINICAL EXAMPLE: Because the body thinks it is being starved, the absorption of nutrients by the small intestine gets very efficient and the body's basal metabolic rate (the number of calories the body burns at rest to maintain normal body functions) decreases to conserve energy. Thus when calories are increased after weight loss, a person regains the weight lost and often more. It takes much more effort to increase metabolic rate to burn more calories than to decrease it. Any caloric restriction below the recommended limits stated above will result in what many call yo-yo dieting and will be counterproductive.

Using the calculations in Box 2.2 may be useful for a healthcare professional or client, or you could use the online calculator at the NIH National Heart, Lung, and Blood Institute website at *www.nhlbisupport.com/bmi*.

One of the most useful tools to achieve weight loss is a dietary journal. Keeping track of everything eaten, the timing of meals and snacks, and the amounts of each food item (which means measuring and weighing), to accurately calculate calories and grams of carbohydrates, protein, and fat and any emotions that accompany eating patterns, is very useful in generating an action plan to change and improve eating habits. Of course, physical activity is a part of any weight-loss program. In order to lose 1 to 2 pounds per week, a person must decrease intake by 500 to 1,000 calories per day or burn that much by increasing physical activity or combine both modalities.

Some weight loss diets advertise a weight loss of 10 pounds or more per week. That is possible in the beginning only because this diet causes water loss and puts a person at risk for dehydration. Eating at least 10 g of protein at every meal helps to prevent the burning of lean muscle mass when trying to lose weight. Muscles burn more calories even at rest,

---

BOX 2.2
Body Mass Index

BMI is body weight in kilograms divided by height in meters squared. To calculate BMI using pounds and inches, perform the following steps:

1. Multiply weight in pounds by 703.
2. Multiply height in inches times itself.
3. Divide the results of step 1 by step 2 and compare with results below.

Example:

1. 170 pounds × 703 = 119,510
2. 5 feet, 4 inches = 64 × 64 = 4,096
3. 119,510 ÷ 4,096 = 29.177 = overweight (see below)

Disease risk based on BMI and waist circumference

Weight category	BMI	Waist circumference	
		≤40 in men	>40 in men
		≤35 in women	>35 in women
Underweight	<18.5	Low	–
Normal weight	18.5–24.9	Low	–
Overweight	25–29.9	Increased	High
Obese	30–39.9	High	Very high
Morbidly obese	≥40	Very high	Extremely high

therefore maintaining or increasing muscle mass is helpful in losing weight and maintaining that loss. Box 2.3 lists advice for weight loss success.

Losing weight can be difficult, but a sign I once saw, "Nothing tastes as good as thin feels," always makes me smile when I think about it. More information about weight loss drugs and surgery for obesity can be found at *www.weightwatchers.com*. Search the site for "The Physics of Weight

---

BOX 2.3
Advice for Weight Loss Success

■ Get accurate measuring cups and spoons. Use smaller plates and bowls.

■ Divide your plate in half and fill with nonstarchy fresh or cooked vegetables. On the other half, put a protein source and a starch source.

■ Substitute herbs and herb blends like Mrs. Dash for salt.

■ Reduce sugar by one-half to three-fourths, and double the amount of spices in recipes.

■ Replace half the fat in baked goods with unsweetened applesauce.

■ Steam mixed veggies such as broccoli, cauliflower, and carrots and top with reduced-fat cheese crumbles, or spritz with spray butter.

■ Roast vegetables such as squash, sweet potato, or colorful peppers to enhance their sweetness and eat more veggies. Try going meat-less once or twice a week.

■ Don't skip meals or go hungry. Snack on fresh fruit and veggies.

■ Eat more whole grains and high-fiber foods.

■ Drink cold water or unsweetened, decaffeinated tea before meals and snacks. You'll burn calories heating it to body temperature and will partially fill your stomach.

■ Brush your teeth and/or chew sugarless gum after dinner to curb evening snacking.

■ Weigh yourself often: every day or every week to test out one or more strategies, for a pat on the back, or to get back on track. Also note how clothes feel (loose is good).

■ Eat more meals at home using grocery store shortcuts and pack healthy lunches.

■ Stop wolfing down meals and snacks. Set a timer for at least 20 minutes, and enjoy the food until the timer rings by putting your fork down between bites. This will help you slow down your eating habits and give your body time to register fullness.

■ Keep a bathing suit or pair of jeans you'd like to fit into in plain sight. Put a picture on the refrigerator of what you'd like to look like. It may keep you from opening it.

Source: Reprinted with permission from Mertig, R. G. (2011). *What nurses know . . . Diabetes.* New York: Demos Health.

Loss," then scroll down to and click on "Bariatric Surgery and Weight Loss" and/or "Weight-Loss Medications."

The Sleep—Weight Connection

Sleep deprivation is common today, but it can make someone sick and fat. Several studies have shown the connection between lack of sufficient sleep and obesity in both adults and children. Inadequate sleep has been linked to lower levels of the hormone leptin, which signals to our brain that we are full. In children, one study showed that inadequate sleep was the biggest contributor to childhood obesity, more so than any other factor (Spruyt, Molfese, & Gozal, 2011). How can a person tell how much sleep he or she needs? Because everyone is different, a good test is to wake up without an alarm clock. Usually when a person wakes up this way, the body is rested. If someone routinely sleeps longer on the weekend, or when he or she does have to be somewhere, that is symptomatic of sleep deprivation. On average, most people need between 7 and 8 hours of sleep every night, although some may wake up after only 4 or 5 hours and feel rested, whereas others may need 10 hours or more. One of the most pleasant ways to lose weight then is to get enough sleep.

OLD FOOD PYRAMID VERSUS 2010 DIETARY GUIDELINES

The 2010 Dietary Guidelines for Americans developed by the U.S. Department of Agriculture (USDA) and the U.S. Department of Health and Human Services is an attempt to individualize the food pyramid. The website *http://mypyramid.gov* provides authoritative advice for anyone 2 years of age and older concerning healthy dietary habits that reduce the risk of major chronic diseases. All anyone has to do is key in his or her age, gender, and physical activity level truthfully and a personalized dietary recommendation based on the 2010 guidelines is produced. It details the kinds and amounts of foods in each food group to eat each day, provides examples and serving sizes of each food in the food groups, as well as encouragement to improve dietary choices and make lifestyle changes in small incremental steps. "My Pyramid Tracker" provides a means to monitor a person's progress. Before nurses and other healthcare professionals can truly understand how to help someone else modify his or her diet and increase healthy choices, they need to go to this impressive site and see how their own diet measures up to the recommendation for age, gender, and physical activity.

Thankfully, the diabetic (ADA) diets of the past are gone. What healthcare practitioners need to remember is that the diet appropriate for a client with diabetes is a nutritious, well-balanced diet full of choices, including sugar. It is a diet that meets all of the recommendations from the American Heart Association, the American Cancer Society, the ADA, and the 2010 Dietary Guidelines for Americans. It is full of vitamins, minerals, antioxidants, flavonoids, and other nutrients that everyone needs to stay healthy. The 2010 Dietary Guidelines were released on June 15, 2010, by the Dietary Guidelines Advisory Committee, which researched and consolidated nutritional data over the past 5 years. These guidelines, an update from the 2005 guidelines, focus on the prevention of obesity and chronic disease and advise Americans to do the following:

- Minimize time spent in front of the television and computer screens.
- Eat more home-cooked meals to lower the sodium and *trans*-fat content of the foods eaten.
- Consume more fruits, vegetables, and whole grains, and decrease consumption of processed foods.
- Minimize consumption of added sugars, as in sweets and regular sodas; refined grains, such as white bread and white rice; and sodium. Avoid adding sugar and salt at the table, and minimize the amount added in cooking.
- Increase physical activity for everyone, not just the overweight. All age brackets benefit from becoming more active. Some physical activity is better than none, and more is even better (U.S. Department of Agriculture [USDA], 2010).

To view the full text of the 2010 Dietary Guidelines, go to *www.cnpp.usda .gov/dgas2010-dgacreport.htm.*

CLINICAL EXAMPLE: Someone is always telling me that I cannot eat this or that because I have diabetes. My answer to them is usually, "If I can't eat it, maybe you shouldn't eat it." I might also add, "If I can give myself sufficient insulin to control blood sugar as your pancreas does, all that will happen is that we will both gain weight."

CARBOHYDRATE COUNTING

If insulin administered should match the amount of carbohydrates ingested, then counting carbs is a worthwhile endeavor. The foods that have the greatest effect on blood sugar include the items in the bread/ cereal food group, the fruit group, the milk group, and starchy vegetables such as peas, corn, lima beans, potatoes, and dried or canned beans, and sweets, of course. The amount of each is also important. The following is a practical guide to counting grams of carbohydrates.

The bread/cereal/starch group equals 15 g of carbs per serving:

Bread	1 slice
Pasta	½ cup (cooked)
Dry cereal	1 oz (¼ to 1½ cups based on the type of cereal)
Cooked cereal	½ cup or 1 packet of instant
Starchy vegetables	⅓ to ½ cup (cooked)
Potato with skins	½ potato measuring 2¼ × 4¾ inches, or ½ cup slice/mash/canned

The fruit group equals 15 g of carbohydrates per serving:

Fresh fruits	1 medium piece or ½ grapefruit, 1 cup strawberries, ½ cup blueberries, ½ banana, or 1 small banana
Fruit juice	⅓ to ½ cup (2.7–4 oz)
Frozen fruit	See nutrition label for serving size
Canned fruit	See nutrition label for serving size (Use only if canned in fruit juice)

The milk group equals 12 g of carbohydrates per serving:

Milk	1 cup
Yogurt, plain	¾ cup or 6 oz

Nonstarchy vegetables have 5 g of carbohydrates per ½ cup cooked or 1 cup raw. I usually eat as much of this food group as I want to avoid getting hungry. Meats and fats have no carbohydrates unless cooked or mixed with something that does. Counting carbs has gotten much easier with food labels and their listed nutritional contents. As stated earlier in this chapter, a serving size is identified at the top of the food label. If a serving size is doubled, the carb grams, as well as all other entities on the label, must also be doubled.

CLINICAL EXAMPLE: Because I have listed serving sizes for whole fruit and fruit juices, I need to differentiate between the two. *Fruit juice* usually has very little fiber and is already in liquid form, so it is absorbed very quickly and raises blood sugar within a few minutes. Juice is ideal for raising blood sugar when someone is experiencing hypoglycemia, but otherwise clients should choose the whole fruit or frozen fruit without added sugar. Whole fruit has fiber and its breakdown to a liquid form by the stomach burns calories before it can be absorbed. Blood glucose rises much more slowly when fruit is eaten, especially after a meal. Healthy, low-carb juices to drink include tomato and V8 juices, although they have a moderately high sodium content. For a list of the lowest carb fruits and vegetables, as well as for other suggestions for snacks, lunches, and dinner ideas, visit *www.dlife.com/food*.

How many carbs should a person eat? The following are some suggestions, depending on total calories (Neithercott, 2011):

Women: 45 to 60 g per meal

Men: 60 to 75 g per meal

Snacks: 15 to 30 g up to two snacks per day as needed

I have not written about the glycemic index as a way of counting carbs, because I find it cumbersome. It is much easier for me to remember the grams of the various food groups and keep a rough idea of their serving size than to look up every product on the glycemic index. My other objection to using the glycemic index is that some high-fat foods are on the low end of the index because the fat content blunts the blood sugar spike. For more information on the glycemic index, go to *www.carbs-information.com/glycemic-index-food-chart.htm*.

To help put everything in this chapter together, it is helpful to have a food count book that lists calories, carbohydrates, protein, fat, sodium, and fiber per serving size. It should include fresh foods as well as brand names. Nutrients of foods from fast food and chain restaurants can be found on their websites. You can suggest to your clients to be prepared with healthy options before eating out. They can also create a personalized menu using foods from the list at *www.changingdiabetes-us.com*, or go to *www.mypyramid.gov* for answers to questions, and let this helpful site plan meals for them. It might also be useful to have a cookbook and only use recipes that list serving size and nutrient content, especially calories and carb and fiber grams.

If you or your clients have been following the debates on healthcare in Washington, you know that it will take awhile to unravel all that is in this massive bill. However, one thing tucked into this bill that might be helpful when eating out at fast food and other chain restaurants is a requirement that calorie counts be on menus, menu boards, and even drive-through menu boards. The FDA has written new rules that must be followed by any restaurant that has 20 or more locations in the country. Other nutritional information besides calories will have to be posted somewhere else in the restaurant. The requirements will be enforced by the FDA with possible criminal penalties for noncompliance. The new rules can be found at *www.fda.gov/NewsEvents/Newsroom/PressAnnouncements/ucm249471.htm*

ALCOHOL: PROS AND CONS

Many people think that anyone with diabetes should not drink alcoholic beverages. Clients may ask the nurse or a healthcare practitioner about this, so you need to know what to tell them. Several studies in both men and women have shown that moderate drinking, no more than one to two drinks per day, can reduce the risk of heart disease and stroke by 30% to 50% by increasing the HDL cholesterol levels and preventing clot formation in arteries (Cheskin et al., 2011). *Johns Hopkins White Papers: Nutrition and Weight Control* (Cheskin et al., 2011) lists the following recommendations with regard to alcohol:

1. If you currently do not drink alcohol, do not start.
2. If you are a man, limit yourself to one to two drinks per day and cut this in half if over the age of 65. It is more difficult to detoxify alcohol with age.
3. If you are a woman, limit intake to no more than one drink per day and only half that amount if over the age of 65.
4. The type of alcoholic drink does not matter. Wine (red or white), beer, and spirits affect cardiovascular health the same.
5. Heavy alcohol consumption (defined as more than two drinks per day) can cause or worsen hypertension, cardiovascular disease, stroke, liver disease, or porphyria, a rare, genetic metabolic disease.
6. Some people should not drink. Anyone with high triglyceride levels, uncontrolled hypertension, pancreatitis, and liver disease or who has had problems with alcohol in the past should not drink.
7. Alcohol can also interfere with many medications. (Individuals should discuss this with their prescribing healthcare practitioner or a pharmacist first.)
8. Do not drink and drive or operate heavy machinery (Cheskin et al., 2011).

Alcohol can be part of the diet for a person with diabetes as long as it is used in moderation and the calories and carbohydrates (if any) are accounted for. Alcohol delivers 7 calories per gram and is metabolized like a fat. One drink is defined as a 12-oz beer, a 5-oz glass of wine, or 1.5-oz glass of distilled spirits.

CLINICAL EXAMPLE: Beer, sweet wines, and after-dinner liqueurs have carbs that need to be counted. Clients with diabetes should not mix alcohol with anything that has carb value, such as fruit juices or regular soft drinks, for the same reason. Refer them to Baja Bob's website for his sugar-free drink mixers at *www.bajabob.com* if they are looking for some tasty mixers that come in bottles or in single-serving packets. No alcohol is required.

Alcohol can cause hypoglycemia, so it should always be consumed with food. The reason for this is that alcohol is detoxified in the liver. If hypoglycemia occurs, alcohol prevents the liver from responding to the glucagon (secreted by the pancreas) by releasing stored sugar, so one's blood glucose may drop dangerously low. In addition, because the behavior of someone experiencing low blood sugar is often mistaken for drunkenness, a diabetic with alcohol on his or her breath may not be treated appropriately, potentially resulting in brain damage and even death from severe hypoglycemia.

SICK-DAY MANAGEMENT

When someone has diabetes and is sick, this can become a big problem. He or she needs to know how to handle issues with glycemic control before the need arises in order to prevent further illness from hypoglycemia or hyperglycemia. Testing blood sugar every 2 to 4 hours when sick is a must even if the person has type 2 diabetes. If a blood sugar is high, clients must stay hydrated with diet or noncaloric drinks such as water, broth, sugar-free tea or coffee, and sugar-free gelatin or popsicles. If a blood sugar is normal or low, then small amounts of regular soda or fruit drinks need to be consumed. Good advice is to start drinking fluids slowly 1 to 2 hours after vomiting or diarrhea. If this causes more vomiting or diarrhea, wait another 1 to 2 hours. Table 2.2 gives more examples of food to eat during an illness.

If insulin or a secretagogue medication has already been administered, glucose tablets or gels should be available to prevent or treat hypoglycemia. The following items each equal about 10 to 15 g of carbohydrates and are appropriate to treat a low glucose level.

Food Item	Amount
Sugar packets	2 to 3 packets
Fruit juice	½ cup (4 oz)
Soda (not diet)	½ cup (4 oz)
Hard candy	3 to 5 pieces
Sugar or honey	4 tsp
Glucose tablets	3 to 4 tablets
Glucose gel packets	1 packet

Clients need to test first before assuming their blood glucose level will drop. Often an illness or infection will stress the body enough to release hormones that will raise blood sugar.

Medical nutrition management for clients with diabetes can be an adventure in good health for the whole family if approached in a positive manner. Since my diagnosis, my whole family has benefited from a healthier diet

TABLE 2.2
What to Eat or Drink During an Illness:
Foods That Have 15 Grams of Carbohydrates

FOOD ITEM	AMOUNT
Fruit juice	½ cup
Fruit-flavored drink (not diet)	½ cup
Soda (regular, not diet)	½ cup
Gelatin (regular, not sugar-free)	½ cup
Popsicle (regular, not sugar-free)	½ cup
Sherbet	½ cup
Saltine crackers	6 crackers
Bread	1 slice
Milk	1 cup
Soup	1 cup
Ice cream (regular)	½ cup
Applesauce	½ cup
Pudding (regular)	¼ cup
Macaroni, noodles, rice	⅓ cup (cooked)
Potatoes, beans, cereal	½ cup (cooked)

Source: Reprinted with permission from Mertig, R. G. (2011). *What nurses know . . . Diabetes*. New York, NY: Demos Health.

because I never prepare anything I should not eat. The emphasis should be on making changes gradually and keeping some favorite foods in the diet for eating on occasion as long as blood sugars are well controlled.

REFERENCES

American Diabetes Association. (2011). Standards of medical care in diabetes—2011. *Diabetes Care, 34*, S11–S61.

Center for Science in the Public Interest. (2004, October 25). *CSPI warns consumers about Frito-Lay "Light" Chips with Olestra*. Retrieved April 12, 2011, from www.cspinet.org/new/200410251.html

Cheskin, L. J., Roberts, C., & Margolis, S. (2011). *Johns Hopkins White Papers: Nutrition and weight control*. New York, NY: Remedy Health Media, LLC.

Collazo-Clavell, M. (2009). *Mayo Clinic: The essential diabetes book*. New York: Time, Inc.

Consumer Reports Health.org. (2010, August). *Where does sodium hide and how to limit it*. Retrieved October 10, 2011, from http://www.consumer reports.org/health/healthy-living/diet-nutrition/diets-dieting/12-ways-to -cut-salt-from-your-diet/overview/index.htm

Mertig, R. G. (2011). *What nurses know . . . Diabetes.* New York, NY: Demos Health.

Neithercott, T. (2011, March). Are carbs the enemy? *Diabetes Forecast.* Retrieved from http://forecast.diabetes.org/carbs-enemy

Spruyt, K., Molfese, D. L., & Gozal, D. (2011, January 24). Sleep duration, sleep regularity, body weight, and metabolic homeostasis in school-aged children. *Pediatrics.* Retrieved April 16, 2011, from http://pediatrics.aappublications .org/cgi/reprint/peds.2010-0497v1

The Hershey Company. (n.d.). *Types of chocolate products.* Retrieved November 24, 2010, from http://www.hersheys.com/nutrition/chocolate.asp

U.S. Food and Drug Administration. (n.d.) *How to understand and use the nutrition facts label.* Retrieved April 13, 2011, from www.fda.gov/food/labelingnutrition/consumerinformation/ucm078889.htm

U.S. Department of Agriculture. (2010). *The 2010 dietary guidelines for Americans.* Retrieved April 21, 2011, from http://www.cnpp.usda.gov/DGAs2010-DGACReport.htm and www.cnpp.usda.gov/Publications/DietaryGuidelines/2010/DGAC/Report/D-5-Carbohydrates.pdf

Warshaw, H. S., & Boderman, K. M. (2001). *Practical carbohydrate counting.* Alexandria, VA: American Diabetes Association.

THREE

Treatment: Physical Activity

What can be done at ANYTIME, will be done at NO TIME.
  —Old Scottish Proverb

I have decided to use the term *physical activity* interchangeably with *exercise* because exercise also has a negative connotation for many people. Just like the word *diet, exercise* seems to portray punishing athletic endeavors: long, boring, and sweaty walking, running, or weight lifting at the gym. Physical activity, on the other hand, means physical movement, the kind that gets you out of bed in the morning and keeps you moving throughout the day. It is important to remind ourselves and our clients that it all counts toward keeping our muscles toned and our bones strong. What we all need is more of it.

I was in Chicago recently, visiting my daughter and her family, and was amazed to see fewer obese children and adults than in my own suburb of Richmond, Virginia. The population in this and, I presume, other large cities is very dense, with most people living in high-rise apartments and condos. Space to park a car is at a premium, and gas prices are terribly high. Most Chicagoans walk to stores, restaurants, friends' homes, and often to work. At the very least, they have to walk to the closest mass transit facility. Avoiding stairs is also often not an option, because public transportation may include walking up to the elevated subway or down to the subway, and most people live in walk-up apartments or condos. During my visit, we ate out a lot, so I was shocked when I returned home to find that I had lost weight. What a refreshing turn of events!

CLINICAL EXAMPLE: I am now walking from my home to the drugstore, library, and anywhere else that is a mile or so away instead of always getting in my car. Walking saves gas and I notice more of what is going on near where I live. Of course, this is presuming there is no inclement weather, but my experience in Chicago has increased the amount of walking that I do. This takes a little planning and time, so I just do not head for my car every time I need to run an errand. As healthcare professionals, we must be able to give evidence that we take our own advice seriously.

WHAT COUNTS AS PHYSICAL ACTIVITY

Physical activity is anything that gets your arms and/or legs moving. If someone does it for at least 20 minutes and it gets their heart and lungs working harder, we call it *aerobic exercise*. It conditions both the heart and lungs so they are in better shape to work more efficiently, even at rest. If a person works on separate muscle groups, such as the upper arms, thighs, or abdomen, we call it *weight training*, and it is an example of *anaerobic*, or passive, exercise. What about stretching muscles and increasing flexibility? Yes, that is exercise, too. Isometrics, in which you use your own body to push and pull against something, also is a form of exercise, called *resistance training*. Even relaxation exercises can benefit muscles and increase stamina. What about work around the house or in the yard? It all counts and burns calories. Table 3.1 lists some examples.

TABLE 3.1
Calories Burned per Half-Hour of Work

ACTIVITY	CALORIES BURNED
Making the bed	68
Doing laundry	73
Washing dishes	78
Ironing	78
Dusting	85
Cooking	85
Washing the car	102
Washing windows	102
Sweeping	112
Vacuuming	119
Scrubbing floors	129
Gardening	136
Raking	146
Yard work	170
Mowing the lawn	187
Rearranging furniture	204
Shoveling snow	204
Carrying 15 pounds up or downstairs	289

Note: These statistics, from www.caloriesperhour.com, are for a 150-pound, 35-year-old woman doing 30 solid minutes of everyday chores around the house.

Types of Exercise

In case you or your client is wondering exactly what to do to increase physical activity level and why, the following discussion should be of interest. You don't need to be a physical therapist to recommend that your clients practice some or all of the following exercises. If you do suggest any, be sure your clients know why they should do these exercises at home—they are more likely to practice them.

Aerobic Exercise

The 2010 Dietary Guidelines for Americans, published by the U.S. Department of Agriculture (USDA), state that most people should aim for a minimum of 30 minutes of aerobic exercise per day on most days. Aerobic exercise is defined as any physical activity that increases the heart and respiratory rates and causes a person to break a light sweat (USDA, 2010). This includes walking inside or outside, dancing alone or with a partner, using an aerobic DVD, swimming, water aerobics, low-impact aerobics classes, ice or roller skating, tennis (even hitting the backboard), biking inside or outside, mowing the lawn, gardening, housework, and so on. Weight-bearing exercises to keep calcium in bones and prevent osteoporosis consist of all of these except exercises in water, because water exercises, although aerobic, do not put pressure on the long bones of the arms or legs and so are not *weight-bearing.* This is why they are good for people with arthritis, but these clients also need to do some other exercise, such as weight training, to help bones stay strong.

Children and teens should aim for at least 60 minutes of exercise a day (USDA, 2010). Some of this time could take place during an active gym class or actively playing during recess at school. This never used to be a problem because most kids enjoy being physically active. As long as excessive TV, video, or computer games and other sedentary pursuits don't take over their playtimes, children will be active. With the dangers today of abduction and physical harm comes the problem of trying to keep our children safe by confining them to the house even when we are present. Parents need to find alternatives to the naturally active play that used to be part of growing up. Interactive PlayStation, Xbox, Wii exercise games, and other computer/TV technology are fun ways to get children and adults to be more active. Other suggestions to make to parents who need to get their children moving more include enrolling them in after-school day care, YMCA programs, or other supervised activities, as well as many other possibilities. Actively playing with children or grandchildren after work not also takes thought and creativity but may be the solution to physical inactivity for both the child and the adult. For me, playing ring-around-the-rosy and other active games with my 3-year-old grandson meets all the criteria for aerobic activity.

CLINICAL EXAMPLE: A large study of overweight adults with prediabetes, The Diabetes Prevention Program (DPP), set out to determine whether lifestyle modification could prevent or delay the onset of diabetes. Lifestyle modifications in this study included weight loss of 7%, maintained for the 3-year study, and a minimum of 150 minutes of physical activity a week, or 30 minutes on 5 days a week. The participants in this study reduced their risk of developing type 2 diabetes by 58%, and those aged 60 years and older decreased their risk by 71% (DPP, 2002). If this sounds like too much physical activity for your clients, suggest that they start slowly, with 10 minutes of physical activity, adding 5 to 10 minutes per day every week or so, until they have reached 30 minutes or more. Exercise doesn't even have to be done all at one time. Three 10-minute periods can also be useful. A study done in Australia of middle-aged clients with prediabetes showed that those who build up to 10,000 steps a day and kept it up for 5 years lowered their body mass index (BMI), had less belly fat, and improved their insulin sensitivity, thus preventing type 2 diabetes. The participants in this study used pedometers to count their steps (Dwyer, 2011).

Strength (Resistance) Training

Increasing muscle tone, strength, and size requires that people lift more weight than they are used to. The more muscle tissue we have, the more calories we burn per hour, day and night. Combining resistance training and aerobic exercise during a 9-month study of sedentary men with type 2 diabetes demonstrated that the combination reduced A1c (see Chapter 5) the most compared with either used separately (Church & Sigal, 2010).

1. Bicep curls: Advise clients to start with 1- or 2-lb weights in each hand, and slowly raise hands, palms up, toward shoulders then slowly lower them to sides.
2. Triceps: Raise the weights over head and slowly lower them behind the head and neck to strengthen the triceps.
3. Arm and shoulder muscles: Raise the weights with straight arms to the side to.
4. For legs: Hooking them under a heavy piece of furniture and, with knees loose, contract thigh muscles slowly, and try to lift. Hold for a count of 10 and then relax slowly.
5. Squats can be done using an exercise ball or beach ball against a wall. With the back on the ball and feet well in front of the body, lean back and lower your body to a sitting position, rolling the back against the ball for stability. If the knees go over the toes when bent, move the feet farther away from the wall.
6. Abdominal muscles: Lie on a mat on the floor with knees bent and soles of feet on the floor. Place hands, palm down, under small of back.

Contract abdominal muscles and press small of back against hands while rolling head and shoulders a few inches off the floor. Hold for a count of 10 and then slowly lower head and shoulder back to floor.

Do eight repetitions of each exercise, pause for 1 minute, and do eight more. Do them slowly, and take deep breaths throughout. When doing two sets of eight becomes easy, either increase the number of repetitions to 12 per set or increase the weights. Remember to move slowly; increase the weights slowly; and, above all, skip a day before exercising the same muscles. It takes 36 to 48 hours for muscles to rebuild, so alternate days for strength training arms and legs. The muscles of the abdomen rebuild in 24 hours, so abdominal exercises can be done every day (Mertig, 2011).

Stretching or Flexibility Exercises

The movements involved in stretching and flexibility exercises help joints remain flexible and injury free during any kind of exercise. Joints and muscles need to be warmed up before stretching, so do some low-intensity walking, arm movements, or sitting and then standing for a few minutes to get the blood flowing. Never stretch a cold muscle. Then focus on stretching each muscle that will be used in whatever aerobic activity planned.

1. For feet and ankles: Stand on the edge of a stair tread and go up on tiptoes, then let heels slowly drop slightly below the tread. Repeat a few times, holding onto the banister or wall.
2. For calves and Achilles tendons: Stand at arm's length from a wall with palms on the wall and fingers toward the ceiling. With left knee slightly bent, place right leg behind, with heel and foot flat on the floor. Bend left knee until you feel a stretch in the calf and Achilles tendon of the right leg. Hold for 10 to 30 seconds. Switch legs and repeat.
3. For thighs: Put one hand on the wall and with the other hand grasp the foot on same side. Pull the heel toward buttocks and hold for 10 to 30 seconds. Feel the stretch in front of thigh. Switch legs and hands and repeat.
4. For hamstrings (back of thigh): Stand behind a chair far enough away so you can bend at the hips and place hands with arms straight on back of chair. Hold for 10 to 30 seconds. Feel the stretch in the back of the thigh.
5. For hips and lower back: Lie flat on back. Bend both knees and clasp them with hands or forearms. Pull knees toward shoulders while exhaling. Hold for 10 to 30 seconds, breathing normally. Feel the stretch in the lower back.
6. For shoulder and upper back: Lie on back, with head on a pillow and legs out straight or with a rolled towel under knees. With arms at your side, bend elbows so fingers point to the ceiling and palms face

forward. Slowly roll arms toward the floor until you feel the stretch in your shoulders. Hold for 10 to 30 seconds. Raise forearms slowly off the floor so fingers point to the ceiling again, then return them to your side.

7. For sides: Stand or sit and reach upward with one arm and hand while the other reaches down the other side of the body. Hold for 10 to 30 seconds. Feel the stretch along the rib cage, back of arm, and waist. Repeat with the other side.

8. For triceps: Bend one arm behind the back and hold it in that position with the other hand at the elbow. Pull toward the opposite side until you feel the stretch along the back of your upper arm. Hold for 10 to 30 seconds and repeat with the other arm.

9. For neck and upper back: Slowly move chin to chest and hold, then bend neck backward and hold. Bend neck sideways with ear toward each shoulder and hold. Turn head so you are looking over each shoulder in turn and hold.

Repeat these stretches after exercising. This is probably the most important time to stretch, to prevent the exercised muscles from getting tight (Mertig, 2011).

Balance Exercises

Aging is the number one reason for poor balance in most people. However, people with diabetes may have a few more issues to contend with, such as neuropathy causing tingling and numbness in feet and uncorrected vision problems, like cataracts and retinopathy. (See Chapter 6 for more about diabetes-related complications.) Poor balance can lead to falls, causing fractures and possibly head injuries. There are many ways to improve balance, including practicing Tai Chi, yoga, and Pilates in addition to walking and general strength training. Clients can also practice the following exercises to improve their sense of balance. If needed, they can hold on to a wall or a chair for more stability.

■ Heel-to-toe walking: Place the heel of one foot in front of and touching the toes of other foot for 12 steps. Repeat two to four times.

■ Standing on one foot: Stand on one foot for 30 seconds. Change foot. Repeat two to four times.

■ Standing calf raises: Go from standing flat to on your tiptoes and hold briefly. Repeat 8 to 12 times. Rest and repeat.

■ Hip extensions: While holding on to the back of a chair, slowly raise your right leg in back of you to about 45 degrees or higher without bending the knee. Bend the upper body at the waist. Hold briefly and slowly lower leg. Repeat 8 to 12 times with each leg. Rest and repeat.

■ Side leg raises: Holding onto a chair, slowly raise right leg out to the side as far as you can. Keep knee straight. Hold and then slowly lower foot to the floor. Do this 8 to 12 times. Repeat with the left leg. Rest and repeat with each leg.

■ Chair stands: Sit on the front of a sturdy chair with feet flat on the floor. With arms crossed over chest and hands on shoulders, stand up slowly and then return to a sitting position. Do 8 to 12 repetitions. Rest and repeat (Mertig, 2011).

The American College of Sports Medicine recommends doing balance, flexibility, strength training, and aerobic exercises at least twice a week (Coltrera & Slon, 2010).

Relaxation Exercises

Exercises that relieve tension and promote calm are important for all of us. I have been doing some of these before falling asleep since I learned them in childbirth classes many years ago. There are many ways to clear the clutter from our brain and the tension from our muscles so we can unwind and relax. Diabetes increases the stress your client experiences every day. The following are some suggestions you could provide to help:

■ Mindfulness: Practice this while doing a repetitive task such as walking, swimming, or any other active exercise. First focus on doing deep breathing—in through the nose and out through the mouth—and the slow rise and fall of the chest and abdomen. After a few minutes, notice the bigger picture beyond your own body while continuing your slow, rhythmic breathing. Notice the sounds and smells around you. Feel the breeze and note the interplay of light and shadow.

■ Meditation can be a source of inner strength and a peaceful way to unwind at the end of a stressful day. Most people need to close their eyes to avoid distraction. Setting aside a special time and place may help. Turn off your phone (land or cell) and get in a relaxed position (e.g., in bed, in a lounger with your feet up and supported). Start with thinking of a peaceful scene (e.g., clouds, the beach, a field, Grandma's house, etc.). Try to recapture the smells you remember or think might be there. Take deep, calming breaths in through the nose and out through pursed lips to slow down your breathing to half the normal rate (eight to ten breaths/minute). Say or think a word or phrase over and over again, like a mantra. Some that come to mind include "I am calm," "I am relaxed," "I am strong," "I can do this," and so on. When you feel distracted, concentrate on your deep breathing until you banish the distractions from your consciousness. This takes practice, but it is worth doing, even for 10 minutes. It is a great way to prepare for sleeping or get rid of stress in the middle of the day.

■ Stretching exercises can also be relaxing if you note how your muscle and joints feel as you move them through their range of motion and feel the stretch in the appropriate muscles.

■ Progressive muscle relaxation exercises involves alternately tensing and relaxing groups of muscles throughout the body while doing deep breathing in through the nose and out through the mouth. It helps to focus on how each muscle group feels when contracted and when relaxed. These exercises are best done lying down on a mat or a bed in a comfortable position. Start with the muscles of the face and progress to the feet or start with feet and ankles and move to the face and scalp. I usually start from the top down, but most guided relaxation tapes start from the feet up. As you feel each group of muscles relax, visualize the stress of the day leaving your body while you sink deeper into your mat or mattress. The upper body exercises can be done at work multiple times a day to relieve tension.

Each exercise described in this chapter thus far requires practice and repetition to get the maximum benefit. Basic tips for everyone include starting wherever they find themselves in the physical activity category, from a couch potato to a marathoner. Then slowly take it to the next level. As clients become more comfortable with each activity, they can increase duration, intensity, weights, or other parameters. Start low and increase slowly. If for any reason an individual has to stop an exercise for longer than a week, he or she should resume at a level below where he or she stopped and progress slowly from there. Overdoing anything may cause pain and injury. Remember, the goal is to develop the lifelong habit of increased physical movement (Mertig, 2011).

BENEFITS OF EXERCISE

The benefits of physical activity are numerous and well documented. Physical activity has the following effects:

- It helps to control weight by increasing muscle tissue and decreasing fat production because the calories consumed are burned more efficiently by the body. Increased muscle mass (lean tissue) increases basal metabolic rate (the rate at which calories are burned at rest) so more calories are burned all day long and even while sleeping.
- It increases the efficiency of the heart and lungs by increasing demands on their functions, thus exercising the heart and respiratory muscles and increasing the depth of respirations needed to sustain aerobic activity. This decreases resting heart and respiratory rates. In fact, in a prospective study from 1970 and 2005, cardiorespiratory fitness in women decreased mortality irrespective of BMI, waist circumference, or percentage of body fat (Farrell, 2010).
- It increases bone density by providing weight-bearing and muscle tension on long bones (legs and arms). This prevents calcium from leaving bones and improves absorption of calcium from the gut. Any outdoor activity increases the manufacture of vitamin D from sun exposure and vitamin D enhances the absorption of calcium. Adequate sun exposure

in light-skinned individuals may take place in as little as 10 minutes. Dark-skinned individuals may need 60 minutes or more.

- It improves balance and stability because leg muscles are increasingly able to correct posture on uneven terrain and keep a person from falling. That is more and more important the older one gets.

- It improves digestion and elimination in the gastrointestinal tract by increasing peristaltic waves and blood flow to the stomach and intestines, thus preventing indigestion and constipation.

- It relaxes blood vessels, thus lowering blood pressure and improving blood flow and oxygenation to all body organs, including skin (the largest organ in the body) and brain.

- It lowers cholesterol levels by increasing HDL (the good cholesterol) and decreasing low-density lipoprotein (LDL) (the bad cholesterol) and triglycerides (Colberg, 2010).

- It improves sleep patterns by increasing blood flow to muscles, thus removing lactic acid buildup. Strenuous exercise should not be done within 3 hours of sleep time, however, because lactic acid may remain in muscles causing stiffness and pain.

- It enhances the body's immune system, not only by helping a person sleep better and more soundly but also by protecting one from the common cold and from some cancers. Light to moderate consistent exercise causes a temporary boost in the production of macrophages, the cells that gobble up bacteria and viruses. However, too much intense exercise can decrease immunity system function. Stress hormones such as cortisol and adrenaline are produced during extreme exercise, such as running in a marathon or triathlon training. These stress hormones raise blood pressure, blood sugar, and cholesterol levels as well as suppress the immune system (Johnson & Knopp, 2009).

- It increases a sense of well-being by providing a productive means of getting rid of excess negative emotions, such as anxiety, anger, frustration, and so forth. On the other hand, it increases positive feelings of empowerment and pride in accomplishing a set goal.

- It even increases libido and performance. Researchers at Harvard Medical School noted in a long-term study that men who exercised 30 minutes a day were 41% less likely to have erectile dysfunction compared with sedentary men (Bacon, 2003). Moderate exercise helps decrease the formation of arterial plaque, thus increasing blood flow to all areas of the body, as noted earlier. For women, the increase in libido is probably due to the increased sense of well-being and positive mood also mentioned earlier.

- If the above is not incentive enough for clients with diabetes, add the fact that physical activity helps to lower blood sugar. Because physical activity makes muscle more sensitive to insulin, glucose is used at a much faster rate.

Studies of sedentary individuals have shown that those who engage in regular, low-intensity workouts, such as a 10-minute leisurely stroll, boosted their energy levels by 20% and decreased their feelings of fatigue by 65% compared with individuals who remained sedentary (Puetz, 2008). This is even more important as we age. So, when you or your clients come home tired from a too-long and stressful day at work, don't sit in front of the TV to relax and unwind. Change into comfortable clothes and supportive shoes and go for a walk, or actively play with your children or grandchildren.

HOW MUCH AND HOW OFTEN?

The U.S. Department of Health and Human Services (USDH) 2008 Physical Activity Guidelines for Americans urge most adults to get at least 150 minutes of moderate aerobic activity or 75 minutes of vigorous exercise, or a mixture of each, every week (USDH, 2008). That works out to 20 to 25 minutes of moderate activity or 11 minutes of vigorous exercise, or some combination of the two, per day, divided up in any way that works for the individual.

CLINICAL EXAMPLE: The differences among light, moderate, and vigorous activity depend on how well a person can breathe, sweat, and talk while exercising. Therefore, it is different for everyone and changes as one becomes more fit. During light exercise, you can breathe and talk easily and are not sweating yet. (Of course, in the South, where I live, sweating depends on the weather and whether you are inside or outside.) With moderate exercise you are working harder, breathing faster, and definitely sweating but are still able to talk. (If you are alone, try talking on a cell phone to assess this.) If you indulge in vigorous exercise, you are breathing and sweating hard and find you can talk only in short bursts, if at all. Another way of measuring intensity is to calculate the number of steps per minute. If you are walking slowly, that translates to about 80 steps per minute. Moderate walking is the equivalent of 100 steps per minute, whereas brisk walking is around 120 steps per minute, and race walking is more than 120 steps per minute (Coltrera & Slon, 2010).

What about pulse rates? There are several ways to look at how fast an individual's pulse rate should be to qualify as aerobic exercise. The easiest method for men is to take their age and subtract it from 220. For women, multiply age by 0.88 then subtract that number from 206 (Gulati et al., 2010). The result of either equals a person's maximum heart rate, which can prove dangerous and should *not* be the pulse rate goal. Take that number and multiply it by 65% (0.65) and 85% (0.85) to find a safe heart rate range. *At least* 50% to 70% of maximum is what the American Diabetes Association (ADA) recommends for most people with diabetes (ADA, 2011). The lower end of the range (65%) strengthens the heart, lungs, and circulatory system, and the upper range (85%) improves endurance (Gulati et al., 2010).

As soon as you stop your activity, place your index and middle finger at the side of your neck or over the thumb side of the inside of your wrist and count beats for 15 seconds. Then multiply by 4. An alternative is to count your pulse for 10 seconds and multiply by 6. This will give you your heart rate per minute after exercising. Heart rate should be checked before cooling down or stretching because, depending on fitness level, the pulse may drop back to normal quickly. It is important to take one's pulse to ensure the activity is strenuous enough to reach the target heart rate but not so vigorous as to overstress the heart. Persons are probably exceeding target heart rate if they have difficulty catching their breath.

CLINICAL EXAMPLE: Personally, I try for 20 to 30 minutes of walking per day, more or less, with a heart rate of roughly 70% of my maximum, with some strength training and stretching every other day. I am working on adding more balancing exercising to my day to strengthen my core muscles and prevent falls in the future.

It is extremely important that we give ourselves permission to not be perfect. We all have good days and some not-so-good days; however, setting realistic goals and scheduling the time are more important than what type of activity we end up doing. As my 92-year-old Swedish friend tells me every time I call her, "Every day I wake up in the morning is a good day." Healthcare professionals and clients alike need to be our own positive influence and find someone like my friend to inspire us.

HOW TO INCREASE PHYSICAL ACTIVITY

The following are some tips to help fit more physical activity into anyone's life:

- Get up earlier to go for a run, a walk, or a bike ride. In fact, why not watch or listen to the morning news while riding a stationary bike?
- Use part of a lunch break to walk or exercise.
- Eat dinner a little earlier or later to fit in some exercise before relaxing for the day.
- Join a gym or a neighborhood sports team. Athletic talent is not usually required.
- Run or walk around an inside or outside track on the way home from work.
- Exercise a dog or actively play with children or grandchildren.
- Vacuum, clean the tiles in a bathroom, scrub floors, or perform other household chores. These are very productive activities even if not the most fun things to do. Listening to music or an audio book can make the time fly by.

■ Perform any physical activity that is appealing and worth the time and energy it takes to do it.
■ Make or schedule the time to add to or increase activity level.
■ Add 10 minutes to a walk around the block, to improve endurance.

Making physical activity a daily routine is as important as going to work or getting to an appointment. Making it a family affair gets the kids active and teaches them that physical activity is important in a well-rounded person. And make it fun. If an incentive to set a specific time for physical activity is needed, reread the Scottish proverb at the beginning of this chapter.

POTENTIAL PROBLEMS WITH EXERCISE

There *is* a downside to physical activity for anyone on insulin or oral medications that make the pancreas secrete more insulin. That problem is hypoglycemia. Tell clients that low blood sugar can be avoided or minimized, however, by adhering to the following advice:

1. The best time to be active is about 30 minutes to 1 hour after a meal. Unless the activity is prolonged (more than 60 minutes) or very strenuous (swimming 50 laps of an Olympic-size pool) or the meal is loaded with fats and protein (10-ounce steak, large order of fries), abdominal cramps will not occur.
2. When exercise occurs more than 2 hours after eating, a blood sugar check is in order. If it is less than 120 mg/dl, consider eating or drinking something that has about 15 to 30 mg of carbohydrates, such as a piece of fruit, 6 ounces of orange juice, or an 8-ounce glass of milk. It might be better to take less insulin prior to a meal that precedes planned exercise if the goal for exercising is to lose weight.
3. If blood sugar is over 250 mg/dl or especially over 350 mg/dl, check urine for ketones, and postpone exercise until blood sugar is less than 250 mg/dl and *ketonuria* is gone. Taking rapid-acting insulin and waiting 30 minutes or so should also help (Scheiner, 2004). When blood sugar is high, it means that the body does not have enough insulin to keep it in the normal range by helping the blood glucose enter cells. This includes muscle cells, which store glucose as glycogen. When muscle tissue is not fed glucose to perform physical activity, it dumps stored glycogen into the blood so the muscle cells can burn this glucose. Unfortunately, this use of glucose does not happen because there is insufficient insulin to transport the blood sugar into these cells. The end result after exercising with a high blood sugar can be an even higher blood sugar and a very sluggish feeling. When cells cannot get to glucose, fat is burned for energy, resulting in blood and urine ketones.
4. Always carry glucose tablets when taking insulin or oral medications that increase pancreatic secretions (secretagogues). If *hypoglycemia unawareness* (see Chapter 5) is a problem, exercise with someone who is aware of symptoms of hypoglycemia and can get help if the need

should arise. Carrying a cell phone to call for help is also good advice and wear an ID bracelet that states you have diabetes.

5. If insulin injections are used, avoid injecting into fatty areas of extremities used during exercise. For example, if brisk walking, jogging, swimming, or skiing is involved, avoid injecting insulin into the fat over upper thighs and buttock muscles. If lifting weights or heavy housecleaning is anticipated, avoid injecting into the back of upper arms. Exercise increases blood supply to active muscles, which causes vasodilation of smaller blood vessels in the subcutaneous fatty layer directly above the muscles. If insulin has been injected there, it will be absorbed into the bloodstream much faster than anticipated. This, along with the fact that exercise increases insulin sensitivity of muscles and other tissue, makes hypoglycemia even more likely.

6. Check blood sugar a couple of hours after exercising, because an intense workout may cause hypoglycemia for several hours. Making the body more insulin sensitive has its drawbacks if the usual amount of insulin or oral agent is taken and exercise is added. It may be wise to discuss with the prescribing healthcare practitioner how to decrease medication on days when planned exercise is prolonged and/or strenuous in order to prevent hypoglycemia (Scheiner, 2004).

7. Before starting an exercise program, check with a physician who may order an exercise stress test to see how the heart and blood pressure respond. If diabetic complications are part of the picture, see Table 3.2 for common restrictions and alternative suggestions. Also see Chapter 6 for further discussion of chronic complications.

8. Adequate hydration is important for everyone, whether they exercise or not. However, it is extremely important for all individuals to drink water before and after exercising. If physical activity is very strenuous or prolonged, fluid intake during exercise is important to prevent dehydration from excessive perspiration. Water is the best choice for fluid replacement. Sports drinks contain calories, sugar, and electrolytes, which are usually needed only by endurance athletes.

9. Inspect feet after exercise to check for blisters and/or reddened areas. This is especially important for those with peripheral neuropathy who may not feel an injury or with peripheral artery disease. Adequate circulation is needed to heal and prevent infection even with a minor wound. Any bruising or injured skin and tissue should be examined by a physician immediately so it can be treated to prevent infection and further trauma to the area.

10. It goes without saying that good supportive shoes and comfortable clothing are a must. Checking the inside of shoes for worn areas or small items, such as a stone, that may cause discomfort or injury is important for everyone. My nondiabetic husband once realized his foot was sharing a shoe with an insect and now always looks before sliding his feet into shoes.

TABLE 3.2

Diabetic Complications and Exercise

COMPLICATION	EXERCISE TO AVOID	RATIONALE	CHOOSE INSTEAD
Peripheral neuropathy	Jogging, brisk walking, climbing	May cause foot trauma, turned ankle, falls	Swimming, stationary bike, rowing machine
Autonomic neuropathy	Strenuous or prolonged exercise	Decreased cardiovascular response, postural hypotension	Walking, swimming, treadmill
Proliferative retinopathy	Jogging, skiing, body contact sports. Any jarring or rapid head movement. Heavy lifting. Any use of Valsalva breath holding	May cause retinal detachment or vitreous hemorrhage	Walking, swimming, stationary bike
Nephropathy	Strenuous or prolonged exercise	May increase proteinuria. Does not affect progression of renal disease	Walking, swimming, exercise equipment for mild to moderate intensity and duration
Cardiovascular disease, including congestive heart failure (CHF) and hypertension	Heavy lifting. Any use of Valsalva breath holding, strenuous or prolonged exercise	May cause angina, arrhythmias, and increased blood pressure if not well controlled	Swimming, treadmill, stationary bike

People with diabetes need to be reminded that healthy lifestyle choices are a must for everyone and not an imposition as a result of having diabetes. Increasing physical activity is important for individuals of any age. All adults should *try* to achieve the recommended 10,000 steps a day. This is a goal, not an absolute. Inexpensive pedometers and aerobic monitors are easily found in drug and variety stores. Recording activity level is both empowering and motivating. Some monitors equate steps taken with calories burned and miles walked. Because every step counts, a step counter may provide the encouragement to take the stairs instead of the elevator or to walk to do errands, especially if today is turning out to be a low-step day. Giving examples of how physical activity impacts *our* life in so many positive ways can be the incentive a client needs to *just do it!*

REFERENCES

American Diabetes Association (ADA). (2010). Standards of medical care in diabetes—2010. *Diabetes Care, 33,* S11–S61.

Bacon, C. G., Mittleman, M. A., Kawachi, I., Giovannucci, E., Glasser, D. B., & Rimm, E. B. (2003). Sexual function in men older than 50 years of age: Results from the Health Professionals Follow-up Study. *Annals of Internal Medicine, 139*(3), 161–169.

Church, T., & Sigal, R. (2010). Aerobic exercise plus resistance training helps control type 2 diabetes. *Journal of the American Medical Association, 304,* 2253–2262, 2298–2299.

Colberg, S. R., Sigal, R. J., Fernhall, B., Regensteiner, J. G., Blissmer, B. J., Rubin, R. R., . . . Braun, B. (2010). Exercise and type 2 diabetes: The American College of Sports Medicine and the American Diabetes Association: Joint position statement. *Diabetes Care, 33,* 2692–2696.

Coltrera, F., & Slon, S. (2010). *Exercise: A program you can live with.* Boston: Harvard Health Publications.

Dwyer, T., Ponsonby, A. L., Ukoumunne, O. C., Pezic, A., Venn, A., Dunstan, D., . . . Shaw, J. (2011). Association of change in daily step count over five years with insulin sensitivity and adiposity: Population based cohort study. *British Medical Journal, 342,* c7249. Retrieved March 25, 2011, from http://www.bmj.com/content/342/bmj.c7249.full

Farrell, S. W., Fitzgerald, S. J., McAuley, P. A., & Barlow, C. E. (2010). Cardiorespiratory fitness, adiposity, and all-cause mortality in women. *Medicine and Science in Sports and Exercise, 42*(11), 2006–2012.

Gulati, M., Shaw, L. J., Thisted, R. A., Black, H. R., Bairey Merz, C. N., & Arnsdorf, M. F. (2010). Heart rate response to exercise stress testing in asymptomatic women: The St. James Women Take Heart Project. *Circulation, 122,* 130–137.

Johnson, R., & Knopp, W. (2009) Nonorthopaedic conditions. In J. C. DeLee, D. Drez, Jr., & M. D. Miller (Eds.), *DeLee and Drez's orthopaedic sports medicine* (Chapter 3, 3rd ed.). Philadelphia, PA: Saunders Elsevier.

Mertig, R. G. (2011). *What nurses know . . . Diabetes.* New York, NY: Demos Health.

Puetz, T. W., Flowers, S. S., & O'Conner, P. J. (2008). A randomized controlled trial of the effect of aerobic exercise training on feelings of energy and fatigue in sedentary young adults with persistent fatigue. *Psychotherapy and Psychosomatics, 77*(3), 167–174.

Scheiner, G. (2004). *Think like a pancreas.* New York, NY: Marlowe & Company.

The Diabetes Prevention Program (DPP) Research Group. (2002). The Diabetes Prevention Program (DPP). Description of lifestyle intervention. *Diabetes Care, 25*(12), 2165–2171.

U.S. Department of Agriculture (USDA). (2010). *The 2010 dietary guidelines for Americans.* Retrieved June 21, 2010, from http://www.cnpp.usda.gov/DGAs2010-DGACReport.htm

U.S. Department of Health and Human Services (USDH). (2008). *Physical activity guidelines for Americans.* [Article online] 2008. Retrieved March 26, 2011, from www.health.gov/paguidelines/guidelines/default.aspx

FOUR

Treatment: Medication

A man too busy to take care of his health is like a mechanic too busy to take care of his tools.
—Spanish Proverb

When lifestyle changes, such as healthy eating, weight loss, and exercise, are not enough to normalize blood sugars, there is always medication. The classifications of oral agents and types of insulin have expanded exponentially in the past 15 years. Diabetes is big business, and pharmaceutical companies both in the United States and around the world are leading the pack to cash in. Besides new medications, we now have combinations of medications that complement each other in one pill as well as newer and faster-acting insulins and injectable noninsulin products. So much has happened so quickly that it is confusing and difficult for healthcare professionals to keep up. By the time you read this, there will be newer, more powerful, and useful drugs on the market. The companies that make these medications and their Web addresses are listed in the Resources section at the end of this book so you can do further research. It will be several years before the patents of the newer drugs expire and their generic equivalents are available. That means that the newest, more potent, and often best medications are very expensive. Many of the pharmaceutical companies have programs for providing their new drugs for free or at reduced cost to people, who meet certain criteria, so if clients can no longer afford their necessary medications, refer them to one of the following websites:

1. Partnership for Prescription Assistance, www.PPARx.org, 1-888-4PPA-NOW (1-888-477-2669)
2. National Diabetes Information Clearing House (NDIC), http://diabetes.niddk.nih.gov/dm/pubs/financialhelp/
3. Free Medicines: http://freemedicine.com/index.htm, 1-573-996-3333
4. Access to Wellness: www.access2wellness.com/a2w/index.html, 1-866-317-2775
5. Astra Zeneca: http://www.rxassist.org/
6. SelectCare Benefits Network: www.scbn.org/index.html, 1-888-331-1002

To receive assistance from one of these groups, clients must be referred through their prescribing healthcare practitioner. Letting a client know this service exists may start the ball rolling. In addition, an Internet search of any drug trade name or generic will result in a list of websites with information for patients and healthcare professional. For older drugs, try searching www.webmd.com.

ORAL ANTIDIABETIC MEDICATIONS

Oral medications that help to lower blood glucose levels do so in a number of different ways. They may stimulate the pancreas to increase its production of insulin, decrease insulin resistance in cells and tissue so a person's own insulin production works better, or slow intestinal absorption of carbohydrates so the rise in blood glucose takes place over a longer period of time, giving the body's own insulin time to move it out of the bloodstream. There are also many combinations of different drugs to accomplish more than one of these actions.

Medications That Increase Insulin Production

Secretagogues are drugs that make the pancreas increase its production of insulin. Four classes of secretagogues are currently in use: (1) sulfonylureas, (2) meglitinides, (3) D-phenylalanine derivatives, and (4) dipeptidyl peptidase-4 (DPP-4) inhibitors. They are prescribed only for persons with type 2 diabetes because in type 1 diabetes a person's beta cells are destroyed so they can no longer produce insulin. Insulin, at least currently, cannot be given orally because the stomach acids would destroy it before it can be absorbed. Because these secretagogues all work a little differently, I discuss them separately.

Sulfonylureas

Sulfonylureas were the first and only oral antidiabetic drugs for type 2 diabetics for many years. Most first-generation sulfonylureas still on the market are rarely used. I've listed the most common of these, Diabinese, in Table 4.1. As you can see, second-generation drugs are more potent and, therefore, can be given at lower dosages. They also have fewer side effects than the first-generation drugs, although hypoglycemia is still a possibility when meals are omitted or delayed or exercise is prolonged. They may also cause weight gain, water retention, and sometimes flushing with alcohol use; however, this is less common than with Diabinese, a first-generation sulfonylurea. The weight gain is an especially vexing problem, because increased weight increases insulin resistance. Water retention can also increase blood pressure, which is often a part of the diabetic picture. Sulfonylureas should only be prescribed for type 2 clients who are able to increase their beta cell production of insulin. Because type 2 diabetes is a progressive disease, eventually the beta cells will have no more to give, and different drugs, including insulin, may be added or substituted to bring blood glucose into normal range. Sulfonylureas are also mild sulfa drugs that may not be appropriate for anyone with an allergy to sulfa products. The following is a list of newer sulfonylureas along with their generic names in parentheses. Drug names marked with an asterisk are currently available in generic form, with more to be added as patents expire:

Glucotrol (glipizide*) and Glucotrol XL (glipizide ER*)
DiaBeta (glyburide*)
Glynase PresTab (micronized glyburide*)
Micronase (glyburide)
Amaryl (glimepiride*), a third-generation sulfonylurea

Sulfonylureas can be taken alone or combined with nonsecretagogue drugs such as metformin, alpha-glucosidase inhibitors, or thiazolidinediones (TZDs).

Meglitinides
The only drug approved by the Food and Drug Administration (FDA) to date in this class is repaglinide (Prandin). Its mechanism of action is similar to sulfonylureas; however, it acts much more rapidly. Therefore, it should be taken right before a meal. It increases insulin production dependent on carbohydrates from this meal. This increases the flexibility of meal planning and decreases incidence of low blood sugar because it should not be taken unless a meal is to be eaten within 30 minutes. It can be taken alone or combined with metformin, alpha-glucosidase inhibitors, or TZDs.

D-Phenylalanine Derivatives
The only FDA-approved drug in this class is nateglinide (Starlix), which acts similarly to Prandin in that it stimulates a rapid release of insulin from the beta cells, thus controlling blood sugars after meals. It is taken right before a meal, so the side effect of hypoglycemia is rare. Because it is metabolized and partially excreted by the liver, its duration of action can be prolonged in people with significant liver disease, resulting in an increased risk of hypoglycemia. This drug can be taken alone or in combination with metformin to enhance insulin sensitivity.

Dipeptidyl Peptidase-4 (DPP-4) Inhibitors
This is the newest class of drugs that increase the amount of insulin produced by the pancreas, but this increase occurs after meals, when blood glucose tends to be high. They are usually taken once or twice a day, with or without food, at the same time of day. These drugs can be taken alone or in combination with metformin but should not be taken with another secretagogue, such as those listed earlier. Side effects include

low blood sugar if meals are skipped. These drugs may also cause a stuffy or runny nose, sore throat, headache, painful, burning urination, stomach pain, nausea, vomiting, diarrhea, and bloating. Three examples of DPP-4 inhibitors currently on the market in the United States are (1) Januvia (sitagliptin), (2) Onglyza (saxagliptin), and (3) Tradjenta (linagliptin), and a combination drug, Janumet (sitagliptin and metformin).

Tradjenta, manufactured by Boehringer Ingelheim and Eli Lilly, was FDA approved on May 2, 2011, as a stand-alone drug or in combination with metformin (Glucophage), glimiperide (Amaryl), and pioglitazone (Actos). It is taken once a day for controlling glucose levels in type 2 diabetes by stimulating the release of insulin in a glucose-dependent manner (the higher the glucose level, the more insulin is released) and decreasing the levels of glucagon in the circulation.

Galvus (vildagliptin), another DPP-4 GLP-1 and GIP inhibitor, manufactured by Novartis has been granted Market Authorization in Europe and Novartis is waiting for FDA approval. Galvus is available in 50 mg tablets to be given twice a day with metformin or a TZD or one tablet in the morning when taken with a sulfonylurea. It also comes in a combination pill with metformin called Eucreas. Both may be approved soon in the United States.

Medications That Decrease Insulin Resistance

Biguanides

Drugs in this class act primarily to decrease the liver's release of glycogen into the blood, in response to inappropriate secretion of glucagon from the pancreas, thus increasing blood sugar. They also improve cellular insulin sensitivity, both problems in type 2 diabetes. Metformin (Glucophage) was the first nonsulfonylurea to be added to the arsenal of oral agents to treat type 2 diabetes. Side effects that decrease over time include diarrhea, bloating, and nausea. They can be minimized by taking the lowest dose and titrating upward until glycemic control is achieved. The most problematic adverse effect is *lactic acidosis*, which is rare but can be fatal. Lactic acidosis is a form of acidosis caused by decreased oxygenation of cells. Lactate is cleared from blood, primarily by the liver, with the kidneys (10% to 20%) and skeletal muscles to a lesser degree. All metformin formulations, including the newer ones and combinations with metformin in them, have a black box warning for this reason. Clients with liver or renal disease should not take these drugs. When taken alone, Glucophage does not contribute to weight gain or cause hypoglycemia. It may even lower LDL cholesterol (the "bad" cholesterol) and triglyceride levels, which are both problems that may occur in type 2 diabetes. This drug can be used alone as a *first-line agent* to improve glycemic control, or it can be combined with sulfonylureas, meglitinides (Prandin), D-phenylalanine derivative (Starlix), alpha-glucosidase inhibitors (Precose and Glyset), TZDs (Actos and Avandia), or insulin. Seven combination pills are currently

TABLE 4.1
Oral Antidiabetic Medication

GENERIC NAME	TRADE NAME	DOSE RANGE	DIRECTIONS	PEAK	DURATION	TARGET ORGAN	COMMENTS
Sulfonylurea (secretagogue)							All: may be used alone or in combination with metformin, thiazolidinediones (TZDs), and alpha-glucosidase inhibitors. Hypoglycemia may be prolonged. May cause water retention, weight gain. With alcohol may cause flushing.
First generation							
Chlorpropamide*	Diabinese	100–500 mg	Take with breakfast	2–4 hr	24–28 hr	Pancreas	
Second generation							
Glipizide*	Glucotrol	2.5–40 mg	1–2X/day AC meal	1–3 hr	12–24 hr	Pancreas	
	Glucotrol XL	2.5–20 mg	Take with breakfast	6–12 hr	24 hr		
Glyburide*	DiaBeta	1.25–2 mg	1–2X/day AC meal	2–4 hr	24 hr		
	Micronase	1.25–2 mg	1–2X/day AC meal	2–4 hr	24 hr		
Glyburide (micronized)*	Glynase PresTab	3–12 mg	1–2X/day AC meal	2–4 hr	24 hr		
Third generation							
Glimepiride*	Amaryl	1–8 mg	Take with breakfast	2–3 hr	18–24 hr	Pancreas	
Meglitinide							
Repaglinide	Prandin	0.5–4 mg	Take before each meal	1 hr	2–4 hr	Pancreas	Alone or in combination with other nonsecretagogues. Less chance of hypoglycemia
D-Phenylalanine Derivative							
Nateglinide*	Starlix	60–120 mg	Take before each meal	1–2 hr	2–3 hr	Pancreas	Alone or in combination with other nonsecretagogues. Less chance of hypoglycemia

(continued)

TABLE 4.1 (Continued)

GENERIC NAME	TRADE NAME	DOSE RANGE	DIRECTIONS	PEAK	DURATION	TARGET ORGAN	COMMENTS
DPP-4 Inhibitors							
Sitagliptin	Januvia	100 mg	Take 1 daily with or without food	1–4 hr	Unknown	Pancreas and liver	Used alone, no weight gain or hypoglycemia. May cause stomach discomfort and diarrhea.
Saxagliptin	Onglyza	2.5–5 mg	Take 1 daily with or without food	2 hr	Unknown		Fluid retention with TZDs. Respiratory infection, sore throat, muscle pain, headache.
Linagliptin	Tradjenta**	5 mg	Take 1 daily with or without food	1.5 hr	Unknown		
Vildagliptin	Galvus ***	50–100 mg	1 or 2X/day				Not yet FDA approved.
Biguanides							
Metformin*	Glucophage	500 mg	2–3X/day AC meals	2–4 hr	8–12 hr	Liver and muscles, fat	Used alone, no weight gain or hypoglycemia. May be used with all other classes of antidiabetic drugs including insulin.
Metformin (long-acting)	Glucophage XR	500 mg	Take with PM meal	4–8 hr	24 hr		
	Glumetza	500 mg	Take with PM meal		24 hr		Side effects: nausea, diarrhea, decreased appetite.
	Fortamet	500–1000 mg	Take after PM meal		24 hr		
Metformin (liquid)	Riomet	500 mg/5 ml	Take 5 ml daily	2.5 hr	24 hr		
Thiazolidinediones (TZDs)							
Pioglitazone	Actos	15–45 mg	Takes 4–6 weeks to take effect	3 hr	16–34 hr	Muscles, fat, liver	May cause heart failure (Avandia). May be used with all other classes of antidiabetic drugs including insulin.
Rosiglitasone	Avandia	2–8 mg	1–2X/day with or without meals				

Drug	Brand	Dose	Timing	Onset	Duration	Site	Notes
Alpha-Glucosidase Inhibitors (starch blocker)							
Acarbose*	Precose, Prandase	50 mg	Take just before eating each meal	Rapid	4 hr	Small intestine	Used alone, no weight gain or hypoglycemia. May be used with all other classes of antidiabetic drugs, including insulin. Causes gas and bloating.
Miglitol	Glyset	50 mg					
Dopamine Agonist							
Bromocriptine–QR	Cycloset	2–6 tabs (each tab 0.8 mg)	Take in AM with food and within 2 hr of waking	Rapid	24 hr	Brain and central nervous system	Does not cause weight gain. May cause nausea, vomiting, fatigue, dizziness, headache
Combination Agents							
Glipizide/metformin*	Metaglip	5 mg/500 mg	Take with meals	See each drug	See separate drugs	See separate drugs	See separate drugs
Glyburide/metformin*	Glucovance	5 mg/500 mg	Take with meals				
Rosiglitazone/metformin	Avandamet	4 mg/500 mg	Take with meals				
Rosiglitazone/glimepiride	Avandaryl	4 mg/1–4 mg	Take with 1st meal				
Metformin/pioglitazone	Actoplus Met	500–850 mg/15 mg	1–2X/day with food				
Metformin/sitagliptin	Janumet	500–1000/50 mg	BID with meals				
Metformin/repaglinide	PrandiMet	500 mg/1–2 mg	BID with meals				
Pioglitazone/glimepiride	Duetact	30 mg/2 mg	With or without food				
Metformin/saxagliptin	Kombiglyze XR	500–1000 mg/2.5–5 mg	Take with PM meal				
Metformin/vildagliptin	Eucreas***						Not yet FDA approved.

*Available as a generic.

**FDA approved May 2, 2011.

***Approved for use in Europe in early 2008. Novartis is awaiting FDA approval.

available: (1) Glucovance* (metformin and glyburide), (2) Metaglip* (metformin and glipizide), (3) Avandamet (metformin and Avandia), (4) Actoplus Met (metformin and Actos), (5) Janumet (metformin and Januvia), (6) PrandiMet (metformin and Prandin), and (7) Kombiglyze XR (metformin extended release and Onglyza). As the rate of type 2 diabetes increases, more drug companies will add to the available combinations. Combination drugs increase ease of use and compliance as well as cost. However, the two separate medications may currently both be available as generics, but the new combination will not be available as a generic for several years after they come on the market.

Metformin alone or in any of its combinations can interfere with the absorption of vitamin B_{12}, which is needed for red cell production and to keep nerve cells healthy. This could complicate a diagnosis of peripheral neuropathy. Clients should be advised to continue getting lab work done yearly, which should help identify anemia, and notify their healthcare provider if they begin to lose sensation in their feet or hands so a B_{12} deficiency or peripheral neuropathy can be differentiated.

Newer drugs in the same class as Glucophage include Glucophage XR, Glumetza, and Fortamet, which are extended-release formulations of metformin for the treatment of type 2 diabetes. They are actually metformin derivatives that may have fewer side effects than metformin and are taken only once a day. Riomet is a liquid formulation of metformin for children with type 2 diabetes and those who have difficulty swallowing pills. The following is a list of drugs currently available in the biguanides class. Those marked with an asterisk are available in generic form. Generic names are in parentheses:

> Glucophage (metformin*) and Glucophage XR (metformin ER*)
> Glumetza (metformin extended release)
> Fortamet (metformin extended release)
> Riomet (metformin oral solution)
> Glucovance* (metformin and glyburide)
> Metaglip* (metformin and glipizide)
> Avandamet (metformin and rosiglitazone)
> Actoplus Met (metformin and pioglitazone)
> Janumet (metformin and sitagliptin)
> PrandiMet (metformin and repaglinide)

Thiazolidinediones (TZDs)

This group of drugs, better known by some as "glitazones" or TZDs, includes pioglitazone (Actos) and rosiglitazone (Avandia). They act by decreasing cellular resistance to insulin, thus improving control of blood sugars. The overweight population of type 2 diabetics may improve glycemic control by adding one of these drugs to lifestyle changes of weight loss, healthy diet, and increased physical activity. They can also be taken with sulfonylureas, meglitinides (Prandin), metformin (Glucophage or as

Avandamet), alpha-glucosidase inhibitors (Precose or Glyset), or insulin. The FDA recommends that liver function tests be done before and during treatment with this class of drugs since the first one, troglitazone (Rezulin), was withdrawn from the market in 2000 because of reports of rare incidents of liver failure and related deaths. The two newer drugs, Actos and Avandia, are much less toxic to the liver, but patient selection must be appropriate. If a patient's liver enzymes increase, the drug is usually discontinued for this individual. TZDs can also cause fluid retention and rapid weight gain independent of fluid retention. Clients at risk for congestive heart failure should probably not take these drugs. All clients taking these drugs need to be monitored for cardiac function and weight gain, ruling out fluid retention as the cause. Medications in this class, including combination drugs, have a black box warning concerning heart failure and heart muscle ischemia.

Because many clients with type 2 diabetes also may be taking drugs to lower cholesterol, the name of their antihyperlipidemic should be documented to prevent a drug interaction.

CLINICAL EXAMPLE: Cholestyramine (Questran) inhibits the absorption of TZDs as well as other drugs and should not be taken at the same time. Also it may take several weeks or months to see the full effect of Actos or Avandia, so blood sugars should be monitored at least once per day and recorded to alert the prescribing healthcare provider. If insulin or a secretagogue is taken during this time, the dose may need to be lowered as the TZD kicks in.

In June 2010, two teams of researchers, after conducting studies with large numbers of patients, concluded that Avandia increases the risk of heart disease, heart failure, stroke, and death in people who take this drug to help control diabetes. On September 23, 2010, the FDA put severe restrictions on the use of Avandia. Any healthcare professional prescribing this drug must state that everything else has failed to control blood sugars and that clients sign a release stating they understand the substantial risks to the heart this drug poses (USFDA, 2010). If a client takes Avandia alone or in a combination drug, the healthcare provider will probably switch the client to another diabetes drug soon. Actos, the only other TZD on the market, affects a different set of genes and is currently considered safe.

Two new combination drugs called Avandaryl and Duetact are on the market. These drugs combine Avandia or Actos and glimeperide, a third-generation sulfonylurea (trade name Amaryl). They have the same precautions concerning liver function that all glitazones have and should be administered with the first good meal of the day to minimize hypoglycemia from Amaryl. The above-mentioned FDA restrictions on Avandia also applies to Avandamet.

Medicines That Slow Intestinal Absorption of Carbohydrates

Alpha-Glucosidase Inhibitors

The two drugs in this class, acarbose (Precose; called Glucobay in Europe and Prandase in Canada) and miglitol (Glyset), work in the small intestine to delay the digestion of carbohydrates (starches and sucrose) and decrease the peak postprandial (after meal) glucose levels, allowing insulin production to better match glucose absorption in clients with type 2 diabetes. They can be taken alone or in combination with sulfonylureas, repaglinide (Prandin), metformin (Glucophage), TZDs (Actos or Avandia), or insulin. When taken alone, these drugs do not cause hypoglycemia, but when taken with other agents that do cause low blood sugar, such as sulfonylureas and repaglanide, only glucose (in the form of glucose tablets or gel) or fructose from 100% fruit juice will be affective in treating the hypoglycemia.

The most common side effects are gas, diarrhea, and cramps. These diminish with time and are minimized by starting at the lowest dose and gradually increasing it, if needed, to control blood sugars. Because of these side effects, this drug may not be appropriate for anyone with irritable bowel syndrome.

CENTRAL ACTING MEDICATIONS

So far, central acting medications only include one drug classification, which is responsible for several actions to improve blood sugars and A1c.

Dopamine D_3 Agonist

The newest drug classification to be added to the list of antidiabetic oral medication is the dopamine agonist group. The first drug in this class is Cycloset (bromocriptine-QR) manufacturing by Santarus. This classification of drugs is typically used to treat Parkinson's disease and certain pituitary tumors, and was once used to block the pituitary glands release of prolactin after childbirth for those women who chose not to breastfeed. Dopamine agonists increase dopamine, a neurotransmitter in the brain, which helps to improve glycemic control independently of insulin production by increasing insulin sensitivity and lowering postprandial glucose levels. The FDA in 2009 approved bromocriptine in a lower dose than for Parkinson's for treating type 2 diabetes (Saudek & Margolis, 2011). Cycloset has been available since November 2010, but is not as yet widely used. The dosage is started with one 0.8 mg tablet and can be increased by one tablet every 7 to 28 days to a max dose of 6 tablets or 4.8 mg based on client response. It should be taken at the same time each day with a meal and within 2 hours of waking. Side effects include dizziness, drowsiness, nausea, sweating, and orthostatic hypotension. The client should not drive or operate heavy machinery until drug effects are known. It may be taken alone or with other antidiabetic agents, such as sulfonylureas and metformin, but dosage of these drugs may need to be lowered. Food interactions include grapefruit, grapefruit juice, and sometimes alcohol. Because it is metabolized in the liver by the cytochrome P450 (CYP) 3A4 isoenzyme, it may have drug-to-drug interactions with other drugs that either enhance or inhibit this CYP450 isoenzyme. Bromocriptine-QR meets the new FDA mandated cardiovascular safety requirements for type 2 diabetes while lowering A1c to less than 7% often within 24 weeks (Cornell & Bryk-Gandera, 2010).

INJECTABLE ANTIDIABETIC MEDICATION

Insulin

The body needs insulin 24/7. When the islet cells of the pancreas perform as intended, a small amount of endogenous (originating from within the body) insulin is secreted constantly to allow some glucose to enter cells for cellular function. When we inject exogenous (originating outside the body) insulin for this purpose, we refer to it as background or *basal insulin*. As the normal islet cells sense a rise in blood sugar from a meal or snack, the beta cells produce more endogenous insulin to keep blood sugar within the normal range. We can give *bolus* doses of exogenous insulin prior to eating to mimic this activity when pancreatic function is compromised. The purposes of insulin therapy are (1) to maximize glycemic control while minimizing the risk of hypoglycemia and (2) to effectively mimic the body's physiologic need for insulin in both a basal and a bolus amount.

Tight glycemic control, especially using insulin, has been shown in several clinical trials to prevent or delay the onset of complications caused by hyperglycemia. The unintended consequence of keeping blood sugars at near-normal levels is hypoglycemia. The pancreas, when it is healthy, does a much better job at figuring this out than the human brain, even when aided by a glucose meter and multiple insulin injections or the use of an insulin pump. However, with effort and the right combination of medications and insulins, clients with type 1 and type 2 diabetes can achieve close to normal glycemic control as measured by hemoglobin A1c with minimal hypoglycemic events. A1c is a blood test that measures the average percentage of blood glucose over a 2- to 3-month period. See Chapter 5 for more on glycemic control.

Obviously, all type 1 diabetics take a basal insulin that keeps their body functioning between meals and throughout the night and a bolus insulin dose before meals. Basal insulins can be composed of

1. One or two doses per day of a long-acting insulin,
2. Two doses of an intermediate-acting insulin, or
3. Various basal rates with rapid-acting insulin using an insulin pump.

Bolus doses of insulin to cover episodes of hyperglycemia and meal or snack carbohydrate amounts, on the other hand, are given as needed.

This is much easier to do with an insulin pump, but it also can be managed by giving injections of rapid-acting insulin prior to a meal or snack. Additional insulin can be added or subtracted on the basis of the current blood sugar level. For instance, a person might start with an insulin coverage scale of rapid-acting insulin to take care of a higher-than-normal blood sugar prior to meals based on insulin sensitivity (how many mg/dl will each unit of insulin lower blood sugar).

CLINICAL EXAMPLE: One unit of insulin might decrease blood sugar by 40 mg/dl or 50 mg/dl or 60 mg/dl or more. Each individual is different. Also, a set ratio of units of insulin to grams of carbohydrates (see "Carbohydrate Counting" in Chapter 2) would be added to the insulin coverage scale amount to minimize the effect of the carbohydrates in a meal or snack on blood sugar. Examples of insulin to carbohydrate ratios might resemble one of the following:

1 unit of insulin for every 10 g of carbohydrate
1 unit of insulin for every 12 g of carbohydrate
1 unit of insulin for every 15 g of carbohydrate
1 unit of insulin for every 20 g of carbohydrate

This ratio may be different at each meal or may remain the same. If this sounds difficult, it can be. The troubling aspect of working all of this out is that each person responds to food and insulin differently, so it is a matter of trial and error. Because each person is different, a client has to be self-reliant and willing to experiment. Only those committed to their long-term survival with the desire to live as normal a life as possible will be willing to handle this challenge. It also helps to have a diabetes educator on a client's diabetes team who is willing to assist with troubleshooting any problems and answer a person's many questions.

Insulin therapy for clients with type 2 diabetes is becoming more common. Because hyperglycemia has such devastating consequences over time, glycemic control needs to be achieved as soon as possible. Insulin should not be thought of as a last resort in type 2 diabetes or as an indication that all attempts with oral agents or the new noninsulin injectables have failed. It should never be used as a threat or punishment for people who may be labeled *noncompliant* with weight loss and lifestyle changes. It can be the treatment of choice for some clients with type 2 diabetes soon after diagnosis. According to the ADA, insulin should be used in treating type 2 diabetes when

1. Hyperglycemia is severe at diagnosis,
2. Glycemic control is not achieved with lifestyle changes and combinations of oral meds,

3. Uncontrolled hyperglycemia is caused by infection, acute injury, surgery, heart attack, stroke, or other cardiovascular incident,
4. The above incidents cause ketonemia and/or ketonuria and uncontrolled weight loss,
5. Liver and/or renal disease complicate metabolism and excretion of oral antidiabetic medications, or
6. Pregnancy is a contraindication to the use of some oral antidiabetes drugs (ADA, 2003)

The ADA recommends that the use of insulin be viewed in the same light as all oral agents for those with type 2 diabetes and that more clients be started on insulin alone or in combination with metformin or other nonsecretagogues sooner rather than later (ADA, 2011). If glycemic control is delayed, the risk of developing chronic complications is increased. The sooner blood sugars are controlled, the better.

Types of Insulin

Insulin was discovered in the early 1920s and at that time consisted of a short-acting insulin distillate from the pancreas of dogs. Children with type 1 diabetes needed injections every 4 or 5 hours, even during the night. In the 1940s, protamine was added to regular insulin to make neutral protamine Hagedorn (NPH) insulin and zinc was added to regular insulin to make lente insulin. This slowed the onset, peak, and, most importantly, duration of insulin and decreased the number of injections needed per day.

Prior to 1985, insulin came from the pancreases of cows and pigs and was marketed as beef, beef-pork, or purified porcine insulin. Porcine insulin was the closest in molecular structure to endogenous human insulin. The use of insulin from different species gave rise to allergic reactions, immunologic suppression of this insulin's action, and the fear that there would not be sufficient animal pancreases to meet the increasing need for insulin therapy. Most insulin used today in the United States is called *human insulin* and is manufactured in a laboratory using recombinant DNA technology. The problem with this human insulin is that if enough regular insulin is given to keep 2-hour postprandial blood sugar under 140 mg/dl, it often causes a low blood sugar 3 to 4 hours later. The minimum 30-minute delay in eating after the insulin dose is often a problem as well. Regular insulin, although the shortest acting insulin we had for decades, just does not match the increase in blood sugar generated by a typical meal. Its duration of action is also too long, causing frequent between-meal hypoglycemic reactions. To mimic the around-the-clock action of the body's insulin, intermediate and long-acting insulins were developed as previously described. Until 2005, NPH, lente, and ultralente insulins were available from both major companies that manufacture insulin in the United States: Eli Lilly and Novo Nordisk. Both have stopped making lente and ultralente because the rapid- and long-acting insulin analogs have supplanted their use. Each company also makes combination vials of NPH and regular human insulins for use in syringes and with their cartridge-filled pens. Wal-Mart also sells Novalin R, Novalin N, and Novalin 70/30 under their own brand, ReliOn.

How to Measure and Inject Insulin

Insulin syringes come in several sizes: (1) a 1 ml with a 100-unit capacity; (2) a low-dose syringe, with a 50-unit capacity, and (3) the smallest, with a 30-unit capacity. Advise clients to use the smallest syringe that will accommodate the amount of insulin prescribed and always check the expiration date on any refrigerated insulin vial. Vials in use should be kept at room temperature and remain potent for 28 days, after which they should be discarded. Inspect vials in good lighting and at eye level for changes in insulin appearance, such as discoloration, swirling cloudiness (NPH should be uniformly cloudy), or crystallization. If NPH or a mixture of regular and NPH clumps or separates in the syringe, throw out the vial. It has probably been frozen and thawed.

In order to draw up liquid from a vial, individuals must first inject the same amount of air into the vial to overcome the vacuum. If a client is mixing rapid-acting or regular (clear) insulin and NPH (cloudy) insulin in the same syringe, they must avoid getting any cloudy solution into the clear. This will slow the action of rapid-acting or regular insulin. Because of this, clients need to be taught to give the mixed insulin immediately or the amount of regular or rapid-acting insulin in the same syringe will also be slowed. Clients should be taught to follow these steps:

1. Wipe both vial ports with an alcohol swab.
2. Draw up air into the syringe to match the amount of rapid-acting or regular insulin and inject it into the vial of regular insulin. Remove the syringe from the vial.
3. Next, draw up air into the same syringe to match the amount of NPH insulin and inject it into the vial of NPH insulin being careful not to touch the NPH insulin with the tip of the needle. This can best be done by keeping the vial base down on a flat surface. Remove the syringe from the vial.
4. Return the syringe to the vial of rapid-acting or regular insulin and draw up the correct amount of this insulin. Remove the syringe containing rapid-acting or regular insulin from this vial and tap the side of the syringe to move any bubbles to the top (needle end). Remove bubbles being careful not to lose any insulin. If any insulin is removed, go back to the vial and replace to the correct amount.
5. With this syringe, return to the vial of NPH and add the correct amount of NPH insulin to the rapid-acting or regular insulin in the syringe. The total amount should equal the amount of rapid-acting or regular insulin plus the amount of NPH insulin. Give this mixture immediately.

Give the injections in the fatty areas of the abdomen, avoiding a 1-inch area around the navel, the back of the upper arm (use a door jamb or other surface to roll the fat forward so you can see it), the front of the thigh, and the upper part of the buttocks. Rotating between areas with each injection, leave about a 1-inch space between injection sites.

CLINICAL EXAMPLE: If a client administers more than one injection a day, he or she should make a plan to rotate between sites based on how much time there is between an injection and eating. Absorption of insulin injected into the abdomen is the fastest and next fastest is from the arms. The thighs have a slower absorption rate, and the slowest absorption is from the buttocks.

To help them plan a rotation schedule, suggest clients use the right side one day and the left the next day. Giving injections in the same area over and over again will create scar tissue and decrease the absorption rate after a while. Also teach clients to avoid injecting into the area that will be exercised soon afterward.

CLINICAL EXAMPLE: Clients should not inject insulin into the fat over the thigh muscles if they plan to walk or run afterward. Exercise will increase the blood supply to thigh muscles and increase the absorption rate for the fatty tissue above, thus potentially causing a low blood sugar.

To inject insulin into the subcutaneous tissue, instruct clients to pinch up the fat and angle the needle from 30° to 90°, depending on the depth of the fat. For more information about insulin injection sites, refer clients to www.lillydiabetes.com/content/insulin-injections.jsp.

To minimize anxiety, advice given by the ADA to parents and caregivers of children who need to begin receiving insulin includes the following:

- Take deep breaths and exhale slowly.
- Give the child bubbles to blow before and during the shot to help him or her breathe deeply.
- Sing a favorite song or tell a silly joke.
- Play pretend doctor. Let the child give a pretend shot to a stuffed animal or to you first.
- Talk about the best thing that happened that day.
- Don't stall—getting it over means getting on with some fun!
- Kiss the site before and after—then give each other a big hug.
- Praise the child for being so brave. (ADA, n.d.)

More advice can be found at www.diabetes.org/living-with-diabetes/parents-and-kids/everyday-life/shots-and-checks.html.

The following information concerning proper disposal of insulin syringes, pen needles, lancets, and pump insertion needles (anything sharp) should be taught to clients and children using them:

1. Get a red biohazard container for this purpose from the health department if required by state or local laws or
2. Use a narrow open, opaque, nonpierceable container, such as a bleach bottle. When this container is three quarters full, seal the cap shut with glue or layers of duct tape.
3. Never throw used needles, even with caps on, into the trash for IV drug users to find or trash handlers to stick themselves with, causing fear of HIV or other infectious diseases.

Insulin Analogs

Insulin analogs are not human insulin: they are better. By rearranging some amino acids on human insulin's protein molecular structure, a faster onset and peak and a shortened duration have been achieved. The result is an insulin that more closely matches the rise of blood sugar caused by a meal or snack. There are three rapid-acting insulin analogs in current use: (1) insulin lispro (Humalog), (2) insulin aspart (Novolog), and (3) insulin glulisine (Apidra), all of which can be used for bolus dosing and also can be used in insulin pumps or combined in a syringe with NPH or in pens with intermediate-acting insulin analogs for basal coverage. All rapid-acting insulin analogs can be used in treating type 1 and type 2 diabetes and injected or administered via insulin pump. All insulin analogs require a prescription and client education regarding their use, especially if the client has had experience with short-acting regular insulin. Regular and NPH insulins as well as their various combinations do not require a prescription, although for health insurance coverage, one may be needed. Some states require that a person sign for insulin sold without a prescription to provide a record.

If rearranging amino acids can accelerate the action of human insulin, why can't different arrangements prolong the action? The first truly long-acting basal insulin was made by doing just that a few years ago. We now have two such basal insulin analogs: (1) insulin glargine (Lantus) and (2) insulin detemir (Levemir). These analogs are described as "peakless" and may be used in addition to rapid- or short-acting insulin in treating type 1 and type 2 diabetes. They may also be used as a basal insulin with secretagogues or other oral agents for type 2 glycemic control. Both Lantus and Levemir require a prescription. Clients must be taught NOT to mix them with other insulins in the same syringe. Therefore, a client must be willing to give two separate injections when using a basal insulin analog in conjunction with rapid- or short-acting insulin. Both types of

TABLE 4.2
Types of Insulin

TYPE	TRADE NAME	ONSET	PEAK	DURATION	COMMENTS
Rapid-acting analogs					
Insulin lispro	Humalog (Eli Lilly)	5–15 min	30–90 min	2–4 hr	All: prescription required. Inject before each meal. May be mixed with NPH and intermediate-acting insulin analogs. Give immediately after mixing.
Insulin aspart	NovoLog (Novo Nordisk)				
Insulin glulisine	Apidra (Sanofi-Aventis)				
Short-acting					
regular insulin	Humulin R (Eli Lilly) Novolin R (Novo Nordisk)	30–60 min	2–3 hr	3–6 hr	All: Inject 30 min before meals. May be mixed with NPH insulin. Give immediately after mixing.
Intermediate-acting					
NPH insulin	Humulin N (Eli Lilly) Novolin N (Novo Nordisk)	2–4 hr	4–12 hr	12–18 hr	All: May be mixed with rapid or short-acting insulins and given immediately after mixing.
Long-acting insulin analogs					
Insulin glargine	Lantus (Sanofi-Aventis)	2–4 hr	None	20–24 hr	All: Prescription required. Cannot be mixed with other insulins. Can be injected anytime during the day but should be given at about the same time each day.
Insulin detemir	Levemir (Novo Nordisk)				

(continued)

TABLE 4.2 (Continued)

TYPE	TRADE NAME	ONSET	PEAK	DURATION	COMMENTS
Mixtures					
70% NPH/30% R	Humulin 70/30%	30–60 min	Dual	10–16 hr	Very convenient and useful for those with difficulty mixing insulins in same syringe. No prescription required.
	Novolin 70/30%	30–60 min	Dual	10–16 hr	
	Novolin 70/30% Penfill	30–60 min	Dual	10–16 hr	
	Novolin 70/30 Innolet	30–60 min	Dual	10–16 hr	
70% aspart protamine/ 30% aspart	NovoLog 70/30% Flexpen	5–15 min	Dual		Prescription required
75% lispro protamine/ 25% lispro	Humalog Mix 75/25%	5–15 min	Dual	10–16 hr	Prescription required
50% NPH/50% R	Humulin 50/50	30–60 min	Dual	10–16 hr	No prescription required

Note difference between Novolin 70/30% and NovoLog Mix 70/30%.

Many of the above insulins come in cartridges for reusable pens or in prefilled disposable pens. See www.diabetes.org/living-with-diabetes/treatment-and-care/medication/insulin/insulin-routines.html and click on pdf of available insulin pens from Eli Lilly, Novo Nordisk, and Sanofi-Aventis, makers of the insulins listed above.

insulin may, however, be given at the same time, but in separate syringes. Both insulin glargine and insulin detemir improve fasting blood sugars and reduce the variability of peak action association with NPH and intermediate-acting insulin analogs. They can both be administered to children as young as 6 years of age with type 1 diabetes.

Eli Lilly makes a premixed insulin, Humalog Mix 75/25, with 75% lispro protamine suspension and 25% insulin lispro and a Humalog mix 50/50. Novo Nordisk's premixed insulin, NovoLog 70/30, contains 70% aspart protamine and 30% insulin aspart. All analog mixtures require a prescription and are available in vials for syringe use and cartridges for each company's insulin pens, manufactured for client convenience. To learn more about the various types of human insulins and analogs currently available, see the Eli Lilly and Novo Nordisk websites listed in the Resources section in the back of this book and visit the ADA's Consumer Guide 2011 to see all of the available insulin pens at http://forecast .diabetes.org/magazine/features/consumer-guide-2011.jsp.

Insulin Pumps

Until there is either a cure for diabetes or an affordable, reliable, internal artificial pancreas, an insulin pump is the next best thing. Characteristics of a person who would do well pumping insulin include someone

1. On intensive insulin therapy (three or more injections per day) but not meeting glycemic goals
2. Able and willing to make appropriate insulin adjustments based on frequent blood sugar testing
3. Well motivated to learn pump technology and able to follow through and make the necessary changes
4. Desirous of or requiring a more flexible lifestyle with regard to meals and exercise
5. Willing to be tethered via tubing to a small box housing a continuous flow of rapid-acting insulin (e.g., the OmniPod, which is wireless and disposable)
6. With added incentive to control blood sugar prior to and during pregnancy
7. Having adequate health insurance to help with cost
8. Perhaps most importantly, with a take-charge personality willing to do whatever it takes to make it work

Pumping insulin is definitely worth the hassles involved.

CLINICAL EXAMPLE: When I was put on my first insulin pump after working at blood sugar control for 10 years with four to five injections a day, I felt like I finally had my life back. I could eat and exercise when I wanted without worrying about when my intermediate-acting insulin was going to peak. When the insulin analogs became available, insulin decision making became even easier. I could eat what I wanted when I wanted, within reason, just like anyone else. However, monitoring blood sugars to set basal rates throughout the day and night meant pre- and postprandial testing, as well as testing two or three times during the night to set up appropriate basal rates. Pumping insulin is not the answer for everyone. It takes effort, willingness to experiment, and the ability to follow through in order to use an insulin pump successfully. Blood sugars usually level out so that the roller coaster ride of highs and lows, often in the same day, rarely occurs. Blood sugars are more predictable, and food, physical activity, and insulin doses finally make sense.

Deciding to use an insulin pump does have its aggravations. Pump alarms for low volume, low battery, and "no delivery" are important safety precautions but they can be annoying and, at times, embarrassing. However, they can usually be set to vibrate. The "no delivery" alarm must be tended to very quickly because very high blood sugars and diabetic ketoacidosis can ensue in a matter of hours. Most pumpers use rapid-acting insulin analogs in their pumps, which have a very short duration of action (see Table 4.2). Tubing, reservoirs, and insulin must be readily available at work and at home, as well as anywhere the client might be, for this potential emergency. A low battery alarm is less problematic because most pumps will continue to function for 8 or more hours. A pump rarely malfunctions, but the 1-800 number on the back of the pump is manned 24/7 to help a person troubleshoot problems and reprogram the pump, if needed. It is probably wise to keep an up-to-date written record of all basal rates so they can be reset. If there is a delay in fixing any glitch, syringes and insulin must be available as backup.

That brings me to the "stuff" that pump users need to carry with them. Anyone diagnosed with type 1 or type 2 diabetes should carry medication that must be taken with meals as well as a glucose monitor, strips, a lancing device and lancets, tissues, a log book, and spare batteries for the monitor. Most monitors come with convenient carrying cases for that purpose. Additionally, anyone on insulin should have available unexpired insulin, syringes, and alcohol swabs. Pumpers also need extra reservoirs and tubing, fresh pump batteries, and any other paraphernalia needed to change the insulin setup and/or insertion site. There are coolers, pouches, and carrying cases for this purpose. Supplies can also be carried in a purse, backpack, fanny pack, or briefcase. If not refrigerated, insulin at room temperature will maintain its potency for at least 28 days. Clients should be told not to freeze or leave insulin in 90° weather, for example, in the glove compartment of a car, not even in the spring or fall.

Most people who use insulin pumps use the abdomen as their insertion site, upper abdomen for men and lower abdomen for women. However, all appropriate subcutaneous sites for insulin injection, such as the anterior thigh, back of the upper arm, and upper buttocks, can be used. The insertion site should be changed every 2–3 days to prevent irritation and infection. Pumps can be removed for bathing, swimming, contact sports, and sexual activity for up to 2 hours if blood sugars are well controlled. Clients need to know to test their blood sugar when they reconnected their pump and give an appropriate bolus dose, if needed.

Persons using insulin pumps need a support system, both professionally and personally. A supportive diabetes educator and/or endocrinologist can help to troubleshoot any pump and/or blood sugar difficulties. Selected family members, friends, and/or coworkers should be informed as to how they can help in meaningful ways. This may mean that they demonstrate their concern by asking about blood sugars/meal preferences, providing privacy, and a regular soda or other fast-acting sugar source when hypoglycemia is a problem, or doing none of the above except when specifically asked. Wearing an insulin pump is a serious financial and personal commitment to controlling blood sugars and managing diabetes while decreasing hypoglycemic episodes and increasing lifestyle flexibility. Insulin pumps are appropriate not only for people with type 1 diabetes but also for those with type 2. Children as young as 1 year can also be managed well with an insulin pump (Fox, Buckloh, Smith, Wysocki, & Mauras, 2005). Parents can set lock-out controls so that young children cannot change settings. See Chapter 8 for more discussion about children with diabetes.

V-Go Disposable Insulin Delivery Device

In December 2010, the FDA approved the use of Valeritas' V-Go insulin delivery system for use with Eli Lilly's Humalog rapid-acting insulin. The V-Go is the first simple, fully disposable device for the delivery of basal-bolus insulin therapy for adults with type 2 diabetes. The V-Go provides a continuous preset basal rate of insulin and allows for on-demand bolus dosing around mealtimes, thereby providing an alternative to taking multiple daily insulin injections. The devise can hold 30 to 40 units of insulin to be delivered in a 24-hour period. A new device is loaded with the correct amount of insulin every day and attached to the body with an h-patch.

On March 1, 2011 the FDA also approved the V-Go devise for use with Novo Nordisk's NovoLog rapid-acting insulin. Visit www.valeritas.com for more details.

Other Injectable Diabetes Medication

Two new types of subcutaneous injectable medications have been recently added to the arsenal of drugs to control blood sugar: (1) pramlintide (Symlin), a synthetic amylin hormone, and (2) a group of drugs classified as *incretin mimetics* (Table 4.3).

Amylin Hormone Analog
Pramlintide is a synthetic amylin hormone that is normally produced by the beta cells of the pancreas, as is insulin. Pramlintide injections given with meals that contain at least 250 calories and 30 g of carbohydrates should not

cause hypoglycemia or weight gain, as insulin does, and may even promote weight loss. It is prescribed for those who have type 1 diabetes as well as those with type 2 diabetes treated with mealtime insulin. It should be given with rapid-acting insulin at meals but cannot be mixed in the same syringe. The amount of rapid-acting insulin given before a meal by either client or caregiver may need to be lowered by 50%. Symlin comes in 60-mcg (for type 1 diabetics) and 120-mcg (for type 2 diabetics) prefilled SymlinPens. Because Symlin is dosed in micrograms, it should never be withdrawn from the pen into an insulin syringe, which is marked in units. This could result in a higher dose. Pens should be refrigerated but never frozen. The pen in current use should be kept cool (under 77°F). Discard an opened pen after 30 days even if it still contains medication. The SymlinPen comes in packages of two per box, requires a prescription, and is light sensitive, so keep it in the box in which it came. Like all pen delivery systems, needles are sold separately and are screwed onto the pen at the time of delivery. Very short needles are available for injection in the fatty layer under the skin just as insulin is. After injection of the medication, the needle should be removed from the pen and the pen returned to the box and placed into the refrigerator or cooler. The benefits of Symlin include the following:

■ It decreases after meal elevations of blood glucose. When a client is using this drug, he or she should be instructed to test the blood sugar before meals, 2 hours after meals, and at bedtime to check on its effectiveness.
■ It smoothes out blood sugar levels throughout the day, with fewer blood sugar swings.
■ It improves A1c test results.
■ It helps clients need less insulin.
■ It helps clients feel full sooner at meals, so they may eat less. This may help with weight loss.

Obviously, this drug is not for everyone. Symlin has been approved for use for people with both type 1 and type 2 diabetes using rapid-onset insulin as a premeal bolus dose, who are not achieving glycemic control on their present regimen, and are well motivated to follow directions carefully. The most common side effect is nausea, which improves after a few weeks. The dose is started low and is gradually increased until the desired effect is achieved.

Incretin Mimetic

The second new class of injectable medications for treating type 2 diabetes is called an *incretin mimetic*. This is a synthetic version of the human incretin hormone GLP-1 (glucagon-like peptide-1) that is secreted in the small intestines, but it lasts longer. The first drug in this class is Byetta (exenatide), which helps the body to self-regulate glycemic control. It enhances insulin secretion only when blood sugar is elevated and decreases insulin production as blood sugar normalizes (Clark, 2006). According to its manufacturers, Amylin Pharmaceuticals and Eli Lilly, this drug is for persons with type 2 diabetes who are taking metformin or a sulfonylurea or both without achieving glycemic control. Byetta is used in conjunction with these medications, although the dose of metformin and/or the sulfonylurea may need to be reduced. Byetta is dispensed in prefilled 30-day supply pens of 5 mcg or 10 mcg, depending on which dose is prescribed. It is given twice a day as a subcutaneous injection (like insulin) within 60 minutes of eating breakfast or dinner.

The GLP-1 hormone is structurally similar to glucagon but acts very differently. Whereas glucagon from the alpha cells of the pancreas causes the release of stored glucose from the liver to prevent low blood sugar, the GLP-1 hormone

1. increases insulin secretion, but only when glucose is elevated (e.g., after meals);
2. suppresses inappropriate glucagon secretion (a problem in type 2 diabetes);
3. promotes a feeling of satiety, which may decrease food intake; and
4. slows gastric emptying, thus decreasing the spike of postprandial blood sugar (another problem in type 2 diabetes).

The most common side effect is nausea, which decreases over time. Byetta pens should be stored in the original carton (protected from the light) and in the refrigerator. Once in use, the pen should be refrigerated or kept cold, but never frozen. After 30 days, the pen should be thrown away even if it still contains medication. The pen needles should be attached right before use and properly discarded after use. Leaving needles on the pen may cause leaking of medication or air bubbles.

The newest incretin GLP-1 mimetic is Victoza (liraglutide), made by Novo Nordisk and approved by the FDA in January 2010. It also comes in an injectable pen form, like Byetta, but is given only once a day and has fewer side effects. If nausea is present, it goes away sooner. Both Byetta and Victoza can lead to pancreatitis, an inflammation of the pancreas that is painful and may be life threatening. They should not be prescribed for clients who have had pancreatitis, gallstones, a history of alcoholism, or high triglyceride levels, because these conditions make them more likely to develop pancreatitis.

Eli Lilly, Amylin Pharmaceuticals, and Alkermes have received approval for their once-a-week injection of exenatide, Brydureon, by the European regulators but are still waiting for FDA approval. Brydureon, a long-acting exenatide, if approved in the United States, could be given as a once-weekly subcutaneous injection instead of the twice-a-day injection of Byetta.

For people with type 2 diabetes, there are six areas of dysfunction causing elevated blood glucose levels, which can be addressed with medication. The dysfunctions occur in the following areas:

1. The pancreas (problems with low insulin secretion and increased glucagon output)
2. The liver (responds to glucagon with increased gluconeogenesis)
3. Peripheral tissues (insulin resistance)

TABLE 4.3

Noninsulin Injectable Diabetes Medications

GENERIC NAME	TRADE NAME	DOSAGE RANGE	DIRECTIONS	PEAK	DURATION	TARGET ORGAN	COMMENTS
Human Amylin Analog							
Pramlintide	Symlin	Type 1 DM:15–60 mcg SymlinPen Type 2 DM: 60–120 mcg SymlinPen	SQ injection BID with meals of at least 250 cal and 30 g carbs. Cannot be combined with insulin in same syringe	19–21 min	Unknown	Pancreas and stomach	Can be used by type 1 and type 2 diabetics Side effects: nausea, vomiting, fatigue, loss of appetite, headaches, dizziness, sore throat
Incretin Mimetics							
Exenatide	Byetta	5–1 mcg from prefilled pen	SQ injection BID within 60 min of AM and PM meal	2 hr	Unknown	Pancreas and stomach	Used only with type 2 diabetics. Side effects: Nausea, diarrhea, vomiting, pancreatitis, thyroid tumors
Liraglutide	Victoza	0.6–1.8 mg from prefilled pen	SQ injection once a day, with or without food	8–12 hr	24 hr	Pancreas and stomach	
Exenatide* (long-acting)	Brydureon		SQ injection once a week				

*Approved for use in Europe. Awaiting FDA approval.

4. The gastrointestinal (GI) tract (increased motility and decreased sense of fullness)
5. Adipose tissue (mostly visceral fat)
6. The brain (decreased dopamine causing overstimulation of hepatic glucose production, increased peripheral resistance, and a redistribution of fat).

"By the time a patient is diagnosed with T2DM, they have most likely had the disease for 9 to 12 years and only 20% to 50% of pancreatic beta-cells are functional" (Cornell & Bryk-Gandera, 2010). They can use secretagogues to maximize the production of insulin from these beta cells but, as a client once correctly stated "It's like whipping a tired horse." Eventually the beta cells can no longer respond. Thankfully there are other drugs to reduce glucagon release to stop the liver from dumping stored sugar (metformin, exenatide, and liraglutide); to increase peripheral sensitivity (TZDs and metformin); to slow stomach emptying (acarbose, miglitol, exenatide, and liraglutide); to increase weight loss by increasing a sense of fullness (exenatide, liraglutide, and pramlintide); and to decrease visceral fat and drugs to increase dopamine in the brain, which increases insulin sensitivity, lowers postprandial glucose levels, and decreases visceral fat (bromocriptine-QR). By adding one or more of these drugs, including long-acting insulin analogs, which could take the pressure of the beta cells still functioning, people with type 2 diabetes, may be able to preserve beta-cell function so these cells can produce insulin for a long time. However, type 2 diabetes is a chronic, progressive disease, which changes over time. This usually means that doses of medication that have been working may need to be increased and new and different drugs may need to be added, including insulin unless weight is lost and physical activity increased.

HOW TO DISPOSE OF MEDICATION SAFELY

All clients, whether or not they are diagnosed with diabetes, should be asked at some point what they do with unused medications.

CLINICAL EXAMPLE: You might ask: "What if your healthcare practitioner prescribes a medication but it doesn't work for you, or you have a reaction to it? What do you do with it?" Many people flush unused pills, capsules, and liquid meds down the toilet or sink drain. The environmental impact of this practice is huge. First, it pollutes lakes and rivers as well as drinking water. It can potentially poison wildlife, plants, and the food we eat. If they do nothing and keep these meds at home, they pose a poison risk for small children. Teenagers may be tempted by narcotics or other drugs found in parental medicine cabinets. Some people throw drugs in the trash, where others, including animals, may find them and ingest them. Also, personal information is on the label, available for those interested in identity theft. Clients should be told not to give medication to friends or relatives who might be taking the same drug. This may not really be the same medication, or the same dose, and prescribers need to be aware of what their patients are taking so they can accurately supervise the therapy.

So what should a person be advised to do? To help dispose of unused medication properly; the National Community Pharmacists Association has launched a "Dispose My Meds" campaign. More than 800 community pharmacies in 40 states have already joined this effort. People can bring the drugs to a participating pharmacy, and it will send these medications to a medical waste disposal facility. Clients can also get a postage-paid envelope from the pharmacy so they can mail the meds without leaving home. This includes any unused drugs, not just ones for diabetes. Go to www.dispose-mymeds.org for more details on the consequences of improper disposal of medication and to find a participating pharmacy near where an individual lives or works. Several states and communities have started Community Medication Take-Back programs, collecting a huge number of solid and liquid outdated and unwanted medications. These drugs are then incinerated by state and local facilities licensed for that purpose (Lauer, Kettell, & Davis, 2010). Nurses, veterinarians, and all healthcare professionals should be at the forefront of this potential environmental disaster.

Clients should also be warned never to put medication into a container other than the one it came in from the pharmacy. In addition, keep drugs out of the sight and reach of children, and avoid taking medications in front of children, because they tend to mimic adults. When giving children medication, even vitamins, avoid calling them "candy." Taking any kind of medication for adults or children is serious business.

NEW DIABETES MEDICATIONS ON THE HORIZON

There are a lot of hassles with the treatment of diabetes and a lot of things can be improved to make life easier. However, diabetes management has come a long way in just the past 15 to 20 years. As far as I'm concerned, the sky is the limit. Until we have a cure for both type 1 and type 2, let us celebrate the research that has brought and will continue to provide easier and better ways to control blood glucose levels.

How a New Drug or Product Gets Approved

There are an estimated 220 million people with diabetes worldwide and almost 26 million people in the United States. Pharmaceutical and manufacturing companies take this target consumer population very seriously. Scores of new antidiabetic drugs, including new insulins and unique deliveries of such medication, as well as treatments for diabetic complications, are under investigation as you read this book. Many never come on the market, such as a nasal insulin from 10 years ago. Some take decades, such as the now-promising inhaled insulin. Some, after considerable experimentation, receive FDA approval only to be recalled because of adverse reactions, as was the case with the first TZD on the market, Rezulin. The process from development to availability encompasses many phases, some of which involve healthy individuals as well as those who have the disease.

Before conducting investigational trials with human subjects, scientists research new treatments in test tubes and experiment on animals, usually mice or rats, to test hypotheses about the potential use of this or that chemical combination. If they discover a promising chemical compound to treat any number of potential causes of a disease or its complications, they refine the process and then may move on to larger animals. After more refinement as to dosage, timing, method of delivery, safety, and side effect profiles, they may start clinical trials using human subjects. Phase I trials use small numbers of healthy, paid adult volunteers of both genders and most races so researchers can test the effects of an experimental drug or treatment to further refine safety, dose range, and side effects and to evaluate whether there are unintended consequences in humans, such as liver, kidney, or other potential problems. The subjects are evaluated often and are taken off the protocols if any negative reactions occur.

If all goes well in Phase I, the drug or treatment goes into Phase II testing. This usually occurs in a few research medical centers in the United States and abroad and involves a small number of clients with the disease, in this case, type 1 or type 2 diabetes. These paid volunteers must meet certain criteria. They usually receive free exams, medical care, and experimental medication or treatment to get a better drug or treatment profile and to see whether the experimental treatment works as intended in the human subjects for which it was developed. A further refinement of safety issues and dosage also occurs. This may take weeks or months, but in the end the drug or treatment is either ready for Phase III or it is scrapped or returned to the drawing board. The drugs or treatments that get to Phase III are tested in double- or triple-blind clinical trials at medical centers across the country and worldwide involving large numbers of volunteers for which the experimental drug or treatment was intended. The subjects are divided into a control group, which may be given a placebo or current therapy, and an experimental group, which receives the item to be tested. This phase compares the experimental treatment with currently available treatments and/or a placebo. To prevent the placebo effect the study has a double-blind control, in which neither the volunteers nor those conducting the experiment know who is receiving either the investigational therapy or a placebo.

Everything is numbered, and records are evaluated by a third party not involved in the actual experiment. Volunteers receive frequent free medical care, treatment, and instructions; records are kept; and the length of the trial is variable, from weeks to months to years. Volunteers may be lost to follow-up or taken off the protocol because of unforeseen occurrences that may or may not have anything to do with the experimental treatment. However, the trial subject numbers are so large that minor subject loss really does not alter the data. Only after all of the data from animal studies through Phase III are completed is a new drug application (NDA) submitted to the FDA. The FDA evaluates the drug or treatment and all of the data submitted by the manufacturer and either approves it, approves it provisionally and asks for more data on specific concerns, or rejects it. At any time along this path an idea may be stopped, reformulated, or continued. Once an experimental drug or treatment has been FDA approved it enters Phase IV, in which it can be prescribed to individuals fitting the criteria for which it was designed. At this point, prescribers are still submitting data on side effects and other information from the clients using this newly approved drug. This phase may go on for years and may lead to a drug being taken off the market if there are reports to the FDA of significant adverse reactions, such as with Rezulin,

---

Four Phases of Investigational Drug Studies

PHASE I

Small numbers of healthy volunteers (as opposed to volunteers afflicted with the disease or ailment that the drug is meant to treat). Purpose is to determine the optimal dosage and pharmacokinetics of the drug (absorption, distribution, metabolism, excretion). Tests are performed.

PHASE II

Small numbers of volunteers who have the disease or ailment that the drug is designed to diagnose or treat. Participants are monitored for drug effectiveness and side effect. If there are no safety issues, testing-may proceed to Phase III.

PHASE III

This phase involves a large numbers of patients at medical research centers. Large numbers provide information about frequent or rare adverse effects that have been identified in Phase II. Placebos are used to prevent bias. The study is conducted in blinded form so the investigator does not know which group has the actual drug being tested.

NEW DRUG APPLICATION

At this point, the FDA reviews all results the company submits in the NDA. If approved, the company is free to market the drug exclusively.

PHASE IV

Postmarketing studies are voluntarily conducted to gain further proof of therapeutic effects of new drug. When drugs are used in the general population, sometimes severe adverse effects show up.

which caused liver damage. Another reason a drug may be taken off the market is if the manufacturer decides it is not selling well. That is what happened to the first inhaled insulin, Exubera.

Volunteering to be a clinical trial participant can significantly impact the course of treatment for diabetes or any other disease or condition. Disease-free individuals are usually recruited for Phase I trials, and those with the disease are recruited for Phases II and III. Most clients are involved in Phase III. There is a detailed informed consent involved that does not bind the volunteer to remain in the study. If you or a client would like to learn more about new and ongoing clinical trials and participant criteria, visit the National Institute of Diabetes and Digestive and Kidney Diseases home page at www2.niddk.nih.gov/Research/ClinicalResearch/ClinicalTrials and click on "Search for Clinical Trials." You can also check out www.clinicaltrials.gov to find clinical trials by location and condition being studied.

WHAT IS ON THE HORIZON FOR NEW MEDS AND DELIVERY SYSTEMS

What can you expect in the future and when? The following is a list of drugs and delivery systems currently in clinical trials.

For Type 1 Diabetes

- Four inhaled insulins for people with type 1 diabetes.
    1. Stage of development: Afrezza has completed Phase III. Afrezza is an ultra-rapid-acting insulin powder dispersed in the very compact "dreamboat" inhaler. The FDA has asked the manufacturer, MannKind Corp, to do additional trials comparing Medtone dispenser, an earlier inhaler, with the second-generation dreamboat inhaler. Pending the results of these studies, Afrezza may be FDA approved in 2012.
    2. Stage of development: A yet-unnamed product produced by Micro-Dose Therapeutx has wrapped up its Phase I clinical trial. No further information could be found.
    3. Stage of development: Alveair produced by Coremed Inc. is both fast-onset and long-acting. The technology formulates unmodified protein molecules (insulin) into submicron particles that resist enzymatic degradation and promote permeability and absorption. No availability date could be found.
    4. PROMAXX made by Baxter has completed Phase I trials. No further information could be found.

For Both Type 1 and Type 2 Diabetes

- Linjeta is a proprietary more-rapid-acting injectable regular human insulin under development for meal-time use by people with type 1 or type 2 diabetes to improve glycemic control. Biodel has submitted an NDA to the FDA for approval to market Linjeta as a treatment for both type 1 and type 2 diabetes, based upon results from Phase III clinical trials. Linjeta reduced risks of hyperglycemia and hypoglycemia and patients had less weight gain than with other human injectable insulin.

■ Two insulin skin patches for people with type 1 or type 2 diabetes are in clinical trials.
 1. Stage of development: Altea Therapeutics' product, currently known as AT1391, is undergoing Phase I and II clinical trials for both types of diabetes.
 2. Another patch, created by Dermisonics, is in Phase I trials.

■ Four oral insulin medications for people with type 1 or 2 diabetes are undergoing clinical trials. (Insulin currently is not given orally because the gastric juices of the stomach destroy insulin before it can be absorbed by the small intestine. To be successfully absorbed, any oral insulin must overcome this problem.)
 1. Stage of development: Oral-lyn, produced by Generex Biotechnology, is in Phase III clinical trials with type 1 participants. Oral-lyn Rapid-Mist, a split premeal and postmeal buccal insulin spray given with an AM and PM injection of NPH human insulin, is being compared with injected human regular and NPH insulins. Its stated completion date was December, 2010 so we should be seeing the results soon.
 2. Stage of development: Emisphere Technologies has completed Phase I trial on its yet-unnamed oral insulin capsule. It compares this oral insulin with regular human insulin injections. The company has partnered with Novo Nordisk using Emisphere's Eligen Technology to further develop this oral insulin.
 3. Stage of development: Coremed's Intesulin is in its initial trial of diabetic subjects. In a limited number of patients, the data are positive from the delivery of a single gel-capsule. There are no reported gastrointestinal irritations, metabolic abnormalities, or hypoglycemia thus far.
 4. Stage of development: VIAtab by Biodel has completed Phase I trials. VIAtab is an oral formulation of insulin designed to be administered sublingually. This therapy is a tablet that dissolves in minutes when placed under the tongue. In a Phase I study, VIAtab delivered insulin to the blood stream quickly and resembled the first-phase insulin release spike found in healthy individuals.

■ Two new basal insulin analogs are being tested by Eli Lilly.
 1. Stage of development: LY2605541 is a structurally different basal insulin analog now in Phase III trials.
 2. Stage of development: Ly2963016 is a new insulin glargine-like product that also began Phase III clinical trials in early 2011.

■ Merck Pharmaceuticals is working on a glucose-dependent insulin called SmartInsulin, which should help to control both fasting and postprandial blood sugars and reduce the risk of hypoglycemia. It is currently still in animal studies and may soon start human trials; however, this means that FDA approval is likely at least 5 years away. Novo Nordisk and Biodel are also working on their own version of a smart insulin product.

For Type 2 diabetes

- Stage of development: Nastech Pharmaceutical Company, Inc., now called MDRNA Inc., is conducting a study to evaluate the effect of nasal insulin on postprandial glycemic control in type 2 diabetic patients compared with NovoLog. This unnamed nasal insulin is in Phase II trials. Nasulin, developed by CPEX Pharmaceuticals, has been withdrawn from Phase II trials.
- Stage of development: An exenatide nasal spray from Amylin Pharmaceuticals and MDRNA is in Phase II trials. Exenatide (Byetta) is usually given by subcutaneous injection.
- One more new category of drugs in late-stage clinical trials is the SGLT2 molecule (sodium-glucose cotransporter) inhibitor. Three drugs in this drug class in development include (1) dapagliflozin, developed by Bristol-Myers Squibb and AstraZenica, (2) Boehringer Ingelheim's BI107333, and (3) canagliflozin, developed by Johnson & Johnson. These drugs are being studied in type 2 diabetics on metformin without normalizing their blood glucose levels. They could also be given with other oral diabetes meds. They work by inhibiting the SGLT2 in the kidney tubules that causes reabsorption of sugar and sodium that otherwise would be excreted in the urine. The result is that more sugar and sodium are excreted, resulting in lower blood sugar, weight loss, and lower blood pressure. The downside of these drugs is that there is a greater risk of urinary and genital infections due to the higher sugar content of the urine (Bailey, Gross, Pieters, Bastien, & List, 2010).
  1. Stage of development: Bristol-Myers Squibb and AstraZenica have submitted a NDA to the FDA and marketing authorization application to the European regulators for dapagliflozin in December 2010 so, if all goes well, this drug may be available in late 2011.
  2. Stage of development: Boehringer Ingelheim's BI107333 is another SGLT2 inhibitor. It is currently in Phase III clinical trials.
  3. Stage of development: Johnson and Johnson is in the process of conducting Phase I trials on canagliflozin.
- Extended release and ultra-long-acting basal insulins are under development.
  1. Stage of development: Eli Lilly, Amylin Pharmaceuticals, and Alkermes Inc. have positive results from their completed Phase II trials with a new one-a-month, extended-release formulation of exenatide, the active ingredient in the twice a day Byetta injection. It is based on the same Medisorb microsphere technology used in their successful once-a-week exenatide, Bydureon.

2. Stage of development: Novo Nordisk is developing an ultra-long-acting basal insulin called Degludec, which can be given once a day or three times a week in type 2 diabetes. It is being compared with insulin glargine (Lantus) in a Phase II trial. Another Phase II trial using (1) insulin degludec/insulin aspart in a soluble coformulation of the basal analog insulin degludec 70% and insulin aspart 30%, or deglutec 55% and insulin aspart 45% is being compared to insulin glargine. These once-daily formulations provided comparable overall glycemic control to insulin glargine with similar low rates of hypoglycemia, but better post-dinner plasma glucose control.

If you or your clients want to check on the status of a particular drug on the Web, or simply see what is new or under investigation, be sure to put the current year next to your search term. This will move current information to the top of the list using this date.

These are very exciting times for clients with diabetes and the healthcare practitioners who provide care for them. Not only are there many different treatments and medication that help clients normalize blood glucose levels but also the ongoing research mentioned at the end of this chapter gives us all hope that living with diabetes will become easier and more manageable as time goes on. The explosion of new types of insulin and oral and injectable medication to treat the ever-increasing number of people diagnosed with diabetes should continue to proliferate in the years to come. Healthcare professionals must keep themselves updated by attending workshops and/or subscribing to professional journals or free online listservs like Medscape (www .medscape.com) if they are to give competent and effective care to clients with diabetes.

REFERENCES

American Diabetes Association (ADA). (n.d.). *Shots and checks.* Retrieved May 3, 2011, from www.diabetes.org/living-with-diabetes/parents-and-kids/everyday-life/shots-and-checks.html

American Diabetes Association (ADA). (2003). *Insulin therapy in the 21st century.* Alexandria, VA: Author.

American Diabetes Association (ADA). (2011). Standards of medical care in diabetes—2011. *Diabetes Care, 34,* S11–S61.

Bailey, C. J., Gross, J. L., Pieters, A., Bastien, A., & List, J. F. (2010). Effect of dapagliflozin in patients with type 2 diabetes who have inadequate glycaemic control with metformin: A randomised, double-blind, placebo-controlled trial. *The Lancet, 375*(9733), 2223–2233.

Clark, W. L. (2006). Exenatide: From the Gila monster to you. *Diabetes Self-Management, 23*(1), 36–40.

Cornell, S., & Bryk-Gandera, M. (2010). Cycloset (bromocriptine mesylate) tablets: A novel treatment for the management of type 2 diabetes in adults. *Pharmacy Times, 12,* 82–84.

Fox, L. A., Buckloh, L. M., Smith, S. D., Wysocki, T., & Mauras, N. (2005). A randomized controlled trial of insulin pump therapy in young children with type 1 diabetes. *Diabetes Care, 28,* 1277–1281.

Lauer, M. F., Kettell, B. D., & Davis, M. H. (2010). Leftover drugs in the water supply: Don't flush those pills! *American Journal of Nursing, 110*(8), 46–49.

Saudek, C. D., & Margolis, S. (2011). *Johns Hopkins White Papers: Diabetes.* Baltimore, MD: Johns Hopkins University School of Medicine.

U.S. Food and Drug Administration (USFDA). (2010, September 26). *Avandia (rosiglitazone): REMS—risk of cardiovascular events.* Retrieved April 10, 2011, from www.fda.gov/safety/medwatch/safetyinformation/safetyalerts forhumanmedicalproducts/ucm226994.htm

FIVE

Glycemic Control

Control will set you free.
—Anonymous

The bottom line with diabetes treatment is attaining near-normal blood sugars while minimizing hypoglycemic episodes. Several research studies, including the Diabetes Control and Complications Trial (DCCT), which focused on people with type 1 diabetes, and the United Kingdom Prospective Diabetes Study (UKPDS), which studied individuals with type 2 diabetes, have shown significant prevention or delay of chronic complications related to high glucose levels as a result of tight control of blood sugars.

The American Diabetes Association (ADA, 2011) currently recommends the following goals for blood sugar control for both type 1 and type 2 diabetes:

Fasting	70–99 mg/dl
Before meals and at bedtime	70–130 mg/dl
Peak: 1–2 hours after meal began	< 180 mg/dl
Hemoglobin A1c	< 7.0%

Hemoglobin A1c is a measurement of the percentage of glycosylation the average hemoglobin molecule experiences (how sugared it becomes) over a period of 2 to 3 months floating in blood containing glucose. Glucose of varying amounts is present in the blood and "sticks" to hemoglobin. The red blood cells, which contain the hemoglobin, live for about 120 days, so the glycosylated hemoglobin of these red cells represents an average blood glucose level during this time period. To put this in perspective, persons without diabetes have a hemoglobin A1c of 4.0%–5.6% (ADA, 2011). As you can see in Table 5.1, the higher the A1c, the higher is the estimated average blood glucose. Therefore, following nutritional recommendations the week before an office visit, a strategy of some with diabetes in the past used to appear compliant, really does not affect the results. The ADA also recommends that glycemic goals be individualized, especially with children, the elderly, and

TABLE 5.1
Correlation Between A1c Level and Estimated Average
Plasma Glucose Levels on Multiple Testing Over 2 to 3 Months

		ESTIMATED AVERAGE PLASMA GLUCOSE	
A1c (%)	Meaning	mg/dl	mmol/L
4.0–5.6	Normal	68–99	3.75–5.4
5.7–6.4	Prediabetes	100–125	5.5–6.95
6.5	Diabetes	126	7.0
7	OK	154	8.6
8	Fair	183	10.2
9	Poor	212	11.8
10	Poor	240	13.4
11	High risk	269	14.9
12	High risk	298	16.5
13	Very high risk	326	18.1

Note: Compiled from information in *Diabetes Care*, Vol. 34, 2011, S11–S61 and using the following conversion formula: A1c = (46.7 + plasma glucose) / 28.7 or Plasma glucose = (28.7 × A1c) − 46.7. To convert mmol/L of glucose to mg/dl, multiply by 18. To convert mg/dl of glucose to mmol/L, divide by 18 or multiply by 0.055. These formulas give approximate results. mg/dl = milligrams per deciliters; mmol/L = milliosmols per liter.

clients who are pregnant or who have frequent and severe hypoglycemia (ADA, 2011). Glucose readings after meals may be particularly difficult to control in clients not on insulin therapy, thus causing a higher A1c average. Additionally, frequent low blood sugars may cancel out high blood sugars, thus lowering the A1c average and creating an artificially appropriate-looking percentage. This is an important point to remember.

CLINICAL EXAMPLE: Prior to using an insulin pump, my A1cs were usually between 5% and 6%. However, I had frequent high and low blood sugars and my lows, especially during the night, were more significant. My seemingly great glycemic control actually indicated that I rode the blood sugar roller coaster most of the time. Since I have been using an insulin pump, my hypoglycemic episodes are very infrequent and any high blood sugars are more noticeable. Thus, my A1cs, usually between 6.8% and 7.3%, are a truer reflection of my glycemic control.

In 2003, the ADA decreased guidelines for normal fasting blood sugar from the 1997 guidelines of 70 to 110 mg/dl to 70 to 99 mg/dl. This increased the span for IGT from 110 to 125 mg/dl to 100 to 125 mg/dl, which is now called prediabetes. The purpose of both changes is to alert more patients and their healthcare providers to the potential damage that can occur prior to the official diagnosis of diabetes at a blood sugar of 126 mg/dl. The hope is that this will be a wake-up call for lifestyle modifications and weight loss, if needed, which should prevent or delay the onset of type 2 diabetes. "Glycemic control is fundamental to the management of diabetes" (ADA, 2011, pp. 16–27). This control is assessed by using client self-monitoring blood glucose (SMBG) records and A1c every 3 to 6 months. Individualizing our approach to teaching and motivating clients to help improve diabetes self-management is covered in depth in Part II of this book.

Acute complications include hyperglycemia and hypoglycemia and are covered in this chapter. Chronic complications are discussed in Chapter 6.

HYPERGLYCEMIA

Technically, higher than normal blood sugar is defined as anything above the levels given at the beginning of this chapter. The glucose levels depend on the timing of food intake from fasting and preprandial levels to 1 to 2 hours postprandial and bedtime levels. Most people with diabetes have no symptoms until blood sugar approaches 250 mg/dl. This is an important point to make with clients who do not routinely monitor their glucose levels. The most common symptoms of hyperglycemia include:

■ Frequent urination of very pale, dilute urine,
■ Thirst from the loss of body fluids in the urine, and
■ Hunger for simple sugars.

Other symptoms may include the following:

■ Headache, sleepiness, difficulty concentrating
■ Visual disturbances from the glucose concentration in the eye fluids and on the lens
■ Dry or flushed skin from dehydration
■ General malaise

These symptoms may be so common that older clients may think they are a normal part of aging. When illness, even the common cold, or other stressors increase blood sugars to 400 mg/dl and higher, *ketoacidosis* can occur. When the body does not have enough insulin to move glucose into cells for energy, the cells turn to fat to provide needed fuel. The metabolism of fat produces fatty acids and ketones that accumulate in the blood and affect the brain, producing the symptoms listed above. The kidneys try to eliminate ketones and glucose, giving rise to *ketonuria* and *glucosuria*.

Testing urine for ketones is confirmation that ketoacidosis is occurring. Other symptoms of this very dangerous condition include the following:

- Shortness of breath
- Fruity smelling breath (more like the acetone smell of nail polish remover)
- Nausea and vomiting

If diabetic ketoacidosis (DKA) persists, the client may lapse into a coma. The blood sugar level that produces a coma is very individualized and can be anywhere from 600 mg/dl to 1,500 mg/dl or higher. This condition occurs mostly with type 1 diabetes and is caused by omitting an insulin dose, eating excessive amounts of carbohydrates, illness, and some medications (see Table 5.2). However, these same conditions, if severe enough, can overwhelm the ability of the pancreas of a person with type 2 diabetes to respond to oral agents by increasing production of insulin. When this happens, even a person with type 2 diabetes can become ketotic. Do not assume that just because someone has type 2 diabetes, he or she cannot develop ketoacidosis.

On the other hand, when ketones are *not* present in an unconscious type 2 diabetic with a high blood sugar, the resulting condition is called *hyperosmolar hyperglycemic nonketotic syndrome (HHNK)*. This may happen in an older client who lapses into a coma from the severe dehydration caused by hyperglycemia (blood sugars over 600 mg/dl). Although this can happen to people with both type 1 and type 2 diabetes, it is more common in those with type 2 diabetes because they do produce some insulin, preventing the burning of fat (ketones). It may follow high blood sugars cause by an illness or an infection. As the body tries to rid itself of the glucose in the urine, the urine is very dilute and copious in amount at first. If the condition that caused the hyperglycemia persists and nothing is done to control high blood sugars, the person gets very dehydrated, the urinary output becomes scant and very dark, and the blood becomes very viscous and concentrated. If the client is not hydrated soon with copious amounts of IV fluids, seizures, coma, and eventually death may ensue. The symptoms of HHNK are very similar to DKA, however, the biggest differences between the two besides ketosis include the type of diabetes and the age of the client.

CLINICAL EXAMPLE: Older clients may not pay as much attention to an illness, thinking it part of the aging process, as someone younger and may not be monitoring blood sugars due to the cost or other issues. It is imperative that family, friends, and neighbors look in on seniors to make sure they are doing well and not in need of medical attention whether or not they have diabetes. What anyone with diabetes, at any age, needs to realize is that the choice to pay attention to blood sugars or not may become a life-or-death decision.

Factors That Raise Blood Sugar

Table 5.2 lists the many factors that affect blood sugar by decreasing the effectiveness of insulin or by increasing the need for insulin to control blood sugar. Many nurses and healthcare professionals are aware that physical stress, such as a heart attack, a stroke, trauma, pain, surgery, or infection, increases blood sugar by increasing stress hormones such as epinephrine and norepinephrine. This reaction represents the old fight-or-flight instinct we inherited from our prehistoric ancestors. We no longer have to fight the saber-toothed tiger or flee from the woolly mammoth, but our adrenal glands secrete these hormones anyway.

Stress hormones are very useful if they are required by the body. For example, what we need in order to fight or flee is sufficient blood pressure (arteries vasoconstrict), increased cardiac output (heart rate increases), sufficient oxygen to hook on to each red cell being pumped out (respiratory rate increases and bronchioles dilate), *and* extra glucose to fuel our brain to think and our muscles to move. Under the influence of stress hormones, therefore, stored glucose is dumped into the bloodstream by the liver and skeletal muscles. During times of physical stress, all clients with diabetes need more insulin even if they are not eating (NPO). Type 2 diabetics who use oral medication to control blood sugars may need rapid-acting insulin during the stressful crisis.

CLINICAL EXAMPLE: Hospitalized clients who have diabetes should have blood sugars monitored before meals and at bedtime by the nurse or the client and recorded by the nurse. The client should be encouraged to monitor glucose levels to verify technique and so the nurse can encourage client problem-solving and/or teach appropriate options if blood sugars do not fall in an appropriate range for this person. In the *Standards of Medical Practice—2011* the ADA recommends that insulin coverage start at 140 mg/dl or greater pre-meal for hospitalized clients. Less stringent glucose targets may be appropriate for patients with comorbid conditions, such as CVD, stroke, or neuropathy (ADA, 2011). However, if the insulin coverage only starts at 200 mg/dl, we need to advocate for our clients to get that lowered to at least 150 mg/dl. Even critically ill patients should maintain blood sugar less than 180 mg/dl. For a client on insulin, glycemic goals should be between 140 and 180 mg/dl for most critically ill patients. This can best be achieved in these clients by use of an IV insulin infusion, which should prevent and/or quickly correct any hypoglycemic episodes by decreasing or stopping the insulin drip (ADA, 2011).

TABLE 5.2
Factors That Affect Blood Sugar

FACTORS THAT INCREASE BLOOD SUGAR	FACTORS THAT DECREASE BLOOD SUGAR
Skipping antidiabetic medication	Too much antidiabetic medication
Overeating, especially carbs	Skipping a meal after taking medication
Significant weight gain	Significant weight loss
Decreased physical activity	Increased physical activity (even several hours later)

Medications
  Corticosteroids
  Thyroid supplements
  Diuretics
  Caffeine (high doses)
  Niacin (high doses)
	Medications
	  Beta-blockers
	  MAO inhibitors
	  Ritalin
	
	Alcohol

Hormones
  Stress hormones (adrenaline)
  Growth hormones
  Cortisol
  Pregnancy hormones (second and
    third trimesters)
  Hormones during menses
  Estrogen
	Pregnancy (first trimester)

Emotions
  Anger
  Depression
  Fear
  Panic
	Stress management

Others
  Excessive sleeping
  Smoking (nicotine)
	Others
	  Heat and humidity
	  High altitude
	  Intense brain activity
	  New or unusual surroundings
	  Socializing
	  Stimulating environment

Poor glycemic control during hospitalization puts patients at risk for infection and poor wound healing (ADA, 2011). The fear of hypoglycemia is what usually drives this inadequate insulin coverage. Testing blood sugars every 4 hours or before meals, if allowed to eat, would demonstrate that hypoglycemia does not occur in a hospitalized, insulin-resistant, type 2 diabetic who becomes even more insulin-resistant with stress hormones. The same hormonal reaction occurs, of course, with the psychological stressors of fear, anxiety, depression, anger, and so forth. These reactions to hospitalization only add to the increase of blood sugar from physical stress. Nurses and mental health professionals may be able to decrease some of the psychological stressors by being good listeners, providing prompt and adequate pain control, and explaining all procedures on the client's level, thus developing a trusting therapeutic relationship. Clients with diabetes who are planning a hospital admission should prepare themselves by reading a new pamphlet by the Joint Commission (JC), a nonprofit organization that accredits healthcare programs in the United States, entitled *Speak Up*. It can be found by visiting the website www .jointcommission.org/speakup.aspx and clicking on *Speak Up: Diabetes— Five Ways to be Active in Your Care at the Hospital* found on the left hand side of the page. There are several others that might be of interest, such as brochures on preventing infection, preventing medication errors, pain management, planning follow-up care, tips for doctor's visits, and more, including a coloring book for children. Clients can watch a video or read/ print a PDF file of each of the brochures. They can also receive free copies of the brochures by calling the toll-free number 877-223-6866.

There are several medications that also increase cellular insulin resistance or that antagonize the action of insulin. The most common is prednisone or any corticosteroid given to control the inflammatory process.

CLINICAL EXAMPLE: Clients dealing with severe asthma, rheumatoid arthritis, systemic lupus erythematosus (SLE), as well as dermatologic, hematologic, and neurologic inflammatory conditions, may be treated with corticosteroids. Even a corticosteroid injected into the spine or a painful joint or given as eye drops can elevate blood sugar in a person with diabetes, sometimes for days. Other problematic hormones that can raise blood sugar include thyroxin, growth hormone, estrogen as part of the menstrual cycle or taken after menopause, and several placental hormones that increase in the second half of pregnancy. Any person not able to increase production of insulin to counter these insulin antagonists will develop hyperglycemia. Other drugs that may increase the need for insulin include some diuretics, such as hydrochlorothiazide (HCTZ), Lasix, and Bumex, and large doses of caffeine or niacin, a B vitamin prescribed in high doses for hypercholesterolemia. In addition, weight gain itself increases insulin resistance, as does excessive sleep (Scheiner, 2004).

Clients with diabetes or prediabetes who smoke should be told that, among the many health reasons to quit, nicotine in cigarettes also increases blood sugar as demonstrated by an elevated A1c. Nicotine inhibits the release of insulin, causing increase in blood sugar levels. Smokers or those trying to quit using nicotine patches, gum, or lozenges who also have diabetes need to monitor blood glucose levels, especially as they withdraw from nicotine's effects (Zhang, Curham, Hu, Rimm, & Forman, 2011). Diabetes medication may need to be decreased to prevent hypoglycemia.

HYPOGLYCEMIA

Anyone with diabetes, especially clients taking insulin or secretagogue drugs (see Chapter 4 for list), can experience low blood sugar. If the intake of carbohydrates does not match the amount of insulin injected or produced by the pancreas as a result of an oral antidiabetic agent, blood sugar will drop. Everyone has his or her own reaction to hypoglycemia. However, most experience the following symptoms:

- Tremors, shakiness, or jerky movements
- Sweating, pale moist skin
- Dizziness, feeling faint, headache
- Excessive hunger, especially for carbohydrates
- Sudden, atypical change in behavior, mood swings, or erratic behavior
- Tingling or numbness around the mouth and/or tongue
- Difficulty paying attention, confusion, sleep
- Visual disturbances, difficulty reading, dilated pupils
- Increased heart and respiratory rates
- Seizures and coma

As you can see, some of these symptoms sound very similar to those of hyperglycemia, especially the visual disturbances, headache, and sleepiness. It is important for clients with diabetes to confirm these symptoms with glucose monitoring so that the meaning is clear. Because the need to treat a low blood sugar is fairly immediate to prevent brain cell damage, clients should be taught that when in doubt, eat. Sometimes, however, the client may correctly interpret symptoms as related to hypoglycemia because he or she has administered insulin and not eaten or has exercised before eating.

Healthcare practitioners of any discipline should ask clients if they experience hypoglycemic episodes, what symptoms they exhibited, and what they do about it. This can be an occasion to praise the client for good problem-solving skills or teach them how to avoid and/or treat low blood sugar events. Treatments for low blood sugar include

Food Item	Amount
Sugar packets	2 – 3
Fruit juice (100% juice, unsweetened)	½ cup (4 oz)
Soda (not diet)	½ cup (4 oz)
Hard candy (not sugar-free)	3 – 5 pieces
Sugar or honey	4 teaspoons
Glucose tablets	3 – 4
Glucose gel packets	1 packet

The last two items can be found over the counter in most drugstores and should be carried by anyone prone to hypoglycemia, including anyone on insulin, regardless of whether he or she has type 1 or type 2 diabetes. Glucose tablets come in 10-tablet tubes and 50-tablet containers used to refill the tubes.

Factors That Decrease Blood Sugar

Chapter 3 provides an explanation of how increased physical activity, including sexual activity, improves cellular insulin sensitivity and decreases insulin needs, perhaps for hours. If the amount of insulin injected is not decreased or more carbohydrates are not ingested, hypoglycemia may result. In the same fashion, the amount of carbohydrates, both simple and complex, must match the amount of insulin secreted by the pancreas or given by injection or pump. With the advent of rapid-acting insulin analogs, clients can wait until a meal is served to decide how many carbs (see "Carbohydrate Counting" in Chapter 2) they plan to eat and then deliver an appropriate amount of insulin. If a client is taking a rapid-acting secretagogue, such as Prandin or Starlix with each meal, he or she can omit taking it if skipping a meal or if no or very few carbohydrate foods are consumed. The problem of needing to eat carbohydrate foods occurs when a client has injected intermediate-acting insulin (NPH) in the morning, which will peak around lunch time, or has taken a long-acting secretagogue (a sulfonylurea or DPP-4 inhibitor) with breakfast, which will increase the amount of insulin secreted by the pancreas all day long. If the carbs do not match the insulin, low blood sugar may result. In the above circumstances just described, the client must be taught to eat meals on time and provide a similar number of carbohydrate grams at each of these meals to prevent glucose levels from going too low—or too high, for that matter.

Drugs that often decrease blood sugar include beta-blockers for hypertension or arrhythmias, MAO (monoamine oxidase) inhibitors for depression, and Ritalin. A good medication history, including over-the-counter and illegal drugs may unearth the cause of unexpected hypoglycemia. Alcohol also lowers blood sugar and should always be consumed with food. The rationale for this is that if a significant drop in blood sugar occurs after ingesting an alcoholic beverage, the liver may not be able to respond to glucagon secreted by the alpha cells of the pancreas, resulting in no stored glucose being released. This can be a potentially dangerous situation. Because many of the symptoms of hypoglycemia resemble drunkenness, the smell of alcohol on the breath may delay the treatment of the hypoglycemia. Other factors that can potentially lower blood sugar include excessive heat and humidity (especially while exercising), high altitudes, and anything that may distract a person from his or her usual routine of checking blood sugar, such as socializing, new or unusual surroundings, a stimulating environment, or intense brain activity (Scheiner, 2004). During these times it is important to monitor blood sugars periodically and often. Table 5.2 summarizes factors that decrease blood glucose.

Hypoglycemia Unawareness

Some people with type 1 diabetes may no longer sense an impending low blood sugar and may simply become unconscious when blood glucose levels are low enough. Because brain cells only burn glucose for energy, they stop functioning and may even die when blood glucose plummets. This very dangerous condition may affect people with long-standing type 1 diabetes, those who have autonomic neuropathy preventing the occurrence of symptoms, such as sweating, tremors, and increased pulse, those who experience frequent (several times a week) or severe ($\leq$ 30 mg/dl) low blood sugars as a result of tight glucose control, or those who are on beta-blockers for cardiac arrhythmias or hypertension. Beta-blockers blunt the effects of epinephrine and norepinephrine in response to a low blood sugar by blocking the beta receptors of the blood vessels, heart muscle, and bronchioles. This is, of course, why they are prescribed for hypertension and arrhythmias but may make the recognition of hypoglycemia by the client much more difficult.

Some people begin to have different symptoms as the years go by and simply fail to acknowledge them as a signal to eat something to raise blood sugars. In any case, frequent blood sugar monitoring is crucial, and eating multiple small meals that should include carbohydrates and protein becomes a necessity. These clients should be advised to alert others with whom they live, exercise, or work that they have diabetes as well as the signs and treatment of hypoglycemia. Having a *Glucagon kit* and teaching others to administer the injection in case of an emergency, such as a coma or inability to swallow juice may become a life-saving measure. Glucagon can be administered subcutaneous, IM, or IV, and the dosage depends on the age and weight of the client. For example:

Infants	0.2 mg/kg with a max of 1 mg over 24 hours
Children less than 20 kg (44 lb)	20–30 mcg/kg or 0.5 mg (0.5 unit)
Adults and children 20 kg or more	1 mg (1 unit)

www.vhpharmsci.com/PDTM/Monographs/glucagon.htm

Injected glucagon causes the liver to release stored glycogen (glucose), which should raise blood sugar within 10 to 15 minutes, enough so a person can eat or drink something. Having this Glucagon kit on hand and teaching others to administer the injection may become a life-saving measure for a client. Watching a good video by Eli Lilly and company, a maker of glucagon, on how to administer this hormone at www.humalog. com/Pages/glucagon-tutorial.aspx?WT.srch=1 can be instructive. The client and a friend, coworker, or family member should watch this video periodically to refresh their memories. When the currently prescribed Glucagon kit expires, they can use it for practice.

THE BLOOD GLUCOSE—SLEEP CONNECTION

In Chapter 2, I discussed the connection between inadequate sleep and obesity. People who are tired usually eat more and exercise less, causing a rise in glucose levels at night, especially if a client eats before going to bed. As stated previously, high blood sugars cause kidneys to try to excrete this sugar and, with it, water causing a person to wake in order to urinate, perhaps multiple times, thus limiting the amount of sound sleep achieved. There is also some evidence that sleep deprivation can cause insulin resistance and give rise to prediabetes in persons not yet diagnosed with diabetes (Donga, et al. 2010).

What about low blood sugar during the night? Most people on insulin have experienced this and report a variety of different symptoms than those they feel during the day. For this reason it is sometimes difficult to recognize and thus treat. Symptoms range from numbness and tingling of the lips and tongue, heart palpitations, and confusion as to where they are even in a familiar setting such as their own bedrooms, what their fingers are feeling (nightclothes, sheets, hands, and face), and the frightening feeling that something is terribly wrong. Unfortunately, they do not have enough blood glucose for brain cells to process the information their senses are sending. This is sometimes described by clients as nighttime terrors.

CLINICAL EXAMPLE: Prior to getting my insulin pump, I experienced many nighttime lows. I would usually wake up from a recurrent nightmare sweating, confused, and frightened. Sometimes I didn't even recognize the lump next to me as my husband who could, if I woke him, provide me with the help I needed. Needless to say, he saved my life and my brain cells on many occasions. For several years neither of us routinely got the sleep we needed. With the insulin pump, that rarely happens.

To prevent or minimize nighttime hypoglycemic episodes, avoid eating anything within a couple of hours of bedtime so its absorption and thus effect on blood sugar can be noted. Always check a blood glucose level before going to bed. If it is over 200 mg/dl, take the corrective amount of insulin, if prescribed, and/or note this in a log book to help explain a higher than normal blood sugar the next morning. Clients may need help troubleshooting why this happened and help preventing morning hyperglycemia. If a nighttime glucose level is below 80 mg/dl, they should be advised to eat something with a carb value of 15 grams, such as a small piece of fruit.

BLOOD GLUCOSE MONITORING

There are many blood glucose meters on the market that rely on electrophoresis to read blood sugar. Most require a drop of blood from the finger; however, alternative sites, such as the forearm or the area of the palm below the thumb, may be used with certain types of meters. The area tested should be washed with warm water and soap to provide a surface free of debris or food residue and to increase the blood supply to the area. To increase the size of the drop of blood, massage the area, let the arm hang down, and/or milk the finger. To ensure accuracy, follow the manufacturer's direction as to coding the meter with each package of strips, if necessary. Strips must be protected from heat and humidity. Periodic testing of strips and meter with the appropriate control solution may be necessary, especially if the glucose reading is in question. When in doubt, throw the package of strips out. If a new package does not solve the problem, call the help-line number on the back of the meter. Most companies will assist with troubleshooting problems and/or send a replacement meter. There are lancing devices and lancets to fit every client's coordination needs and depth of skin, so clients should be encouraged to experiment with others if the one that came with the meter is not satisfactory. Meters today require a very small drop of blood, from 3 ml to 0.03 ml. The resource guide provided by the ADA at http://forecast .diabetes.org/magazine/features/consumer-guide-2011.jsp provides information and comparisons for meters, strips, lancing devices, lancets, syringes, and many other diabetes supplies. This guide is updated each year so change the end of this URL to the current year. Another good source to help evaluate the particulars of meters, including A1c meters and kits, is www.mendosa.com/meters.htm.

Frequent blood sugar monitoring is recommended for both type 1 and type 2 clients. I am frequently asked how often to test, and my answer is "Whenever you need the information." Nurses and other healthcare professionals should advise clients to follow the guidelines in Figure 5.1. Today with all of the devices available, it is inconceivable to me that anyone would persist in wondering what their blood sugar is. If a person feels bad or odd, it is a simple procedure to rule in or rule out blood sugar as a cause. For a long time, insurance companies

1. Carry blood glucose meter and supplies at all times.
2. Test blood sugar often, especially before eating, taking diabetes medication that will increase the amount of insulin in the blood, or going to bed, or after experiencing physical or emotional stress, including physical activity.
3. If using intermediate-acting insulin (NPH) or a long-acting secretagogue, eat on a preset schedule with a predetermined amount of carbohydrates.
4. Take rapid-acting insulin or short-acting secretagogue only immediately before eating a meal with carbohydrates.
5. If hypoglycemia is a potential problem, always carry fast-acting glucose, such as gels or tablets, available at drugstores.
6. Always carry extra supplies needed to correct potential high blood sugar, such as extra insulin and syringes, even if using an insulin pump and other antidiabetic medication if prescribed.
7. Check expiration dates and protect supplies from extremes of heat and cold.

FIGURE 5.1 Rules to Follow for Glycemic Control

did not cover glucose strips (the expensive part of monitoring blood sugars) for type 2 diabetics unless they were on insulin—sort of a penny-wise and pound-foolish approach. Today, several states have passed laws that mandate that insurance companies cover meters, strips, lancing devices, and lancets, as well as diabetes education for anyone diagnosed with diabetes. Many physicians still do not ask their type 2 patients to test blood sugars, or if they do, the testing is very sporadic. In order to understand how food and physical activity affects each individual, that person must test his or her blood sugar. Doing lab work only at a doctor's office visit is really too little, too late. Living with blood sugars in the 200s or higher is causing tissue damage. The sooner hyperglycemia is discovered and treated, the less damage is done.

What should a client do with the glucose monitor numbers? Currently there are many options from low-tech lifestyle changes such as omitting or decreasing the amount of certain foods (e.g., carbohydrates) or increasing physical activity to changing medication regimens to include administration of insulin via syringe or pump. Checking a blood sugar 1–2 hours after eating pizza or taking a 30-minute walk is more convincing to a client than anything he or she can read or hear about from a healthcare professional. Being aware of the increased blood sugar from eating excessive amounts of carbohydrates from the pizza or the normalizing of blood sugar provided by simple exercise is very empowering.

CLINICAL EXAMPLE: Testing blood sugar before meals is important because problem-solving may be needed if levels are either too high or too low. The decisions center on food choices, timing, physical activity, and medication. If glucose levels are too high, a person can take more insulin or oral medication, if prescribed, and/or delay eating for 30 minutes or more, exercise before eating, or minimize the carbohydrates eaten at this meal. It makes no sense to dump more carbs into a system that is already overloaded with blood sugar. If, on the other hand, blood sugar level is too low, eating fast-acting carbohydrates quickly is imperative, medication, especially insulin, and exercise may need to wait until the glucose level is higher. When administering rapid-acting insulin, the amount should be based on current blood sugar, increasing or decreasing the amount if glucose is out of target range, plus an amount to cover the carbohydrates that a person is planning to eat. Less may need to be taken if an individual plans to exercise after this meal. The proof that a client's decisions were correct or not lies in the postprandial blood sugar levels (Scheiner, 2011). Figure 5.2 includes advice as to when a person should monitor blood glucose levels, rationale for doing so, and suggestions concerning how they should handle the monitored results.

The ADA recommends that healthcare practitioners evaluate how clients monitor their blood sugars because the accuracy of self-monitoring is instrument and user dependent. It is important that their technique be checked not only after first being taught how to use a particular monitor but also periodically and when changing to a new monitor. In addition, clients must be taught how to use the data provided by adjusting food intake, physical activity, and/or medications to achieve glycemic targets. These decision-making skills must also be reevaluated and updated periodically to ascertain that clients remain secure in their knowledge and confident in their diabetes self-management (ADA, 2011).

Most people are not convinced to change their lifestyle with scare tactics warning of the development of chronic complications in 10 to 20 years' time. The convincing evidence needs to be more immediate. Glycemic control improves personal well-being right now. It prevents infections, improves health, increases energy, sharpens the mind, and stabilizes emotions. As clients redefine their goals in life based on improved glycemic control in particular and their health in general, they will be encouraged to continue to eat nutritiously, lose weight, if needed, increase physical activity, and follow the resulting blood sugars and periodic A1c percentages. Clients and healthcare practitioners alike must also remember that no one is perfect. Blood glucose numbers are neither good nor bad. They are simply data that help a person make better choices now and in the future.

Monitor blood sugar every day, for the following reasons:
Before giving insulin, to adjust the amount as directed.
Before each meal and at bedtime, to adjust the carbs eaten and/or any medication taken

> If ⩾ 180 mg/dl, eat fewer carbs or take more insulin.
> If ⩾ 80 mg/dl, eat more carbs or take less insulin.

If directed to monitor blood sugar before breakfast only and the blood glucose level is routinely ⩾ 180 mg/dl, follow the instructions above and test again at bedtime.

> If bedtime blood sugar is ⩾ 180 mg/dl, omit a snack and test before dinner the next day.
> If dinnertime blood sugar is ⩾ 180 mg/dl, follow the instructions above and call a healthcare provider for further instructions.

Monitor 2 hours after a meal if any adjustments to carbs, insulin, or medication have been made:

> If ⩾ 180 mg/dl, decrease carbs even more, increase meds, and/or call a healthcare provider.
> If < 180 mg/dl, the adjustments worked.
> If ⩽ 100 mg/dl, cut back on the adjustments.

Monitor before exercise unless a meal has just been eaten:

> If ⩾ 250 mg/dl, wait until blood sugar is lower, or take more insulin.
> If ⩽ 150 mg/dl, eat a 15-gram carbohydrate snack before exercising.

Monitor when not feeling well to rule in or rule out whether this is related to blood sugar level. Because illnesses do affect blood sugar, follow this advice:

> If glucose is ⩾ 250 mg/dl, notify a healthcare provider for instructions.
> If glucose is 80 to 120 mg/dl, then the illness is not related and not affecting glucose level. Repeat the test in 4 hours to check for changes.
> If glucose is < 80 mg/dl and objective signs of hypoglycemia are present, eat or drink 15 grams of carbohydrates. Retest in 20 minutes.
> If blood sugar is still low, eat 15 more grams of carbohydrates.

Source: Reprinted with permission from Mertig, R. G. (2011). *What nurses know . . . Diabetes.* New York, NY: Demos Health.

FIGURE 5.2 When to Monitor Glucose Levels, Why, and What to Do With the Results

Continuous Blood Glucose Monitors

Wouldn't it be nice to know what blood sugars were without sticking a finger? Well, we are not there yet, but three companies so far have products that come close. They provide real-time glucose values, glucose trend information via line and bar graphs, and customized early warning alarms to alert a person that their glucose levels are trending low or high so they can take action by eating (low) or giving more insulin (high) before they get into trouble. This is particularly important if clients' blood glucose levels drop at night while they sleep, or if they have hypoglycemia unawareness. People with type 1 and type 2 diabetes can use them with or without an insulin pump; however, using a continuous glucose monitor (CGM) with a pump makes more sense to me. Because insulin pumps usually have a great deal of memory, and can remind users how much insulin is still active from their last bolus dose based on parameters they have programmed into their pump, it can prevent them from giving more insulin if there is sufficient insulin on board to prevent the high trend from going higher. More information on insulin pumps is provided in Chapter 4.

Here is how these systems work. Continuous glucose monitoring systems (CGMSs) test interstitial glucose levels every 5 minutes or so, depending on the system. This continues for 72 hours or longer, at which time the sensor must be changed, and wirelessly transmits the information to a receiver (cell phone size or smaller) or an insulin pump that displays the results. (Because the CGMS transmits radio wave signals, it must be turned off when flying.) A disposable sensor is inserted via a needle, usually in the abdomen. The needle is removed, exposing a tiny wire that measures glucose levels in the interstitial fluid (around the cells). Because a wire is involved, it must be removed before undergoing an MRI (magnetic resonance imaging). Because the CGMS is not testing blood directly, there is a 15-minute lag time when the sugar in the blood is moving into this tissue fluid. A CGMS does not replace a glucose meter, because periodic finger sticks are needed to calibrate the system and verify a low or a high reading for accuracy (Garg et al., 2004). All CGMSs require a prescription and may or may not be covered by insurance. They are expensive and worth a call to the health insurance company to see what the requirements are. If an insurer covers a CGMS, it may require that a healthcare practitioner justify its use for this client. All CGMSs come with computer software so a user can download monitor and pump information in bar and line graphs to e-mail to their medical provider or print and bring with them to each office visit. This is very helpful for both to troubleshoot any problems, make any treatment adjustments, and evaluate how well a client is doing. Also a CGMS does not have to be used all the time.

CLINICAL EXAMPLE: I use mine when I am likely to have difficulty regulating my glucose levels, such as when I am on vacation, visiting friends or family, or any time I am not in charge of the food being served. I can fairly accurately count carbs (see my discussion of carbohydrate counting in Chapter 2), but this system gives me even more control over blood glucose levels. It warns me that I have given myself too much or too little insulin before I would get this information from my next manually monitored blood sugar. Simply checking blood glucose levels even several times a day just gives a snapshot of the ups and downs of blood sugars at that particular moment. Continuous monitoring provides the whole video throughout the day.

The companies that currently make CGMSs include the following:

1. Metronic MiniMed, maker of the *Paradigm REAL-Time* CGM, which transmits data to their Pardigm insulin pump and the *Paradigm Revel* pump with a built-in CGMS. The Revel is the first integrated system on the market to combine both a pump and a CGMS in one small gizmo the size of a cell phone. More information can be found at www.medtronic.com/your-health/diabetes/device/insulin-pumps/paradigm-real-time-system/index.htm
2. Abbott Laboratories makes the *FreeStyle Navigator* CGMS. It transmits data wirelessly to a receiver or an insulin pump. For further information visit www.diabetesselfmanagement.com/Blog/Tara-Dairman/freestyle_navigator_cgms_approved/
3. DexCom makes the *DexCom Seven Plus*, a CGMS that transmits data to a receiver. Learn more at www.dexcom.com/products/seven_difference
4. Insulet produces the *OmniPod* Personal Diabetes Manager, a disposable, tubeless insulin pump with a manual glucose meter that transmits insulin delivery instructions. For more information check out www.myomnipod.com. It can also be used with any available CGMS, such as the FreeStyle Navigator described in item 2.
5. Animas is the maker of *One Touch Ping*, their latest insulin pump. Currently it must be used with a manual glucose meter that communicates with this pump. Visit their website at www.animas.com/animas-insulin-pumps/onetouch-ping

The last two companies are both working with DexCom and its CGMS so their pumps can display and record data from the DexCom Seven Plus. Both should be FDA approved and available by the middle of 2011. In addition, DexCom and Insulet are in the process of developing an integrated pump/CGM OmniPod system in competition with the Metronic Revel. Metronic, on the other hand, is developing a disposable, tubeless pump like the OmniPod. Metronic also has a very sophisticated integrated system, the Veo that automatically suspends the flow of insulin when its CGMS detects hypoglycemia, an advantage for systems worn by children and individuals with hypoglycemia unawareness. So far Veo is available only in Europe, Canada, and Australia, but Metronic is testing it in the United States and may soon get approval from the FDA.

6. Debiotech has a new insulin pump, the *JewelPUMP*, which is the lightest and thinnest pump on the market today, yet it holds 450 units of insulin, is

disposable, and does not need to be changed for up to 6 days. It is controlled by a touch screen PDA. For more information visit www.jewelpumb.com.

7. Another innovation to make a diabetic's life easier is the *Cellnovo*, the smallest insulin pump so far. It consists of a waterproof, wireless touchscreen made by Cellnovo, which can deliver insulin, adjust bolus doses, monitor glucose, track activity, access a person's journal, check the nutritional information of foods, and so on (Stuart, 2010). www.cellnovo.com/products.aspx.

8. The *t:slim*, another new insulin pump, from Tandem Diabetes Care is thin, the size of a credit card and looks like a smartphone, but holds 300 units of insulin and features a USB-rechargeable power cell. It is not yet available in the United States, but more information can be found at www.tandemdiabetes.com/Concepts.

9. *Solo micropump* currently made by Roche Diabetes Care is small, light, and very discreet for a full-featured insulin pump. It was designed by Medingo in 2009 but bought by Roche in 2010. The company has a planned global launched in 2012. For more information on this product see www.diabetesincontrol.com/articles/newproduct/8187-new-product-the-solo-insulin-dispensing-patch.

10. For the techies among your clients, there are now free apps for recording, storing, analyzing information electronically and more using iPhone, iPod Touch, and iPad, unless otherwise noted, including the following:

   ■ AgaMatrix's app, *WaveSense*, lets you record blood glucose levels, insulin, and number of carbs eaten and view the results in graph or chart format. You can also watch videos on various diabetes topics. Check it out at http://itunes.apple.com/us/app/wavesense-diabetes-manager/id325292586?mt=8.

   ■ *Vree* is a newly launched app from Merck. It lets you record blood sugars, weight, food intake, blood pressure, and medications and graphs results to send to a healthcare provider. Visit http://itunes.apple.com/us/app/vree-for-diabetes/id355923059?mt=8 for more information.

   ■ *OnTrack*, an Android application, can be exported via e-mail to healthcare professionals. For more information visit www.andro-lib.com/android.applicatio.co-gexperts-ontrack- jnim.aspx.

   ■ *Lose It* is an app from iTunes by FitNow for tracking weight loss, after setting goals and daily calorie amounts. Foods and its calories can be found and recorded, as can any physical activity. More information can be seen at http://itunes.apple.com/us/app/lose-it/id297368629?mt=8.

   ■ Calorie Counter by *MyNetDiary* is another meal planning, weight loss app that also includes restaurant menus. For more information visit www.prweb.com/releases/2011/02/prweb5048094.htm.

   ■ An app that might appeal to children, developed by Roche Diagnostics' is the *Glucose Buddy* Iphone App. It can sync phone to an online account to manage data on their website at www.glucosebuddy.com.

   ■ An app from Life Med Media is compatible with the iPhone (OS 3.0 or later), iPod Touch, and iPad. At the iTunes store you can buy and download Diabetes Companion by dLife to track blood sugar, find diabetes-friendly recipes, watch videos from dLifeTV, and get answers to your diabetes questions, all for 0.99. For more information visit www.dlife.com/dlife_media/mobile.

WHAT IS ON THE HORIZON FOR FUTURE GLYCEMIC CONTROL?

New meters are constantly being developed to appeal to a variety of users using traditional and nontraditional sites, and some are even noninvasive. Several of the listed glucose monitoring devices below may need a prescription, and some may still be in clinical trials or awaiting FDA approval for use in the United States. Follow their development using the Web links provided below.

■ Bayer's new *Didget* glucose meter plugs into a Nintendo DS or DS lite game player, which may make this a good choice for children. They even get points for regular recording and keeping blood sugars within preset targets. They also get points for use of the meter in a game, Knock 'Em Down World's Fair, included with the meter. For more information visit the website www.bayerdidget.com/Home.

■ A meter the size of a USB, *iBGStar*, has been developed by Sanofi-Aventis and AgaMatrix. It uses the screen of an iPhone or iPod touch when plugged into either device, which can be used as a log or to view trends and analyze data using the Diabetes Manager app. It is not yet available in the United States or Canada, but more information can be retrieved from www.ibgstar.com/web/ibgstar.

■ *Jazz Wireless* glucose meter from Agamatrix wirelessly transmits blood glucose data from meter to computer using Bluetooth technology. For more information click on www.sinovo.net/Agamatrix-Wavesense-Jazz-Wireless-1473.asp

■ Glucose monitoring technologies in development include some non–finger stick devices, including the *nano ink tattoos* that use reactive dyes and fluorescent beads that change color based on glucose changes in the interstitial fluid under the skin (http://socialhype.com/lifestyle/938-nano-ink-tattoo-that-monitors-diabetes.html) and *soft contact lenses* that change color to show when glucose levels are going too high or too low (http://communications.uwo.ca/com/western_news/stories/nano-composites_could_change_diabetes_treatment_20091216445482).

■ There are also other noninvasive monitors, such as the *GlucoWatch* meter with membranes on the underside that use small electric currents to draw interstitial fluid through the skin and monitor blood glucose values that way (http://my-blood-glucose-meter.com/what-is-a-wrist-watch-blood-glucose-meter).

■ Calisto Medical produces the *Glucoband* glucose monitor, a wristwatch device that uses proprietary technology to noninvasively measure blood glucose levels in the body. It uses a bio-electromagnetic resonance technique to continuously monitor glucose levels after an initial measurement, with the results viewable on an integrated LCD screen in the watch (www.engadget.com/2005/06/13/glucoband-wristwatch-continuously-monitors-your-glucose-levels).

■ *GlucoTrack*, a noninvasive glucose monitor due for release in 2011, manufactured by Integrity Applications Ltd, an Israeli company, uses ultrasonic, conductivity, and heat capacity combined technologies (www.integrity-app.com).

Diabetes and diabetes management have become big business due to the ever increasing numbers of people with diabetes. More and diverse companies are inventing new gadgets and vying for the diabetes community's business. In the future, look for new insulin pumps, CGMS, and systems integrating the two, as well as other diabetes-related paraphernalia. Competition among companies should also make this equipment less expensive.

The most important value of any glucose monitoring device is its impact on diabetes management. Obviously the more data a client has, the better he or she can analyze the information and make appropriate corrections, which should result in greater glucose control, lower A1c percentage, and prevention of both acute and chronic complications. The better the blood sugar control, the more options a client has and the more normal and fulfilling life can be. Control of blood sugars by whatever means necessary and available can leave a person free to enjoy life to the fullest. That should be the goal and the mantra of all diagnosed with diabetes, as well as the nurses and healthcare practitioners who serve them.

REFERENCES

American Diabetes Association. (2003). *Insulin therapy in the 21st century.* Alexandria, VA: Author.

American Diabetes Association. (2011). Standards of medical care in diabetes—2011. *Diabetes Care, 34,* S11–S61.

Donga, E., van Dijk, M., van Dijk, J. G., Biermasz, N. R., Lammers, G.-J., van Kralingen, K., . . . Romijn, J. A. (2010, March 31). Partial sleep restriction decreases insulin sensitivity in type 1 diabetes. *Diabetes Care, 33.* Retrieved April 5, 2010, from www.care.diabetesjournals.org/content/early/2010/03/24/dc09-2317.full.pdf+html

Garg, S., Schwartz, S., & Edelman, S. (2004). Improved glucose excursions using an implantable real-time continuous glucose sensor in adults with type 1 diabetes. *Diabetes Care, 27,* 734–738.

Scheiner, G. (2004). *Think like a pancreas.* New York, NY: Marlowe & Company.

Scheiner, G. (2011, January/February). Strike the spike II: Dealing with high blood glucose after meals. *Diabetes Self-Management.*

Stuart, M. (2010, December). Cellnovo's mobile health approach to diabetes care. *In Vivo: The Business & Medicine Report,* pp. 40–44.

Zhang, L., Curham, G. C., Hu, F. B., Rimm, E. B., & Forman, J. P. (2011). Association between passive and active smoking and incident type 2 diabetes in women. *Diabetes Care, 34*(2). Retrieved April 4, 2011, from http://care.diabetesjournals.org/content/early/2011/02/25/dc10-2087

SIX

Chronic Complications

When one door closes, another opens; but often we look so long at the closed door that we do not see the one which has opened for us.
    —Helen Keller

Most of my previous chapters have emphasized the positive aspects of diabetes self-management and, I hope, will be empowering to you and your clients. Understanding chronic complications, however, is helpful in picking up the early signs and symptoms. Here are some statistics from the Centers for Disease Control and Prevention (CDC) 2011 National Diabetes Fact Sheet that you and your clients might need to understand.

- Adults with diabetes have heart disease death rates two to four times higher than adults without diabetes.
- The risk of stroke is two to four times higher among people with diabetes.
- Of adults with diabetes, 67% have hypertension.
- Diabetes is the leading cause of new cases of blindness among adults aged 20 to 74.
- Diabetes is the leading cause of kidney failure and accounted for 44% of all new cases of kidney failure in 2008.
- About 60% to 70% of people with diabetes have mild to severe forms of nervous system damage. The results of such damage include impaired sensation or pain in the feet or hands, slowed digestion of food in the stomach, carpal tunnel syndrome, erectile dysfunction, or other neurologic problems.
- More than 60% of nontraumatic lower-limb amputations occur in people with diabetes.
- Young adults with diabetes have twice the risk of developing gum disease as those without diabetes.
- People with diabetes are more susceptible to many other illnesses and, once they acquire these illnesses, such as pneumonia or influenza, are more likely to have a worse prognosis than those without diabetes.

It is very important for healthcare practitioners to know something about each of the major complication; the signs and symptoms of each to alert clients so they can get help immediately; and, more importantly, how they can prevent, delay, or treat each condition.

In Chapters 2 through 5, I described in detail how to live with diabetes so clients can feel well and live the life they want to live. Whether it is type 1 or type 2 diabetes that they have been diagnosed with, they probably do not feel bad as long as their blood glucose stays under 250 mg/dl or above 60 mg/dl. However, it is important to point out to them that living with a blood sugar between 200 and 250 mg/dl or higher most of the time can and does cause damage to glucose-sensitive organs, even if they don't feel bad. Having a hemoglobin A1c of 7% means that the estimated average blood glucose over the past 2 to 3 months is 154 mg/dl, an acceptable number, considering the fact that some blood sugars were lower and some higher. However, an A1c of 8% equals an average of 183 mg/dl, an A1c of 9% means 212 mg/dl, and an A1c of 10% equals 240 mg/dl. The good news is that a blood glucose level under 250 mg/dl does not usually make a person sleepy or lethargic, but the bad news is that an A1c over 8% indicates fair to poor blood sugar control (see Chapter 5) and eventually causes organ damage. It may take 20 years, but unless clients were 70 years of age when they were diagnosed, the high blood sugars ought to be of concern to them. They need to be motivated to get as close to an A1c of 7% or below as soon as possible and do whatever it takes to keep it there.

The glucose-sensitive organs I keep talking about include the heart and all blood vessels, the brain, eyes, kidneys, nerves, skin, feet, gums, stomach and intestines, and the immune system. High blood glucose levels are like a poison to most if not all body systems and organs. This chapter will hit the high points of most complications in terms of prevention, symptoms, diagnosis, and treatment. Please remember that prevention and/or delay of complications is a life-long goal of diabetes self-management, but it never motivated me to do what I needed to do on an hourly and daily basis. I work hard at controlling blood sugars so I can feel good today, right now, and live the kind of life I would want to live if I did not have diabetes. Hopefully warning clients of the dire consequences of not caring for their diabetes will not be necessary and should never be used as a threat. With all the medications and gizmos we have today to help normalize blood glucose levels, all that is needed is the willpower to make it happen.

Having said that, know that bad things can happened to good people. This is why emphasizing the prevention of complications should *not* be your first-line plan in teaching diabetes self-management. The purpose of teaching about complications is so that people with diabetes can catch a complication as early as possible. This is what everyone connected with diabetes management should be looking for. Besides my endocrinologist, who is concerned with my diabetes and hypertension, I also see an ophthalmologist who specializes in diseases of the retina, a periodontal dentist who checks for gum disease, and a podiatrist who cuts my toenails and checks my feet for calluses at least once a year or more often. Diabetes is an expensive disease, but nothing takes the place of testing blood sugar levels as often as needed and correcting them when needed to live a long and healthy life.

If you or your clients do any research on the Web for more information, please remember and advise clients to put the current year after the search terms. This will put the most current information first. There is a lot of old outdated material out there.

Diabetes greatly increases the occurrence of macrovascular (large blood vessel) disease, including coronary heart disease, stroke, and peripheral artery disease and microvascular (small blood vessel) disease, including retinopathy, nephropathy, and neuropathy.

HEART AND BLOOD VESSEL DISEASE

Heart disease is the number one killer of adults in the United States, with or without diabetes. Cardiovascular complications will affect 75% to 80% of people with diabetes (Saudek & Margolis, 2011). These complications include atherosclerosis (fatty deposits in arteries), heart attack, hypertension, stroke, and peripheral arterial disease that can lead to decreased circulation of the feet and, potentially, an amputation. The good news is that *none* of this is inevitable, even if a person does have diabetes. Risk factors for CVD include a family history of CVD; smoking; uncontrolled high cholesterol, especially high LDL (the "bad" cholesterol), low HDL (the "good" cholesterol), and high triglycerides; and uncontrolled high blood pressure and high blood sugar.

Coronary Heart Disease

The main reason heart disease, especially a heart attack, can often prove deadly is that men and women do not take symptoms seriously. The following are possible symptoms that should never be ignored:

- Anxiety or intense fear of impending doom, such as feeling like fainting or not being able to catch your breath.
- Chest discomfort or intense pressure, like an elephant sitting on your chest or a squeezing or burning sensation. It does not have to feel like pain.
- A cough that is persistent or wheezing, which can be a sign of heart failure, when the heart is having difficulty pumping out blood to the body and fluid backs up into the lungs.
- Dizziness or lightheadedness and even loss of consciousness from a heart attack or a dangerous heart rhythm.
- Fatigue that is not typical, especially in women.

- Nausea or unusual lack of appetite. During a heart attack, some people actually vomit. Because the heart is having difficulty pumping blood to the body, blood is not going to the stomach, so it cannot digest whatever food is in there.
- Referred pain to other parts of the body, such as the jaw, shoulders, arms, back, neck, or abdomen. Men more often feel pain in the left arm or jaw, whereas women may experience pain in both arms or between the shoulder blades in the upper back.
- Rapid or irregular pulse, especially if accompanied by weakness, dizziness, or shortness of breath, which can mean a heart attack, heart failure, or an arrhythmia.
- Shortness of breath, especially with any of the preceding symptoms, which can mean a heart attack or heart failure.
- Sweating, especially a cold sweat for no good reason, which could be caused by a heart attack.
- Edema, which can mean that heart failure is causing accumulated fluid, often in the feet, ankles, legs, or abdomen, as well as sudden weight gain from retained fluid.
- Weakness, often severe and unexplained, which can precede and accompany a heart attack.

Obviously any of these symptoms can be of no consequence on their own, but that should be diagnosed by medical personnel. Tell your clients to be sure to call 911 if they experience any of these symptoms. Sometimes a person can have a silent heart attack, with no symptoms at all. An ECG, called an EKG by some, can document that one has occurred. Healthcare providers should discuss with such clients options to increase heart-healthy activities to prevent a second heart attack in the future.

CLINICAL EXAMPLE: Clients with heart disease should be advised to avoid holding their breath while having a stool. This is called a *Valsalva maneuver* and is performed by forcible exhalation against a closed airway, usually done by taking a deep breath and holding it while pushing down with the abdominal muscles. This action increases thoracic pressure, making it harder for the heart to pump blood. It also increases overall blood pressure. If constipation is a problem, they can get an over-the-counter stool softener, eat more fiber-rich foods, such as fresh fruits and vegetables, and drink more water. If someone does have to strain, he or she should let some air out slowly, as in hissing, and make this partial breath holding brief.

If a client has angina, it means that they have a coronary artery (or arteries) that is (are) partially blocked, enough to restrict the flow of blood to the heart muscle. Advise a client to get a prescription for nitroglycerin tablets, which should be carried in a moisture-proof, opaque container, and put a tablet under the tongue when chest pain is felt. The tablet will be absorbed very quickly by the blood vessels there. Swallowing these pills will prolong the absorption for 30 to 60 minutes, way too long to prevent worsening consequences. If this happens often, clients can get a prescription for a longer acting nitrate that is taken two or more times a day to keep cardiac vessels open all day, or a nitro-paste or gel patch that is taped to the body during the day. Beta-blocker drugs, which reduce the effects of stress hormones on the heart, can also be used on a regular basis to prevent angina. Calcium-channel blockers can reduce the oxygen needs of the heart muscle by lowering heart rate and reducing the forcefulness of each heartbeat. A newer drug, Ranexa (ranolazine), a fatty acid oxidation inhibitor, gets the heart muscle to switch from burning fatty acids to using glucose for energy. Glucose metabolism requires less oxygen so the heart can pump longer during exercise before symptoms of angina occur (Bennett et al., 2011). Ranexa has even been shown to lower A1c in clients with coronary artery disease and diabetes (Ning et al., 2011). There are other drugs on the horizon in this medication class. Specific cardiac aerobic exercise training can also build up collateral circulation around the partial blockage and can provide improved oxygen delivery to the affected part of the cardiac muscle.

Invasive and surgical procedures for treating angina and preventing a heart attack include angioplasty. With or without a stent (mesh tubing) being placed, and coronary artery bypass surgery. Angioplasty involves a balloon-tipped catheter that is threaded to the site of the narrowed or blocked cardiac artery. The balloon is then inflated to crush the fatty plaque causing the blockage. Often a stent is left behind to hold the artery open. Coronary artery bypass surgery is open-heart surgery done under general anesthesia that requires a hospital stay and weeks to months of rehabilitation, depending on the patient's physical condition prior to surgery and the extent of the surgical procedure. Usually a vein from the leg or an artery from the chest wall is sewn in place before and after the blockage, thus carrying blood around the blockage and bypassing it. No matter what treatment for angina is used, the causes of the blocked cardiac artery or arteries must be addressed to prevent a new blockage from forming. Control over cholesterol, blood pressure, and blood sugar, as well as weight loss and an increase in activity level, are essential elements for the treatment of heart disease. It goes without saying that quitting smoking and/or avoiding inhaled second-hand smoke will improve anyone's ability to survive heart disease.

CLINICAL EXAMPLE: Teach clients to call 911 and chew four 81 mg aspirin uncoated tablets or one 325 mg uncoated tablet, as long as they are not allergic to aspirin, if they think they are having a heart attack. They should also sit or lie down close to the outside door so they can be found easily by the emergency personnel, note the time by pulling out the stem on their watch to stop it or by telling the 911 operator when the symptoms started. If a clot-busting drug or a tissue plasminogen activator is to be used, timing is important. They should try to take deep breaths and stay as calm as possible to increase the blood supply available to the heart muscle. Preventing further heart damage will minimize the possibility that a client will develop heart failure.

Sleep Apnea

Clients should be questioned about *sleep apnea*, a condition in which breathing is interrupted repeatedly during sleep, which can damage both the heart and the brain. It is associated with a higher risk of hypertension, heart failure, and stroke. Often people who have sleep apnea snore, may gasp and choke at night, frequently wake up exhausted because sleep was not restful, may experience headaches from brain cells repeatedly deprived of oxygen, and may have chest pain from periodic decreases in oxygenation, increased heart rate, and constricted blood vessels from an adrenaline surge that occurs when apnea is taking place. Losing weight, avoiding alcohol and sedatives before going to bed (because these relax throat muscles), quitting smoking, and controlling of blood pressure and blood sugar all help to prevent these nightly attacks. If more intense help is needed, or if sleep apnea is severe, a continuous positive airway pressure (CPAP) machine can help. This small apparatus pressurizes air and blows it through a small tube attached to a mask worn at night to keep the airway open and prevent any apneic spells (Mayo Clinic Staff, n.d.).

Atherosclerosis

Cholesterol is needed by the body for healthy nerve function and to make certain hormones and bile salts, and it is the precursor to vitamin D. Every cell membrane in the body contains cholesterol. Cholesterol also functions as a powerful antioxidant, thus protecting the body against cancer and aging. The liver produces cholesterol to meet the body's needs; however, diet and/or familial predisposition can cause cholesterol, particularly the unhealthy LDL cholesterol, to become excessive. High cholesterol levels can be brought under control by decreasing saturated and *trans*-fats in the diet and eating a diet that includes high-fiber foods and foods rich in mono-unsaturated fats and omega-3 fatty acids (see Chapter 2). Keeping blood glucose levels as close to normal as possible also helps (see Chapter 5). In addition, physical activity aids in ridding the body of cholesterol and unhealthy fatty acids to prevent plaque from building up in artery walls.

Cholesterol is a soft, waxy, blood lipid (fat). LDLs can form a fatty deposit (plaque) on the inside of artery walls that often leads to an obstruction in blood flow, causing a heart attack or stroke. HDLs, on the other hand, carry the excess cholesterol out of the body and remove the plaque deposits from arteries, so the higher the HDLs the better. In addition to the measures described earlier, teach clients ways to control stress by deep breathing, putting everything in proper perspective, getting enough sleep, and finding things to laugh about every day. You and they can use a stress ball, or go for a walk (even if only in the hall or up and down the stairs). Talking to someone or journaling about the causes of stress is also useful. According to the American Diabetes Association (ADA, 2011), the cholesterol numbers in Table 6.1 are what you should help your clients aim for.

Everyone who smokes should quit, and anyone who is overweight should lose weight or maintain a healthy weight for their body type (get rid of fat around the waist). If these healthy lifestyle changes do not bring cholesterol numbers under control, medication can be prescribed (Table 6.2). The "statin" drugs are frequently advertised on TV. They are currently the most common drugs used to decrease cholesterol levels. Other medications can also be prescribed, especially if elevated triglycerides and/or low HDLs are a problem. Because they all work differently, more than one classification of drugs can be prescribed to achieve the values listed above.

If triglyceride levels are normal, moderate use of alcoholic beverages can increase HDL and lower LDL. Remember that *moderate* drinking means no more than one drink for women or two drinks for men per day. If a client does not drink, he or she should not start now. Alcohol also raises triglycerides, which may make this plan counterproductive.

Hypertension

High blood pressure is another health concern that can lead to heart disease, stroke, and peripheral artery problems. It also damages the eyes and kidneys. Risk factors for high blood pressure include a family history, membership in certain ethnic groups (African Americans and Native Americans), age (the older we are the greater the risk), and gender (men have a greater risk until age 44; women catch up between age 45 and 54 and then surpass men at age 55 and beyond). These are the risk factors over which we have no control (American Heart Association, n.d.).

TABLE 6.1
Cholesterol Ranges

	ALL ADULTS WITH DIABETES	ADULTS AT HIGH RISK FOR HEART DISEASE
Total cholesterol	<200 mg/dl	<160 mg/dl
LDL ("bad" cholesterol)	<100 mg/dl	<70 mg/dl
HDL ("good" cholesterol)	>40 mg/dl for men >50 mg/dl for women	>60 mg/dl for men and women
Triglycerides	<150 mg/dl	<100 mg/dl

Source: Reprinted with permission from Mertig, R. G. (2011). *What nurses know . . . Diabetes*. New York, NY: Demos Health.
Note: mg = milligrams; dL = deciliters.

TABLE 6.2
Cholesterol-lowering Medication (generic names in parentheses)

CLASSIFICATION	MEDICATION	FUNCTION	SIDE EFFECTS
Statins	Crestor (rosuvastatin) Lescol (fluvastatin) Lipitor (atorvastatin) Mevacor (lovastatin) Prevachol (pravastatin) Zocor (simvastatin)	Blocks the enzyme the liver needs to produce cholesterol, helps lower LDL cholesterol and raise HDL	Increased liver enzymes, headache, muscle aches, abdominal pain, nausea weakness
Fibrates	Lopid (gemfibrate) Tricor (fenofibrate) Trilipix (fenofibrate)	Lowers cholesterol and triglycerides	Fever, nausea, vomiting, weakness
Bile acid-binding resins	Colestid (colestipol) Prevalite (cholestyramine) Questran (cholestyramine) Welchol (colesevelam)	Binds with bile acids in gut and lowers total and LDL cholesterol and triglycerides	Constipation, diarrhea, flatulence, bad taste in the mouth
HMG-CoA reductase inhibitor	Zetia (ezetimibe)	Reduces the absorption of cholesterol or other sterols from the gut	Abdominal pain, back pain, diarrhea, joint pain, sinusitis
High-dose niacin, vitamin B_3, or nicotonic acid	Endur-Acin Niacin SR Niacor Niaspan ER Nicotinex Slo-Niacin	Blocks the breakdown of fats to decrease VLDL and cholesterol and increase HDL	Flushing, rash, itching, nausea, vomiting, gas, increased blood pressure
Omega-3-acid ethyl esters	Lovaza (EPA + DHA or high-dose fish oil)	Decreased triglycerides made in liver	Burping, heartburn, nausea, back pain, rash
Combinations	Advicor (lovastatin + niacin) Pravigard (pravastatin + buffered aspirin) Simcor (simvastatin + niacin) Vytorin (ezetimibe + simvastatin)	See above	See above

Source: Reprinted with permission from Mertig, R. G. (2011). *What nurses know . . . Diabetes*. New York, NY: Demos Health.
Note: HMG-CoA = 3-hydroxy-3-methylglutaryl-coenzyme A; VLDL = very low-density lipoprotein; EPA = eicosapentaenoic acid; DHA = docosahexaenoic acid.

An unhealthy, high-salt diet, obesity, and high stress levels are the factors that we can control. Clients with diabetes are at high risk for hypertension and often develop hypertension at an earlier age than their brothers and sisters without diabetes. A diet high in saturated and *trans*-fats causes narrowing of arteries from plaque, which increases blood pressure. A high sodium intake causes kidneys to hold onto fluid, which increases the pressure on arterial walls. As if that were not bad enough, increased stress hormones cause further constriction of arteries made stiff with fatty plaque. Dietary changes can have a huge impact on blood pressure (see Chapter 2). The DASH Diet (Dietary Approach to Stop Hypertension) consists of low-sodium, high-potassium fruits, vegetables, and whole-grain foods. Wise food guidelines include the following:

1. Eat fresh fruits at each meal.
2. Eat one or two servings of vegetables at lunch and dinner.
3. Switch to low-fat or fat-free dairy products.
4. Eat whole-grain breads and cereals.
5. Eat one-fourth cup of nuts or two tablespoons of a nut butter most days.
6. Choose lean meats (skinless chicken or turkey, lean beef, fish, boiled ham, pork tenderloin).
7. Cook using low-fat methods (baking, roasting, broiling—no butter, grilling, microwaving, steaming).
8. Add little to no salt at the table or during cooking.
9. Try herbs, herb blends, light salt, salt substitutes, and spices instead of salt.
10. Read food labels and choose foods with less than 400 mg of sodium per serving (ADA, n. d.).

Physical activity can also help to lower blood pressure. Three or four 10-minute walks per day can relieve stress, relax blood vessels, and help with weight management or loss. If a client smokes, he or she should quit and avoid inhaling second-hand smoke. Nicotine constricts arteries and thus raises blood pressure. Also, excessive (more than one or two drinks per day) alcohol intake can increase blood pressure. The ADA and the NIH recommend a target blood pressure of less than 130/80 (ADA, n. d.). In Table 6.3 please note the *and*, meaning both numbers are needed to be

TABLE 6.3
Blood Pressure Ranges

	SYSTOLIC		DIASTOLIC
Ideal normal	<120	and	<80
Prehypertension	120–139	or	80–89
Hypertension stage 1	140–159	or	90–99
Hypertension stage 2	160 or higher	or	100 or higher

Source: Reprinted with permission from Mertig, R. G. (2011). *What nurses know . . . Diabetes.* New York, NY: Demos Health.

considered ideal. The *or* means that either number is considered abnormal and in need of lowering using all means possible, including medication.

CLINICAL EXAMPLE: If a person's blood pressure goes up at the doctor's office, it could be due to "white coat hypertension." Have the nurse repeat the reading at the end of the visit. If you are taking a client's blood pressure remember the following: Tell the client not to smoke, exercise, or consume anything with caffeine for at least 30 minutes before getting blood pressure taken. To get an accurate blood pressure a person should sit quietly for at least 5 minutes, with feet on the floor and the arm flexed at the elbow, relaxed, and at the level of the heart (rest arm on a desk or table). Check both arms and, if there is a difference, record the higher pressure (ADA, 2011).

Again, when lifestyle changes are not enough, there is always medication. Often more than one type of blood pressure medication may be needed. Table 6.4 provides a list of the many antihypertensive medications under each classification, with a brief description of how they lower blood pressure, and their side effects:

TABLE 6.4
Antihypertensive Medications (generic names in parentheses)

CLASSIFICATION	MEDICATION	FUNCTION	SIDE EFFECTS
ACE inhibitors	Accupril (quinapril) Altace (ramipril) Capoten (captopril) Coversyl, Aceon (perindopril) Gopten (trandolapril) Lotensin (benazepril) Monopril (fosinopril) Prinivil (lisinopril) Vasotec (enalapril) Zestril (lisinopril)	Inhibits the enzyme that converts angiotensin I to angiotensin II, a strong blood vessel constrictor. Keeps blood vessels dilated to lower blood pressure.	Cough, increased blood potassium, dizziness, headache, rash, metallic taste, weakness
ARBs	Atacand (candesartan) Avalide (irbesartan) Benicar (olmesartan) Cozaar (losartan) Diovan (valsartan) Micardis (telmisartan) Teveten (eprosartan)	Blocks the angiotensin II receptors on blood vessels so they do not constrict.	Dizziness, hypotension, high blood potassium, headache, diarrhea, metallic taste

CLASSIFICATION	MEDICATION	FUNCTION	SIDE EFFECTS
Beta-blockers	Corgard (nadolol) Inderal (propranolol) Levatol (penbutolol) Lopressor (metoprolol) Normodyne (labetalol) Prent (acebutolol) Sectral (acebutolol) Tenormin (atenolol) Timolide (timolol) Toprol XL (metoprolol) Visken (pindolol) Zebeta (bisoprolol)	Blocks beta-receptors on blood vessels so stress hormones cannot cause them to constrict.	Diarrhea, stomach cramps, rash, nausea, vomiting, muscle cramps, headache, depression. May mask symptoms of hypoglycemia
Calcium channel blockers	Adalat (nifedipine) Procardia (nifedipine) Calan (verapamil) Cardene, Cardene SR (nicardipine) Cardizem (diltiazem) Dilacor XR (diltiazem) Nimotop (nimodipine) Norvasc (amlodipine) Plendil (felodipine)	Slows the movement of calcium into the cells of the heart and blood vessel walls, which makes it easier for the heart to pump, and widens blood vessels.	Constipation, nausea, rash, headache, edema, hypotension, drowsiness, dizziness
Diuretics	Hydrodiuril (hydrochlorothiazide) Bumex (bumetanide) Lasix (furosemide)	Makes kidneys excrete more water in the urine, thus decreasing blood pressure.	Fatigue, thirst, weakness, muscle cramps, hypotension
Alpha-blockers	Cardura (doxazosin) Flomax (tamsulosin) Hytrin (terazosin) Minipress (prazosin) Uroxatral (alfuzosin)	Keeps the hormone norepinephrine (noradrenaline) from constricting the muscles in the walls of smaller arteries and veins causing vessels to remain open and relaxed.	Headache, pounding heartbeat, nausea, weakness, weight gain and small decreases in LDL cholesterol. Also used for benign prostatic hypertrophy (BPH)

Source: Reprinted with permission from Mertig, R. G. (2011). *What nurses know . . . Diabetes*. New York, NY: Demos Health.
Note: ACE = angiotensin-converting enzyme; ARB = angiotensin receptor blocker.

If you look at the generic names of the various antihypertensives in this table, you will notice that ACE inhibitors all end in *-pril*, ARBs end in *-sartan*, beta-blockers end in *-lol*, most calcium channel blockers end in *-dipine*, diuretics end in *-ide*, and most alpha-blockers end with *-zosin*. This is an easy way to keep track of what kind of blood pressure medication your clients are taking.

CLINICAL EXAMPLE: Teach clients to understand that hypertension is often called the "silent killer." Unless it rises rapidly, it usually does not have any symptoms until the damage to organs is already underway. If, however, a person suddenly develops any of the following symptoms, consider this an emergency and he or she should seek help immediately:

- Feeling confused or other neurological symptoms
- Nosebleeds
- Fatigue
- Blurred vision
- Chest pain
- Abnormal heartbeat

Of course, these symptoms could be caused by something else other than hypertension, but none of these symptoms should be ignored.

Anyone diagnosed with hypertension should know to avoid oral decongestant medications. They will raise blood pressure whether or not a person is taking an antihypertensive medication. The higher the blood pressure, the harder the heart has to pump to get blood out to the body. If the heart cannot get enough blood to oxygenate the kidneys, the kidneys will produce renin, an enzyme that converts angiotensin I to angiotensin II, a potent vasoconstrictor, causing constriction of blood vessels and raising blood pressure even higher. Renin also sends the false message to the hypothalamus that the body is dehydrated because the kidneys are not being supplied with adequate blood supply. This stimulates secretion of the antidiuretic hormone (ADH) from the pituitary gland, causing the kidneys to decrease urine output. (ADH is made in the hypothalamus and released from the posterior pituitary gland.) This, in turn, also increases blood volume, which increases blood pressure even more.

Stroke (or Brain Attack)

There are two kinds of strokes. The rarer and more fatal kind is a *hemorrhagic stroke* in which a cerebral blood vessel ruptures. Unless the aneurysm or other vessel malformation is discovered early and removed or stented, this is not something anyone can usually prevent. The much more common stroke, an *ischemic stroke*, is caused by a buildup of fatty plaque in the carotid arteries (one on each side of the neck), the main vessels that supply blood to the brain or one or more of the smaller cerebral arteries. When these vessels get blocked or their lumen significantly decreases the blood supply to a part of the brain, a *brain attack* occurs, like a heart attack. The part of the brain without a good blood supply begins to die, as does the heart muscle in a heart attack.

Warning signs of a stroke include brief lapses in brain function, such as confusion, visual disturbances, and difficulties in walking and talking, often called a *transient ischemic attack* (TIA). Symptoms of a stroke depend on which side and which area of the brain is affected. The National Institute of Neurological Disorders and Stroke (n.d.) list the following symptoms of stroke:

- Sudden numbness or weakness of the face, arm, or leg (especially on one side of the body)
- Sudden confusion, trouble speaking or understanding speech
- Sudden trouble seeing in one or both eyes
- Sudden trouble walking, dizziness, loss of balance, or coordination
- Sudden severe headache with no known cause

The narrowing or blockage of arteries in the brain can be seen using a CT scan or an MRI. If a clot is present, "clot-busting" drugs must be given within hours of a stroke, therefore, calling 911 is imperative. Other treatment options include a carotid endarterectomy to remove the fatty plaque buildup, thus restoring blood flow to the brain if this is the problem. Another surgical procedure, a carotid stenting, consists of a tube that is inserted into the blocked or narrowed brain artery. A balloon is then inflated, breaking up the plaque, and a stent, or mesh tube, is left in place. Treatment after a stroke may include rehabilitation therapies to restore function and/or help clients learn new ways of using the parts of the body weakened by the stroke. Therapies may include physical, occupational, and/or speech rehabilitation, as well as psychological counseling. Prevention of future attacks include quitting smoking; avoiding inhaled secondhand smoke; and controlling blood sugar, blood pressure, and cholesterol with healthy meal planning, physical activity, and medication.

Peripheral Arterial Disease

Another area of blood vessel concern includes the arteries of the legs and feet (the ones farthest from the heart). The healthcare provider should be checking the pedal pulses on the top of feet and tibial pulses behind the inner ankle bone.

CLINICAL EXAMPLE: One way for a client to check circulation is to press on the skin over the bone on top of the foot. It should blanch, and the color should return quickly, within 3 seconds, when the finger or thumb is removed. If toenails look healthy and hair is present on toes, tops of the feet, and lower legs, circulation to the feet is probably good. Hair and nails are the first to be deprived of blood supply when circulation diminishes. Since my diagnosis with diabetes, I love looking at my hairy toes and never put polish on my toenails so I can check their color and circulation. Of course, if clients have never had hair on their toes, they should be taught to use the pressing of the skin on the upper feet technique to assess circulation.

Another indication of arterial narrowing in the legs is *intermittent claudication* (cramping) of the calves, thighs, and even buttocks. This pain occurs when walking or exercising the legs and is promptly relieved by stopping the activity. Because the exercised muscle cannot get enough blood supply, it cramps and causes pain that is similar to the angina pain of narrowed coronary arteries.

CLINICAL EXAMPLE: Clients can be taught ways to increase blood supply to the leg muscles, including carrying a cane with a seat while walking until leg pain occurs. Then they should sit until the pain goes away, usually a few minutes, followed by walking some more. Doing this a few times during a walk will help to develop collateral circulation around the blocked or narrowed artery in affected leg muscles. As time goes on, the client should be able to walk farther and farther before pain occurs. This can also be done using a treadmill. In addition, strength training exercises for calf and thigh muscles can also increase collateral circulation.

Medication used to increase circulation to partially blocked arteries of the legs include:

- Pletal (cilostazol), which dilates the arteries supplying blood to the legs and prevents platelets from sticking together and to the plaque narrowing the artery so a clot will not completely block the artery.
- Trental (pentoxifylline), which thins the blood and makes red cells more flexible so they can maneuver around narrowed arteries.
- Plavix (clopidogrel), which helps prevent harmful blood clots that may cause heart attacks or strokes. Peripheral arterial disease increases the risk for heart attacks and strokes.

Surgical correction for intermittent claudication consists of the following options:

1. Percutaneous transluminal angioplasty, in which a catheter with a balloon tip is inserted into the artery. The balloon is inflated to crush the fatty plaque and dilate the blocked artery. Sometimes a stent (thin

wire mesh sleeve) can be inserted to keep the vessel opened. This stent may be coated with an anticoagulating medication to prevent clots from forming in the future.

2. Surgical bypass of the blocked artery can be done using one of a person's own veins or a synthetic Dacron graft, which is attached above and below the blockage. This allows blood to flow around the blocked area, much the same way that coronary artery bypass surgery is done for coronary artery disease.

Poor circulation is also a byproduct of nicotine intake, so if your client smokes, he or she must *stop* and avoid breathing in second-hand smoke.

CLINICAL EXAMPLE: As a nurse, the worst case of circulatory deficits in the feet and legs I ever saw was in a 60-year-old client who smoked and did *not* have diabetes. She eventually lost both legs and died of infection and lack of wound healing. During all of her many admissions for surgery she refused to stop smoking, even though she knew that it would soon kill her.

Prevention for all CVDs is the same. Clients with diabetes must be taught to follow the ABCs:

A1c less than 7%
Blood pressure below 130/80
Cholesterol < 200 mg/dl, LDL <100 mg/dl (better yet, <70 mg/dl), HDL > 40 mg/dl for men and > 50 mg/dl for women (better > 60 mg/dl for everyone), triglycerides < 150 mg/dl (better < 100 mg/dl)

Clients should talk to their medical practitioner about taking an enteric-coated baby aspirin (81 mg) each day to prevent platelets from sticking to plaque in the arteries and forming a clot (ADA, 2011). The enteric coating helps to protect the stomach lining because this preparation does not dissolve until it gets to the alkaline fluids of the small intestine. Recent studies have shown that "aspirin significantly reduced cardiovascular heart disease events in men but not in women. Conversely, aspirin had no effect on stroke in men but significantly reduced stroke in women" (ADA, 2011, pp. S11–S61).

Because type 2 diabetes is a risk factor for heart disease, which oral anti-diabetic medications are better than others at protecting the heart and blood vessels? A recent study done in Denmark reviewed the records of patients with diabetes controlled by a single agent over a 20-year period looking at cardiovascular mortality associated with secretagogues and metformin. The results were published in the *European Heart Journal* online April 6, 2011. Metformin, gliclazide (not sold in the United States), and repaglinide (Prandin) appear to be associated with a lower risk of cardiovascular events when compared with glimepiride (Amaryl), glibenclamide (glyburide in the United States), glipizide (Glucotrol), and tolbutamide. Today metformin is a first-line drug in the treatment of type 2 diabetes and apparently does not cause an increase in cardiovascular complications in this population (Schramm et al., 2011).

CLINICAL EXAMPLE: Clients should quit smoking by any and all means possible and take prescribed medication as directed. If a client can't afford the prescribed medication and generics are not available, they should be referred to any of the programs mentioned at the beginning of Chapter 4. Many pharmaceutical manufacturers provide their nongeneric meds at no or reduced cost to those who meet certain criteria. Clients should be advised never to stop taking prescription meds without talking to their medical professional.

VISION PROBLEMS

By far the most troublesome of all the complications for me is fear of blindness. Having type 1 diabetes for 25 years put me at risk for *retinopathy*, or damage to the retina, the light-sensitive nerve tissue in the back of the eye, and other vision complications.

Retinopathy

Almost everyone with type 1 diabetes, and more than 70% of those with type 2, will eventually develop some degree of retinopathy, often, thankfully, without any loss of vision. Diabetic retinopathy is a microvascular complication that remains the leading cause of preventable blindness in young and middle-aged adults. Control of blood sugar, blood pressure, and blood cholesterol are the keys to prevention and/or progression (Cheung, Mitchell, and Wong, 2010).

Nonproliferative retinopathy is the early stage, when the tiny blood vessels that feed the retina weaken and form bulges that can leak small amounts of blood or fluid into the surrounding tissue. This can begin to happen after 15 years or sooner with type 1 diabetes. Vision at this stage is usually not affected unless the blood vessels around the macula begin to leak. When this happens, *macula edema* develops and central vision is threatened unless treatment begins soon. The *macula* is the site on the retina that focuses on central vision needed to see straight ahead for reading, driving, and doing any close work, such as knitting or needlepoint. Diabetic macula edema is the most common cause of vision loss in people with diabetes. It is important that an ophthalmologist experienced with diabetic retinopathy should be checking each person for progression and particularly for the development of macula edema, probably every 4 to 6 months. Nonproliferative retinopathy can progress very slowly over many years or can rapidly deteriorate with the development of macula edema, depending on control of blood sugar and blood pressure.

Proliferative retinopathy is the next stage, when fragile new blood vessels grow on the retina and out into the gel (vitreous) in the back of the eye as a result of poor oxygenation of the retina caused by high blood sugars and uncontrolled hypertension. These blood vessels can rupture and bleed into this gel, causing blurred vision or temporary blindness. If scar tissue forms on the retina, it can cause a detachment and, if not reattached soon, lead to loss of vision in that area. Vitreous bleeding nearly always indicates abnormal vessels with high-risk characteristics, and laser photocoagulation to prevent bleeding is usually indicated.

CLINICAL EXAMPLE: I recently experienced bleeding into the vitreous of my left eye, which caused the 20/20 eyesight in that eye to deteriorate to 20/400 (the big E on the eye chart). Over the past 12 months, my body has absorbed more and more of the blood in the back of the eye, and my eyesight has improved to the point where I now see 20/25 in that eye without treatment.

To prevent the worst-case scenario from happening, an ophthalmologist should do a thorough exam of the retina through dilated pupils every 6 months to 1 year, depending on the degree of retinopathy. These exams should start after 5 years or sooner with type 1 diabetes and occur at least yearly. Individuals with type 2 should start yearly exams as soon as possible after diagnosis because high glucose levels may have been present for several years and retinopathy may already be developing.

Maintaining tight blood glucose control (Alc <7%), keeping blood pressure under 130/80, and controlling cholesterol levels can help prevent the onset and/or progression of the retinal damage. In the ACCORD-EYE study, the combination of fenofibrate and simvastatin reduced by 40% the rate of progression of diabetic retinopathy compared with simvastatin alone. Other studies are needed to establish the place of lipid-lowering drugs in the treatment of macular edema and the prevention of vision loss (Ansque, Crimet, & Foucher, 2011). A 2009 study showed that being on an ACE inhibitor or an ARB for hypertension can prevent the development of retinopathy by 70% (Mauer et al., 2009). See the types of cholesterol-lowering and antihypertensive medications listed earlier in this chapter.

Treatment of proliferative retinopathy with laser photocoagulation can zap fragile blood vessels before they bleed and cloud vision and can also be used to reattach the retina, if needed, to preserve vision.

These laser treatments are an outpatient procedure and usually do not cause pain.

CLINICAL EXAMPLE: As part of the prevention of further bleeding, my ophthalmologist recently used the laser on parts of the retina of my left eye. All I felt was some mild pressure and a few hours of blurry vision from all of the drops used before and after the procedure. I was afraid I'd move during the procedure, but the nurse held my head firmly against the band at my forehead to prevent that and a contact lens was inserted to stabilize the eye.

If there has been extensive bleeding into the vitreous gel, a vitrectomy can be done. This is also an outpatient procedure in which the vitreous gel in the back of the eye is removed and replaced by a saline solution. Most people notice an improvement in vision and can resume reading and driving. Sometimes the body can absorb the blood if it is not continuous and the situation can resolve itself, as it did in my case.

Prevention is, of course, most important, but next to that are early diagnosis and treatment with laser photocoagulation to eliminate the blood vessels that are leaking or that might in the future. Because I already have proliferative retinopathy, I listen to what my ophthalmologist dictates to his nurse as he is looking into my dilated pupils. When he says "The macula is dry," it is like music to my ears.

Other treatments for macular edema include a series of intraocular injections of anti-VEGF (vascular endothelial growth factor) medication such as Avastin, Lucentis, or Macugen. These injections are done in the ophthalmologist's office and usually improve vision and stabilize the eye from further vision loss. VEGF is a protein that allows the tiny blood vessels of the retina to grow and proliferate. By blocking the action of this protein in the eye, the tiny blood vessels shrivel up and die, thus preventing any further leakage from current vessels. However, new vessels can grow, necessitating repeat injections. A newer treatment, Ozurdex, is a sustained-release drug delivery system. The rod-shaped biodegradable intravitreal implant contains 0.7 mg of dexamethasone, a steroid, and is injected directly into the vitreous using Novadur technology manufactured by Allergan (Irvine, CA), gradually releases dexamethasone for up to 6 months. Biodegradable polymers release the drug as they themselves degrade and are finally absorbed within the body. It is approved by the FDA to treat macula edema caused by retinal vein occlusion but may soon be approved for diabetic macula edema caused by arterial leaking as well. On the horizon is another sustained-release steroid delivery system called Iluvien. It is now awaiting FDA approval and may be marketable in late 2011. This system will last for 24 to 36 months after injection. The "vehicle" that delivers the steroid is tiny and is injected via a 25-gauge needle (Wong, 2010).

CLINICAL EXAMPLE: The gauge of a needle is the measurement of the *bore*, or inside diameter; the smaller the bore, the larger the gauge. This does not tell you anything about the length of the needle, just the inside diameter. For example, blood transfusions are delivered using an 18-gauge (large) needle, and insulin syringes have a 31 or larger gauge (very small) needle. The steroid-delivery vehicle remains in the eye, but it is miniscule. This is a small price to pay for improved vision.

Cataracts and Glaucoma

These conditions are more common in people with diabetes and can develop at an earlier age than in people without diabetes. A *cataract* is a clouding of the lens of the eye and, over time, it impairs vision. Basically, in those of us with diabetes it is caused by an excess level of blood glucose, which sticks to the lens. Today when a cataract is removed, a lens implant that can correct for far vision is inserted. This implant can even correct astigmatism. In the near future it may also make the need for reading glasses after cataract surgery obsolete.

When cataracts are removed and a person also has some form of retinopathy, the risk of a vitreous bleed is increased. The eye surgeon should look at the retina with pupils dilated in all follow-up visits and at least every 6 months thereafter for evidence of vessels on the retina that might bleed.

With *glaucoma* the high fluid pressure within the eyeball can damage the optic nerve (part of the retina), which carries what a person sees to the brain for interpretation. Each time anyone has an appointment with an optometrist or ophthalmologist for an eye exam, eye pressure should be measured. Because this increase in pressure causes no symptoms until the damage is done, everyone, not just people with diabetes, should have this pressure tested at least once a year. Treatment usually consists of eye drops to lower the intraocular pressure. If this is not enough, laser treatment may be necessary to prevent loss of vision. Being proactive in getting eye exams and following through with any treatment necessary is a must, as is tight glucose and blood pressure control, for anyone with diabetes.

KIDNEY DAMAGE (NEPHROPATHY)

The tiny blood vessels, called *capillaries*, of the nephrons, the working units of the kidney, can be damaged from excessive blood glucose levels and uncontrolled hypertension. About 30% to 40% of people with type 1 diabetes and 20% of those with type 2 diabetes will eventually develop some kind of kidney damage (Collazo-Clavell, 2009). The kidneys and their nephrons filter the blood constantly to remove waste products, including metabolized drugs. They also play a major role in fluid and electrolyte balance. Electrolytes, such as sodium, potassium, magnesium, calcium, and phosphorus, regulate the nervous system, make muscles contract and relax, help blood to clot (calcium), and keep bones strong (calcium, magnesium, and phosphorus). When the kidneys can no longer get rid of excess body fluids, blood pressure goes up and the risk of a heart attack, stroke, or eye damage increases. Because everyone with diabetes is at risk for renal disease, urine should be tested for small amounts of protein called *albumin* once a year. The condition, if the urine test shows 30 or greater, is called *microalbuminuria*. This may start to develop as early as 5 to 10 years after diagnosis. If present, it may take another 10 years or so for larger amounts of protein to appear in the urine (*proteinuria*) due to worsening damage to the nephrons. There should be no protein lost in the urine under ordinary circumstances, so proteinuria is a late sign of renal damage (Saudek and Margolis, 2011). Another test that should be done yearly to assess kidney function is a *blood creatinine*. Healthy kidneys should filter this waste product out of the blood. *Renal insufficiency* is a decreased ability of the kidneys to filter the blood. This condition may progress slowly for many years. When the nephrons can no longer get rid of wastes and excess fluid, kidney failure has occurred. At this point, dialysis, either hemodialysis or peritoneal dialysis, or kidney transplantation are the only options.

The strategies to prevent or slow the progression of kidney damage include

1. Tight glucose control (Alc < 7%)
2. Successful treatment of hypertension (< 130/80)
3. Adding an ACE inhibitor or ARB if not already prescribed for hypertension (see the list of medications for hypertension presented earlier in this chapter)
4. Limiting the use of NSAID (nonsteroidal anti-inflammatory drug) pain relievers, lab tests that use contrast dye, and any other medication that can damage kidneys
5. If kidneys continue to fail, limiting protein intake may be needed to decrease the stress on the nephrons (ADA, 2011).

Of the above, the most important strategies to prevent kidney damage are tight blood sugar and blood pressure control. If kidney function is decreased, any medication that is excreted in urine may need a dosage reduction.

Symptoms of kidney failure include fatigue, weakness, headaches, itchiness, nausea, vomiting, loss of appetite, foamy dark urine that is decreased in amount, and fluid retention causing edema, and an increase in blood pressure. Fatigue and weakness come from anemia because the failing kidneys cannot produce erythropoietin, a hormone that stimulates the bone marrow to produce red blood cells. Like insulin, this hormone can be given by injection in the fatty tissue of the abdomen. When the kidneys cannot dispose of waste products or control the levels of electrolytes as they should, a renal diet may be prescribed. This diet limits the intake of protein, fluids, sodium, potassium, and phosphorus. Lists of foods that are high and low in these substances can be found at www.mcw.edu/display/ ClinicalServices/DietforRenalPatient.htm. As soon as renal failure is diagnosed, most people are placed on the kidney transplant list and dialysis is begun.

Hemodialysis

This treatment to filter the blood outside the body is usually done in special dialysis centers, takes from 3 to 5 hours, and is repeated three times per week on one of the following schedules: Monday, Wednesday, Friday or Tuesday, Thursday, Saturday. There is a special shunt, fistula, or graft placed in the arm or leg between a large artery and a large vein. It takes several weeks for this shunt to mature and be ready for the dialysis procedure. A large bore needle is placed in the shunt and attached to a dialysis machine that takes the blood and passes it through a dialysate solution that removes the waste products of the body's metabolism, any drugs and other products broken down by the liver, and excess water, all of which the kidneys would do if they could. The cleansed blood is returned to the body via a needle inserted in the shunt above the outflow needle. Many people feel very weak after this procedure because their blood pressure, which was high from excess water before the procedure, is now low. An alternative to this form of dialysis is *home hemodialysis* offered by some dialysis centers. The person uses a dialysis machine at home after he or she is taught how and can dialyze the blood every day or while sleeping at night. The dialysate is prepared for the client by the dialysis center (Mayo Clinic Health Letter, 2011). Maintaining an intact shunt with either method is very important because there are only a few places in the arms and legs with large enough blood vessels where this shunt can be placed. Heparin is usually used to maintain patency and the shunt should be placed in the nondominant arm. For a healthcare professional who is caring for someone with a hemodialysis shunt, the following rules must be followed:

- Always check the shunt access site for patency before each treatment.
- Keep the access clean at all times and observe for signs of infection, such as redness, warmth, and edema.
- Use the access site only for dialysis, not to draw blood or for any other reason.
- Be careful not to bump or damage the access site.
- Do not put a blood pressure cuff on the arm with the access site.

■ Teach the client not to wear jewelry or tight clothes over the access site.
■ Teach the client to avoid sleeping with the access arm under his or her head or body.
■ Teach the client to avoid lifting heavy objects or put pressure on the access arm.
■ Check the patency of the access site by listening for a "whoosh" with a stethoscope every day and teach the client to feel for a "thrill" or vibration indicating blood flow (Collazo-Clavell, 2009).

Peritoneal Dialysis

This method of cleansing the blood is usually done by the person or a family member at home or at work after careful instruction is given. Peritoneal dialysis requires a surgically implanted flexible catheter in the abdomen through which the dialysate or dialysis solution is delivered. This solution is hung higher than the body, which allows it to flow into the abdomen by gravity. When the bag is empty, it is lowered below the abdomen and the peritoneal fluid passes through the peritoneal membrane (in the abdomen), which filters out the waste products and excess fluid from the body. This fluid flows into the old bag, which is then disconnected and discarded. This procedure is done four to five times every day and takes about 30 to 60 minutes. There are cycler type machines that can be connected for 10 to 12 hours and used at night.

CLINICAL EXAMPLE: Peritoneal dialysis gives the person much more flexibility in scheduling, there are fewer dietary and fluid restrictions, and he or she often feels better because wastes and fluids are removed every day and do not build up. Peritoneal infection is the number one problem with this method of dialysis. To prevent infection, the client must be taught the following:

■ Store supplies in a cool, clean, dry place
■ Inspect each bag of solution for signs of contamination
■ Find a clean, dry, well-lighted space to perform the exchanges
■ Wash hands before handling the catheter
■ Clean the exit site on the abdomen with an antiseptic every day
■ Wear a surgical mask when performing the exchanges

Watch for signs of peritoneal infection, such as:

■ Fever
■ Nausea or vomiting
■ Redness or pain around the catheter site
■ Unusual color or cloudiness in used dialysis solution.

If any of the preceding occurs, the person must call a healthcare practitioner promptly so that the problem can be treated.

Kidney Transplantation

The ultimate remedy for kidney failure is a kidney transplant from a live donor or a person who has donated his organ after death. It may take awhile for a kidney to become available, so dialysis is done as a stop-gap measure. Because people need only one kidney, a close family member or other person whose HLA (human leukocyte antigen) markers match may choose to give one to the person who is in renal failure. When a person with type 1 diabetes needs a kidney, a pancreas, partial pancreatic, or islet cell transplantation may also be done. (See Chapter 1 for more on pancreatic and islet cell transplantation.) Although immunosuppressant drugs have come a long way in recent years in preventing rejection of the transplanted kidney, they must be taken for life, and they may cause the recipient to be unable to fight off common infections and some cancers. Prevention of kidney damage is definitely preferable.

NERVE DAMAGE (NEUROPATHY)

Diseases of the nervous system affect about 60% to 70% of people with both type 1 and type 2 diabetes. Tight control of blood glucose (A1c <7%) decreases the risk of nerve damage by up to 60% (Saudek & Margolis, 2011). Peripheral neuropathy affects nerves of the feet, legs, hands, and arms. Autonomic neuropathy affects the nerves of the autonomic nervous system, which regulates body functions not under our conscious control. None of these conditions is pleasant or easily managed.

Peripheral Neuropathy

Many people with type 2 diabetes are diagnosed when they see a healthcare practitioner for numbness, tingling, or pain, especially in the feet, that often keeps them awake at night. Obviously they have had high blood sugars for many years before nerve damage occurred. Peripheral neuropathy puts a person at risk for other problems of the limbs, especially when combined with poor circulation, as with peripheral artery disease, discussed earlier in this chapter. Continuous high blood glucose levels are toxic to nerve fibers and eventually kill them. When someone's feet are numb, they don't feel a blister or a stone in their shoe. A wound can get infected and, if circulation is impaired, the white blood cells that fight infections and the red blood cells that help an injury heal do not get to the site. A simple blister can be the start of what may end up as an amputation.

In addition to high blood sugars, hypertension, cardiovascular problems, and high cholesterol levels increase a person's risk for developing neuropathy. These problems, if uncontrolled, result in poor circulation that deprives the nerves of oxygen. Controlling blood sugar, blood pressure, and cholesterol with or without medication are the most important things anyone can do to prevent neuropathy or to minimize nerve damage if it is already present. Because nicotine affects circulation, quitting smoking and avoiding inhaled second-hand smoke is equally important.

Nerves are classified as either *sensory nerves* or *motor nerves*. Sensory nerves signal the brain that sand or a rock is in a shoe or that the bottom of the feet are burning when walking barefoot on hot cement around a pool. When nerves are damaged, there is numbness, tingling, burning, and sharp, jabbing pain at, for example, the least touch of the sheets on the toes. These sensations are more noticeable at night because the brain is not so distracted by what is going on. It makes sleeping very difficult.

Motor nerves, on the other hand, send signals to the feet and leg muscles to contract and relax in order to walk, run, or jump. When they are damaged it may be difficult to raise the front of the feet, and a condition called *foot drop* develops. The muscles become weak and don't respond well to loss of balance, so falls are more probable. There is also a lack of coordination and perhaps even paralysis. When muscles are not stimulated they get smaller or atrophy, which increases weakness.

Both sensory and motor involvement can occur in the hands as well, and writing, picking up small objects, and even turning the page of a book can become difficult. Picking up anything even slightly heavy can become impossible if weakness of the hands and forearms is involved.

The good news to point out to clients is if they are feeling the early signs of sensory nerve damage, they can do a lot to improve these conditions by controlling blood sugars and the other causes mentioned earlier. The bad news is that if they don't work at this, these nerves may die and they will feel nothing and not be able to move the muscles in their feet and/or hands. Pain is a protective mechanism that causes us to remove the foot or hand from whatever caused the pain, such as a rock or a nail or a hot stove. When feet, in particular, lose sensation, an ulcer can form and, if left untreated, can become gangrenous and necessitate an amputation of one or more toes, or worse. Healthcare practitioners should be testing for peripheral neuropathy at every visit by using a monofilament to determine whether a client feels where it touches the underside of the foot and placing a tuning fork on the knuckle of the big toe to test for vibratory sensation. Vibratory sensations are the first to go before the sense of light touch as a person experiences neuropathy.

Another thing besides high blood sugars that can lead to neuropathy is a decrease in vitamin B_{12} absorption, causing anemia. The diabetes drug metformin (Glucophage) can decrease the absorption of this important vitamin. Also, as we age we lose some of the cells in the stomach lining that produce intrinsic factor necessary for oral B_{12} absorption. After removal of part of the stomach because of cancer surgery or stomach reduction due to gastric bypass surgery or stomach banding for weight loss, vitamin B_{12} injections may be necessary to maintain nerve cell health and to prevent anemia. A deficiency of vitamin B_{12} should be ruled out before a diagnosis of peripheral neuropathy is made because the B_{12} deficiency can be more easily corrected. As a healthcare professional, you must avoid the assumption that all complaints from someone with diabetes are related to this disease and that nothing can be done to correct the problem.

The following are some treatments to ease the discomfort of sensory nerve damage:

- Pain relievers, such as Extra Strength Tylenol, and NSAIDs, such as ibuprofen and naproxen, help for mild symptoms.
- Antidepressants help ease nerve stimulation, which can reduce nighttime symptoms. Examples include some of the older antidepressants, such as amitriptyline, nortriptyline, and Tofranil (imipramine), and a newer drug, Cymbalta (duloxetine). They should be taken at night because they may cause drowsiness and dizziness.
- Antiseizure medications, such as Neurontin (gabapentin), Topamax (topiramate), Tegretol (carbamazepine), and Lyrica (pregabalin) also quiet nerves. These drugs should also be taken at night.
- Lidocaine patches, which contains the anesthetic lidocaine, can numb the painful areas.
- Alpha-lipoic acid, a common dietary supplement, can be taken orally or by injection to decrease burning pain and paresthesia.
- A transcutaneous electric nerve stimulation or TENS unit is used for pain difficult to control by other methods. Electrodes are placed on the skin over painful areas and a gentle electric current is delivered to mask the neuropathic pain.
- Research is currently in Phase III trials to test the effects of injecting Botox into the skin on top of the feet to relieve pain as compared with an injection of saline (a placebo). Completion date is late 2014 (National Institutes of Health [NIH], March 28, 2011).
- Research on oxcarbazepine, an oral capsule, is in Phase IV trials comparing it with a placebo to treat neuropathic pain. Results should be available in December 2011 (NIH, February 23, 2011).

Foot Care

The most important aspect of taking care of one's feet is to prevent amputations. Regardless of whether someone has peripheral neuropathy and/or peripheral arterial disease, diabetes itself increases the risk of amputation. Of course, if a client has either or both of these complications the risk is compounded. Constant high blood glucose levels slow down one's ability to fight infection anywhere in the body. It is like the immune system and white blood cells are trying to get to the site of infection in a sea of molasses. By the time they get there, the infection may be well established. Their distance from the heart and the small size of their blood vessels makes fighting infections in the feet most difficult. Therefore, checking feet nightly for redness, warmth, bruising, blisters, and any break in the skin is important to teach anyone with diabetes.

CLINICAL EXAMPLE: Teach clients to use magnifying mirrors to see the underside of their feet and toes and in between the toes, because these areas are where most of the problems occur. They should keep mirrors in the bathroom or wherever they are most likely to use them. This may be near the chair where they sit to watch television. Make sure the area is well lighted. Other preventive measures that clients with diabetes need to know to avoid foot trauma include the following:

- Always wear well-fitting shoes that allow for movement of toes, including shower shoes at the gym. Going barefoot can be dangerous for anyone. Glass and stones can cut or bruise feet. Getting athlete's foot from a communal shower or sliding on a wet tub or tile surface can happen to anyone but will have more consequences for those with diabetes.
- Always check inside shoes before putting them on to feel for debris, tears, sharp edges, or worn areas that might cause irritation or injury to feet.
- Wear seamless socks with shoes to absorb moisture and prevent friction, which could cause a blister.
- Never use sharp implements to treat a callus. See a podiatrist instead.
- Avoid electric blankets, heating pads, or foot soaking products, because these can cause burns and irritation to sensitive skin.
- Use good moisturizing lotions on feet and heels to keep the skin from cracking. Avoid putting lotion between the toes because this can encourage fungal growth.
- Call a healthcare practitioner if they notice any symptoms of peripheral neuropathy or any area of irritation or a blister or ulcer, or any signs of infection on their feet. They need to be seen immediately or within 24 hours. If that is not possible, they should go to an urgent care center, especially if they have peripheral neuropathy and/or decreased circulation to their feet.

Charcot's Joint

When a foot has lost most of its sensation, including pain sensation and the ability to sense the position of the joint, muscles also lose their ability to support the joint properly. With an unstable foot, a sprained ankle, inflammation, dislocation, and, eventually, a deformity may follow. This neuropathic joint disease, called *Charcot's joint*, after the doctor who first described it, can be very debilitating. People with peripheral neuropathy are at risk for this complication and need to be on the lookout for any symptoms of inflammation, such as swelling, redness, heat, and a strong pulse as well as decreased sensations of the feet. They should notify their healthcare providers so the foot can be immobilized with a cast to prevent the progression of any deformity. After the cast is removed, they will have to wear a brace when walking to protect the joint from further damage.

Autonomic Neuropathy

Not as common but even more problematic is the nerve damage done to the autonomic nervous system by uncontrolled hyperglycemia. The autonomic nerves regulate body functions that are not under conscious control, such as digestion, heart rate, blood pressure, and bladder and bowel control. Anyone who has autonomic neuropathy probably also has peripheral neuropathy, because the former takes longer to develop. The list of possible problems is long and includes gastroparesis, or slow stomach emptying; neurogenic bladder, or poor bladder control; constipation, diarrhea, or both; rapid or irregular heartbeat; postural drop in blood pressure; difficulty regulating respirations; hypoglycemia unawareness; erectile dysfunction in men; and female sexual dysfunction in the form of frequent yeast infections, vaginal dryness and irritation, decreased libido, and difficulty achieving orgasm. Any of these problems can certainly disrupt a life already complicated by diabetes.

Gastroparesis

This condition occurs in 5% to 12% of people with uncontrolled diabetes (Gebel, 2009). Normally, food is broken down by the stomach in about 3 hours or less, depending on what is eaten. This slurry then moves to the small intestine, where digestive enzymes from the pancreas and the liver (bile) digest the fats, proteins, and carbohydrates and begin the process of absorption of these nutrients, as well as the vitamins and minerals they contain. With gastroparesis, food remains in the stomach much longer and symptoms such as fullness and bloating, abdominal pain, heartburn, erratic blood glucose levels, nausea, and vomiting may occur. Controlling blood sugar levels most of the time should prevent this and other types of neuropathy, but once this complication develops blood glucose levels may rise and fall at unanticipated times, making control difficult. Any medication that delays stomach emptying, such as Symlin or Byetta, may make matters worse. Eating six small meals a day and limiting high-fat and high-fiber foods, which also slow stomach emptying, usually help. Liquid or pureed foods may be needed in severe cases. To increase comfort, medications that cause the stomach to contract, moving food into the small intestine, can be prescribed, as can anti-nausea and anti-gas drugs. As a last resort, a feeding tube may be surgically inserted into the small intestine to bypass the stomach altogether. This will ensure an intake of adequate nutrients, vitamins, minerals, and calories to avoid malnutrition and make it easier to stabilize blood sugars.

Neurogenic Bladder

A neurogenic bladder is one that does not respond to fullness and the need to urinate, so the bladder may not get emptied. This retained urine can grow bacteria and cause a bladder infection that can force infected urine up into the kidneys, causing renal damage from the pressure and the infection. The opposite is also possible, causing urinary incontinence. A person with either problem can be taught to self-catheterize at regular intervals throughout the day. Medication can be prescribed for an overactive bladder as well as for a urinary tract infection, and sometimes surgery can be done to reposition the bladder in women to help with bladder emptying. Both men and women can be taught to use the Credé method (applying manual pressure over the bladder) to enhance emptying.

Hypoglycemia Unawareness

This condition was covered in Chapter 5, but its root cause is autonomic nerve damage brought on by consistently high blood sugars. People who experience this complication have no warning that a low blood sugar is occurring. They do not experience the sweating, shaking, and rapid heartbeat that signal hypoglycemia. This is truly a medical emergency, because if a person does not respond to a very low blood glucose level by eating or drinking something to raise blood sugar, they may have a seizure, become comatose, and/or develop some brain damage. People who develop hypoglycemia unawareness almost always have had type 1 diabetes for many years. They benefit from using a CGMS, described in Chapter 5, and should be recommended for pancreatic or islet cell transplantation.

Sudomotor Neuropathy

This consists of nerve damage to sweat glands. This can cause excessive sweating and dry skin, which can lead to skin infections and dehydration. Conversely, it can also hinder the ability to sweat, causing a person's internal temperature to rise to dangerous levels, resulting in heat stroke. People who experience either of these complications must work at normalizing their blood sugars most of the time, stay hydrated, minimize working or playing in hot weather, and moisturize and check skin for infection daily.

Heat stroke should be treated by emergency medical personnel, who can start an IV line and transport the person to the hospital.

Postural Hypotension

This condition can prevent blood vessels from automatically constricting when a person goes from sitting or lying down to a standing position. Without this narrowing of blood vessels to increase blood pressure, blood drains from the head by gravity, and the person faints. Other symptoms of this problem include increased heart rate, dizziness, low blood pressure, nausea, and vomiting. To counteract these symptoms, affected clients should be advised to change positions slowly when sitting up from lying down or when standing from a sitting position, and stay near the bed or chair until they no longer feel like fainting. Some people wear compression stockings that help venous blood return from the legs into the arterial circulation to increase the blood to the brain, and medications to increase blood pressure are available.

Sexual Dysfunction

This dysfunction can affect both men and women with either type 1 or type 2 diabetes. It is been estimated that about 35% to 75% of men with diabetes will experience at least some degree of erectile dysfunction in their lifetime. Men with diabetes tend to develop erectile dysfunction 10 to 15 years earlier than men without diabetes. As men with diabetes age, erectile dysfunction becomes even more common. Above the age of 50, the likelihood of having difficulties with an erection occurs in approximately 50% to 60% of men with diabetes. Above the age of 70 there is about a 95% likelihood of having some difficulty with erectile function (WebMD, n.d.). Autonomic neuropathy from consistently high blood sugars is only one cause of sexual dysfunction. For men with diabetes, this translates to *erectile dysfunction,* or the inability to have or sustain an erection, especially if combined with poor circulation to the area. In order to have an erection, a man needs to have nervous system stimulation and a rush of blood to the penis. Other health issues that combine to make erectile dysfunction more likely include *hypercholesterolemia,* which clogs the arteries, and hypertension, which constricts arteries, both resulting in decreased circulation to the penis. Prevention involves controlling blood glucose levels, blood pressure, and cholesterol levels. TV ads for Viagra, Cialis, and Levetra help to tell the story; however, the success rate of these medications in men with diabetes is only about 50% to 60%, which is less than in men without diabetes (Saudek & Margolis, 2011). A new oral medication in the same classification, Staxyn (vardenafil HCl), an orally disintegrating tablet for erectile dysfunction was approved in 2010. It is another brand name for the same generic as Levetra. It disintegrates on the tongue without liquid. It works by increasing blood flow to the penis during sexual stimulation. This increased blood flow can cause an erection.

CLINICAL EXAMPLE: Drugs for erectile dysfunction can interact with antihypertensive medication, especially alpha-blockers and medication for angina, such as nitrates, to cause a dangerous drop in blood pressure. Healthcare prescribers need a list of all of a person's medications to check for drug-to-drug interactions. Pharmacists should also check this list.

There are other treatments for erectile dysfunction if oral medication does not work, including injections of medication directly into the blood vessels of the penis. This works in 60% to 80% of men with diabetes. Vacuum constricting devices also have a high rate of success. They help to achieve and maintain an erection. In addition there are also pellets that can be placed into the urethra as well as surgically inserted penile implants (WebMD, 2010). Maintaining good glucose, blood pressure, and cholesterol control, which would prevent the problem in the first place, are better options.

Female sexual dysfunction doesn't get much press but is equally devastating to the women who experience this complication. Nerve damage to the vagina causes decreased lubrication, decreased or absence of orgasm, vaginal infection with odorous discharge, and vaginismus, a constriction of the vaginal walls making penetration painful or impossible. Many women notice that blood sugars are higher or lower than normal the week before the start of their menstrual cycle. Healthcare professionals can suggest that women keep blood sugar records for a couple of months, noting when their period starts. This may help to see this relationship more clearly so that the client can adjust her medication or insulin, diet, and exercise during these times to help even out the hormonal influences. Menopause is another time when women need to rethink how they are managing their diabetes. Emotions also greatly affect blood glucose. For more on this topic, see Chapter 11. To minimize the likelihood of vaginal infections, the client should practice good sexual hygiene before and after intercourse. Also they should use a vaginal lubricant or estrogen cream suggested or prescribed by their gynecologist if vaginal dryness is a problem. A gynecologist may also have suggestions to increase libido.

Reviewing a complete list of prescriptions, over-the-counter medications, and herbal supplements to see whether any of them contribute to sexual dysfunction is the job of pharmacists and any healthcare prescribers. Some have side effects that do. As with all complications, prevention by controlling blood sugars, blood pressure, and cholesterol levels should be emphasized.

From the serious and life-threatening complications to the very disconcerting and annoying ones, high blood sugars can affect every body system. In the following sections, I discuss a few of the non-life-threatening but bothersome conditions that may strengthen a client's resolve to work at glucose control.

TEETH AND GUM PROBLEMS

People with diabetes are at higher risk for developing mouth infections. Bacteria thrive in moist, dark places like the mouth, especially when they have sugar-laden mucous to feast on. The higher a person's blood sugar, the sweeter all their secretions are. Besides controlling glucose levels, clients need to brush their teeth at least twice a day with a fluoride toothpaste that also has a bacteria-killing ingredient. Flossing or using another device to keep food particles from lodging between teeth is also important. Dental cleaning and check-ups at least every 6 months permit a dental hygienist and/or a dentist to clean and check teeth for cavities and plaque formation and gums for *gingivitis,* the red, swollen, bleeding gums that can lead to *periodontitis,* an inflammation and infection of the gums, ligaments, bones, and other tissue that hold the teeth in place. If pockets of infection form beneath the gum line, a specialized dentist can do procedures such as tooth scaling and root planing to get rid of the plaque and infection. Often an antibiotic is needed to treat the infection. Consistently high blood sugars (>200 mg/dl) can lead to periodontitis, but the reverse is also true. Periodontal disease can worsen blood sugar control. If gum disease is not caught early, it can lead to tooth loss.

CLINICAL EXAMPLE: Clients should be advised to use a soft toothbrush when brushing teeth to avoid causing trauma to gums that might leave an open area for bacteria to invade. They should use small, circular motions to remove food and plaque from the gum line and between teeth. When flossing between teeth, they should use a sawing motion from the gum line to the end of the tooth to avoid cutting into the gum line. If they wear dentures, they should rinse them and soak them overnight in a liquid made for that purpose, or use an effervescent tablet in water. Chewing sugar-free gum can help to loosen food trapped between teeth and increase saliva production. It can also help in digestion.

In addition to gingivitis and periodontitis, high blood sugars can cause *thrush,* a fungal infection of the mouth, tongue, gums, and even the throat. It looks like white patches that cannot be brushed away and often hurts when any food or liquid, even water, touches it. There are a few antifungal rinses available that can be swished and swallowed to eradicate this infection. Getting a new toothbrush may also be necessary to prevent reinfection. Another common mouth problem is dry mouth, or *xerostomia.* This can cause constant bad breath and needs to be treated because the normal amount of saliva helps to keep teeth and gums healthy and free from infection. *Canker sores* may also be an indication that blood glucose levels are out of control. Again, clients should be advised to quit smoking, because this makes dry mouth and any gum disease worse. Controlling stress is important because it can make fighting any infection, including periodontitis, more difficult. Blood sugar control really will help clients keep their teeth and their healthy smile.

Clients with diabetes should let their dentist know and bring him or her a list of all their prescriptions, over-the-counter medications, and herbal supplements they take so the oral care they receive is appropriate for them. Chronic inflammation from gum disease is also associated with heart disease, blocked arteries and stroke, lung infections, preterm labor, and worsening memory and math skills (AAP, n.d.).

MUSCULOSKELETAL SYSTEM

Keeping bones, muscles, joints, and ligaments healthy and functional depends on keeping blood sugar levels under control. There are several conditions in this body system that occur more frequently in people who have diabetes than in those without diabetes.

Frozen Shoulder

Frozen shoulder (adhesive capsulitis) is a painful restriction of shoulder movement. The capsule of a shoulder joint includes ligaments that attach the arm to the scapula, or shoulder blade, in the upper back, and the arm to the clavicle or collar bone. The shoulder joint is a ball-in-socket joint, which makes it the most versatile joint in our body. It can rotate 360° (a full circle); can move arms forward, backward, across the chest, and outward away from the body; and allows the arm to reach the back from above and below. The rotator cuff muscles stabilize this joint.

CLINICAL EXAMPLE: Because of all of these useful, everyday movements the shoulder can easily be injured when overly stressed. This happens when a person attempts to lift, push, pull, or throw something heavier than he or she is used to. Constant high glucose levels can cause inflammation of many body parts, including muscles and tendons. When inflammation of the capsule occurs, tendons and ligaments get stiff and swollen, and movement is restricted. When movement causes pain, the natural tendency is to avoid moving that joint. Inflammation in joints that are immobile causes adhesions to form, restricting movement even more.

The key to regaining full range of motion of the shoulder joint is to reduce the inflammation with good blood sugar control, NSAIDs such as ibuprofen or naproxen, or cortisone injections, and physical therapy. Early and aggressive treatment is necessary. This is truly a case of "move it or lose it." If a significant amount of scar tissue has formed, arthroscopic surgery may be needed. Manipulation of the joint under anesthesia to break up the adhesions is another option. Physical therapy and daily exercising of the shoulder joint after either procedure are absolutely essential to prevent more scar tissue and adhesions from forming in response to the irritation from surgery. The body's way of protecting an injured body part is to form a fibrous band of tissue (adhesions, or scar tissue) to protect the body part from further injury. This happens not just in joints but after any surgery.

The importance of controlling blood sugar cannot be overstated. Anyone with diabetes is four times more likely to experience a frozen shoulder, a partial frozen shoulder, or a rotator cuff injury than people who don't have diabetes (dLife, Feb 18, 2010). However, it can also happen to others. I had a partial frozen shoulder several years before I was diagnosed with diabetes. Because I got help early, all I needed was physical therapy and daily exercises, such as wall climbing with that arm and doing deep knee bends while holding on to a doorknob with my back to the door. I still do shoulder stretches most days. See Chapter 3 for examples of helpful exercises for the shoulder joint.

Carpal Tunnel Syndrome

Median nerve entrapment, or *carpal tunnel syndrome*, is often caused by repetitive motion, such as typing or painting, that irritates the tendons around the median nerve at the wrist. This causes the nerve to swell, which makes the bony tunnel space narrower and compresses the nerve. Hyperglycemia can also add to this inflammation. Numbness, tingling, or a burning sensation of the palm side of the thumb and the first three fingers, as well as pain, sometimes in the forearm, are all reasons for a client to seek medical attention. If a person also has peripheral neuropathy of the hands, there are tests to differentiate between the two. If the problem is carpal tunnel syndrome, then resting the affected hand and wrist, often by wearing a splint, especially at night, is very important. NSAID pain relievers and/or cortisone injections to relieve the inflammation and reduce the swelling are an important part of the treatment.

CLINICAL EXAMPLE: The best anti-inflammatory drug is cortisone, a steroid. Even when it is injected into a joint, it often raises blood sugar for 24 to 48 hours. Clients should be advised to check blood sugars more often than usual and limit carbs until the blood sugar problems are resolved. NSAIDs are usually good alternatives, depending on the degree of inflammation. Note that Tylenol is not an NSAID. It works on pain and fever, but not inflammation.

If splinting and drugs don't cure the problem, carpal tunnel release surgery, which widens the carpal tunnel, may be necessary. This is an outpatient procedure done under local anesthesia. If a client does nothing about this problem, the consequence is more than living with pain. The nerve can be permanently damaged and the thumb muscles can atrophy. And, of course, a client with diabetes should be told to control blood sugar to prevent this condition from coming back.

Trigger Finger

Flexor tenosynovitis, also called *trigger finger*, is an irritation and narrowing of the sheath that surrounds the flexor tendon, causing it to catch and release like a trigger. The most common finger affected is the ring finger of either hand, but any finger or the thumbs, for that matter, can be involved. You'd think it would more likely happen on your dominant hand, but I've had two fingers and the thumb of my left hand, and only the ring finger of my right hand, surgically repaired so far.

CLINICAL EXAMPLE: The cause of such minor annoyances is the same as with all other muscle or tendon inflammation. Blood glucose control matters, but how long a person has had diabetes seems to matter more. People whose work or hobbies require repeated gripping actions, such as knitting or crocheting, whether or not they have diabetes, are more susceptible. The first time it happened to me was caused by tightly gripping the steering wheel for a tense 40-minute commute to work on mostly interstate highways. It is more common in women and in anyone with diabetes.

Nonsurgical interventions can include splinting the finger(s) or thumb, especially while sleeping, to prevent a person from curling his or her fingers into a ball. This can also be done by placing the hand, palm down and fingers straight, under the pillow. Gentle finger massage from the palm down the affected finger(s) or thumb and warm soaks may give temporary relief. The use of NSAIDs and cortisone injections may be useful to relieve the inflammation and swelling.

NSAIDs like ibuprofen (Advil, Motrin, etc.) or naproxen (Aleve and others) must be taken with or after food, even crackers; otherwise, they may irritate the stomach lining and, over time, cause a stomach ulcer to form. All of these meds work like aspirin in that they prevent platelets from sticking together and forming a clot. However, if a client is also taking other drugs that prevent clotting, such as Coumadin or Plavix, their body's ability to clot when needed may be compromised, leading to excessive bruising (bleeding under the skin) or, potentially, hemorrhaging.

For a more permanent solution to a trigger finger, an orthopedic hand surgeon may perform a percutaneous (performed through the skin) release of the affected tendon. This is an outpatient procedure done under local anesthesia. For a good picture of a trigger finger check out the Mayo Clinic's website at www.mayoclinic.com/health/trigger-finger/ds00155/dsection=risk-factors, or the American Academy of Orthopedic Surgeons site at http://orthoinfo.aaos.org/topic.cfm?topic=a00024. After the bulky dressing and stitches are removed, clients will need to gently message the palm and finger(s) or thumb and stretch them to get full extension. They should compare the surgical hand with their other hand to see how far back the fingers should go. They should keep working on the operated fingers or thumb several times a day until they look like the ones on the other hand. This can take several weeks to months.

SKIN PROBLEMS

Dry skin is common for people with diabetes, and applications of a good emollient, such as Vaseline Intensive Care, Gold Bond, or Aveeno lotion daily, are very important, especially on the heels and feet to prevent cracking that can open up the skin for bacteria to enter. A person with diabetes should never put lotion in between toes, because this provides a good medium for fungus to grow. With any break in the skin, an antibiotic cream should be applied and the wound covered with a water-resistant adhesive bandage. Once it starts to close, the wound should be left open to air at least at night if it needs to be protected, depending on its location, during the day.

CLINICAL EXAMPLE: Any open wound, even just a crack, cut, or abrasion, should be checked often for signs of infection. Any redness, puffiness, warmth, or oozing should be seen by a medical practitioner immediately. Even a mild infection can easily get out of hand when a person has diabetes. An infection also raises blood sugar, and increased glucose levels make infections worse. Clients should be taught to check blood sugars more often than usual until the situation is resolved.

Diabetic Dermopathy

This condition consists of roundish, slightly indented brown or purplish patches, usually over the shin bones. It may occur after many years with diabetes. It does not hurt and usually does not itch. It may fade with improved blood sugar control but usually does not require treatment.

Acanthosis Nigricans

This skin problem results in the darkening and thickening of skin, especially in creases. The skin may be slightly raised. It is more common in very overweight individuals, often indicates insulin resistance, and usually precedes the diagnosis of type 2 diabetes. Blood sugar control and weight loss may improve this condition.

Necrobiosis Lipoidica

This skin disease occurs in the lower legs and often indicates reduced blood supply to the skin. The skin becomes thinned and reddened. Trauma to the area can cause ulceration. It can be itchy and painful. Good blood sugar control usually prevents it, however, and ulcers need to be treated to prevent infections.

Fungal Infections

Because sustained high blood glucose levels put the immune system in sleep mode, it is easy to see why people who don't control blood sugars are susceptible to infections. Fungi and bacteria need to be fed to grow, and glucose in bodily secretions, blood, and sweat and on the skin is a perfect food. They also like warm, dark, moist areas. Fungi grow well between the toes as athlete's foot, in the groin area as jock itch, in the vagina as a yeast infection, and in the mouth as thrush, as well as in the armpits, under the foreskin, and under the breasts. *Ringworm* is a ring-shaped itchy patch caused by a fungus (no worm involved). Fungi can also grow under nails and around nail beds. Antifungal creams and/or oral antifungal medication may be needed to treat these infections. Blood sugar control is also needed.

Bacterial Infections

If talking to your clients about the last paragraph doesn't gross them out enough, let me list the various bacterial infections that can plague those who are not motivated to live a healthy lifestyle and work at controlling blood sugars. Bacteria that are allowed to multiply on and under the skin can cause boils and carbuncles (deeper and larger than boils), a stye (infection of the glands of the eyelids), folliculitis (infection of the hair follicles), and infections around toenails and fingernails. Staphylococcal skin infections need to be treated with oral antibiotics, good hygiene, and blood glucose control.

Wound Care

When there is a break in the skin anywhere, clients with diabetes need to be worried. A minor wound can be cleansed with soap and water and an over-the-counter antibiotic ointment and a Band-Aid large enough to cover and pad the area. Gauze and paper or surgical tape can also be used. When a person gets a cut, he or she should change the dressing at least once a day, wash the area with soap and water, and dry carefully. Clients should also observe the wound itself for healing. It should go from red or bleeding to oozing pink and then clear fluid as a scab forms. When a scab starts to form, the area should be kept clean and exposed to air unless it needs to be padded to protect it from injury during the day. Teach clients to look for signs of infection, such as the area around the wound getting red, swollen, or hot, or drainage that is green or bright yellow. It may also have an odor, and blood sugars might be higher. If the client notices any of these signs, he or she should see their medical practitioner or diabetes educator as soon as possible.

If a wound is extensive and/or deep, seeing a medical provider or going to an urgent care center is a must. Any infected wound can become a major wound when a person has diabetes. If a person's diabetes is not treated with insulin, he or she may be put on insulin until the wound is on its way to being healed and the infection is gone. If clients usually inject or pump insulin, they will probably need to take a higher dose. They will also need to take an antibiotic by mouth, injection, or IV, which may necessitate hospitalization. Special dressings may be needed and, depending on the wound's location, a cast, special shoes, bedrest, or a special mattress to keep the pressure off the wound or ulcer may be ordered. This is nothing for you or your diabetic client to fool around with.

If, despite all the clients' efforts, they develop a complication or two, they should be reminded that there are lots of treatments, as listed in this chapter, and more on the horizon. They should also be encouraged with the knowledge that what they are experiencing would have happened sooner and been worse if they had not worked so hard at controlling their glucose levels. As a part of their healthcare team you should encourage them to seek help early and work to stay on top of whatever they are confronting. Diabetes management is not an exact science. Human error, whether through carelessness or willful inattention, accounts for most of the ups and downs of blood sugars. However, as long as they continue to work on being as healthy as they can, they should feel good about themselves no matter what the numbers on the glucose meter are. Teach them to look at the meter numbers as a learning experience. If there is no apparent reason for a high reading, they should record it, try to get it down with medication and/or timing and kinds of food (limit carbs at this meal), and move on. Dwelling on it will take away from the joy of living, as will excessive worry about complication. Keeping a log of what, when, and how much they eat; what, when, and how much they exercise; and what their blood sugar levels are will be important in putting the pieces of the puzzle together so they and you can understand how all of these data relate. Successful people of any age, in any walk of life, facing any challenge, medical or otherwise, all have one thing in common: They take the cards they were dealt and play them to the best of their ability. Win, lose, or draw, that meets my definition of success.

This may have been a hard chapter to read. It was a hard chapter for me to write. If you, as a healthcare professional, skipped through and read only those areas about which you had questions, you know where to find more answers. Read more when you or your client have questions or need more information. We are all human and thus certainly not perfect. We all need to keep in mind that doing the best we can under the circumstances is all any of us can ask of ourselves. One of the best things that you and your client can do to keep informed is to join the ADA at www.diabetes. org. For the cost of membership (currently $28 per year) you will receive a monthly subscription to *Diabetes Forecast*, one of the most informative journals I have ever read.

REFERENCES

American Academy of Periodontology. (n.d.). *Periodontal disease, a chronic inflammatory disease, is linked to other health risks.* Retrieved May 17, 2011, from www.perio.org/consumer/mbc.top2.htm

American Diabetes Association. (2011). Standards of medical care in diabetes—2011. *Diabetes Care, 34,* S11–S61.

American Diabetes Association (n.d.). *High blood pressure (hypertension).* Retrieved May 3, 2011, from www.diabetes.org/living-with-diabetes/complications/high-blood-pressure-hypertension.html

American Heart Association. (n.d.). *Understand your risk factors for high blood pressure.* Retrieved May 8, 2011, from www.heart.org/HEARTORG/Conditions/High BloodPressure/UnderstandYourRiskforHighBloodPressure/Understand-Your-Risk-for-High-Blood-Pressure_UCM_002052_Article.jsp

Ansque, J. C., Crimet, D., & Foucher, C. (2011). Fibrates and statins in the treatment of diabetic neuropathy. *Current Pharmacology Biotechnology, 12*(3), 396–405.

Bennett, N. M., Arndt, T. L., Iyer, V., Garberich, R. F., Traverse, J. H., Johnson, R. K., ... Henry, T. D. (2011). Ranolazine refractory angina registry trial: 1-Year results. *Journal of the American College of Cardiology, 57,* 1050.

Centers for Disease Control and Prevention. (2011). *National diabetes fact sheet: National estimates and general information on diabetes and prediabetes in the United States, 2011.* Atlanta, GA: U.S. Department of Health and Human Services, Centers for Disease Control and Prevention.

Cheung, N., Mitchell, P., & Wong, T. Y. (2010). Diabetic retinopathy. *The Lancet, 376,* 124–136.

Collazo-Clavell, M. (2009). *Mayo Clinic: The essential diabetes book.* New York, NY: Time, Inc.

dLife. (2010, February 18). *Frozen shoulder.* Retrieved May 15, 2011, from www .dlife.com/diabetes/information/complications/musculoskeletal/frozen-shoulder.html

Gebel, E. (2009 , October). Feeling full: This nerve disorder can leave your stomach out of sync. *Diabetes Forecast,* 40–41.

Mauer, M., Zinman, B., Gardiner, R., Suissa, S., Sinaiko, A., Strand, T., Drummond, K., Donnelly, S., Goodyer, P., Gubler, M.C., & Klein, R. (2009). Renal and retinal effects of enalapril and losartan in type 1 diabetes. *The New England Journal of Medicine, 361,* 40–51.

Mayo Clinic Health Letter. (2011). Home dialysis: Advances in kidney care. *Mayo Foundation for Medical Education and Research, 29,* 4–5.

Mayo Clinic Staff. (n.d.). *Sleep apnea.* Retrieved May 19, 2011, from www.mayoclinic .com/health/sleep-apnea/DS00148/DSection=treatments-and-drugs

National Institutes of Health. (2011, March 28). *Early administration of Botox® in neuropathic pain due to thoracoscopy or thoracotomy (APTODON).* Retrieved May 15, 2011, from http://clinicaltrials.gov/ct2/show/NCT01325090

National Institutes of Health. (2011, February 23). *Oxcarbazepine for the treatment of chronic peripheral neuropathic pain (IMIOXC).* Retrieved May 16, 2011, from http://clinicaltrials.gov/ct2/show/NCT01302275

The National Institute of Neurological Disorders and Stroke. (n.d.). *Know stroke. Know the signs. Act in time.* Retrieved May 19, 2011, from www.ninds.nih.gov/ disorders/stroke/knowstroke.htm

Ning, Y., et al. (2011). Ranolazine increases beta-cell survival and improves glucose homeostasis in low dose STZ-induced diabetes in mice. *The Journal of Pharmacology and Experimental Therapeutics.* Retrieved May 19, 2011, from http://jpet .aspetjournals.org/content/early/2011/01/11/jpet.110.176396

Saudek, C., & Margolis, S. (2011). *Johns Hopkins White Papers: Diabetes.* Baltimore, MD: Johns Hopkins University School of Medicine.

Schramm, T. K., Gislason, G. H., Vaag, A., Rasmussen, J. N., Folke, F., Hansen, M. L.,...Torp-Pedersen, C. (2011). Mortality and cardiovascular risk associated with different insulin secretagogues compared with metformin in type 2 diabetes, with or without a previous myocardial infarction: A nationwide study. *European Heart Journal.* Retrieved May 8, 2011, from http://eurheartj .oxfordjournals.org/content/early/2011/04/05/eurheartj.ehr077.abstract

WebMD. (2010, July 30). *Erectile dysfunction treatments for men with diabetes.* Retrieved May 8, 2011, from www.webmd.com/erectile-dysfunction/treatments-people-diabetes

WebMD. (n.d.). *Erectile dysfunction guide.* Retrieved May 20, 2011, from www .webmd.com/erectile-dysfunction/guide/ed-diabetes

Wong, R. V. (2010, March 17). *Iluvien: New drug for diabetic macular edema.* Retrieved May 20, 2011, from www.retinaeyedoctor.com/2010/03/iluvien-new-drug-for-diabetic-macular-edema

PART II

Diabetes Self-Management

What I wanted most as a newly diagnosed diabetic was a set of rules to help me live with this chronic illness. As I left the doctor's office that day of diagnosis, I wondered what in the world I could fix for dinner that evening. Because I was diagnosed as an outpatient, I had not benefitted from a consultation with a registered dietitian. So I bought a diabetic cookbook. By dinnertime I had decided that what we usually ate was going to have to do. At my next office visit, I asked to see a dietitian and was told my insurance would not cover this as an outpatient. I told my doctor that he had two choices: he could teach me what I needed to know about my diet or he could request a dietary consult. So for a fee of $16 per hour, I consulted first with one, then a second registered dietitian, learned the standard instructions, and then picked their brains for rationale and "what ifs" and received answers to most of my early questions. It has since occurred to me that if I had not insisted on that dietary consult to help me learn what I needed to know, I might still be floundering and overwhelmed. The second thing that occurred to me after this experience was that the rest of my education was up to me. What a scary thought, but at least I had a head start.

After about a year and a half into my life as a diabetic, a wonderful thing happened. I was asked, along with many others in Richmond, Virginia, who had type 1 or type 2 diabetes, to participate in a research project to see if diabetics could be trained to be better guessers of blood sugars, both high and low. At that point, glucose monitors were just becoming popular and affordable (but not small and not yet covered by insurance). I jumped at the opportunity. Toward the end of the 6-week session, the participants and I were communicating with each other more than the researchers were. I asked if the other participants wanted to continue to meet as a support group. The response was overwhelming. Because I needed a support group and there was none in my area, I started one. I led this group for 7 years, well after it had met my personal needs. I learned how desperate people and their families are for any advice and education, as well as an opportunity to share their story. This all came about by dumb luck, but if it weren't for dumb luck, some of us would have no luck at all.

In the American Diabetes Association's latest *Standards of Medical Care in Diabetes—2011*, the following quote gives healthcare professionals direction: "People with diabetes should receive medical care from a physician-coordinated team. Such team may include, but is not limited to, physicians, nurse practitioners, physician assistants, nurses, dietitians, pharmacists, and mental health professionals with expertise and a special interest in diabetes. It is essential in this collaborative and integrated team approach that individuals with diabetes assume an active role in their care" (ADA, 2011). From this stated intent of the American Diabetes Association that diabetes care is not the business of the medical provider alone, it is clear that the client with diabetes is, or should be, an integral part of this team. In order for this to happen, all healthcare practitioners must be informed about diabetes and help the client and/or his family become as knowledgeable as possible about diabetes self-management. Healthcare professionals are also in a unique position to help clients with diabetes get a better handle on controlling their diabetes. Here are a few examples of how each of you can empower them.

Nurses see clients with diabetes in hospitals, clinics, long-term care facilities, physician's offices, and multiple other point-of-care facilities. You can make a huge difference in people's lives if you let them tell their stories. Ask them about their diabetes and how this disease affects how they live; their medications and how they take them; when they test blood sugars and what they do with the results; and a number of other questions suggested in the following chapters. Ask questions before you make assumptions and before you start teaching so you can individualize your care and this teaching. You may have a client like me who has a lot of answers or you may be assigned one who knows very little. We both need you to help us put the pieces of the current puzzle together so we can understand how whatever brings us to you affects our diabetes and vice versa.

Social workers and psychologists might treat depression, anger, guilt, or other psychological problems in clients who also have diabetes. In fact, diabetes may be the cause of these emotions or these strong emotions may complicate diabetes management by increasing glucose levels or decreasing a client's energy or willingness to monitor food choices, participate in physical activity, and check blood sugars. A review of the client's diabetes management and how emotions relate to control might be a good starting point in dealing with both problems.

Dentists, dental hygienists, and periodontists understand the connection between diabetes and gum disease, dental caries, and mouth infections. You may have a golden opportunity to increase a client's knowledge base about diet, exercise, and how to handle hyperglycemia, which may motivate him or her to work harder at glycemic control. By detailing the connection between high blood sugars and dental problems, gum infections, and eventual tooth loss, the client may be motivated to prevent further dental problems by controlling blood sugars.

Opticians, optometrists, and ophthalmologists often see clients with diabetes before and after they begin to have problems with diabetic retinopathy. By asking your clients how often they test blood sugars, what these glucose levels usually are, and what they do about them may illicit many issues with regard to the client's understanding of diabetes management. A few suggestions about counting carbohydrates and including exercise in their daily regimen might increase a client's understanding about the connection between high blood sugars and possible decreasing vision.

Podiatrists and other foot care specialists have a ready-made invitation to improve glycemic control in clients with diabetes by asking these clients open-ended questions about how their lives are impacted by this disease. Everyone has a different answer to that question, which usually illicit factors that get in the way of diabetes self-management. These may range from lack of knowledge to fear of complications and beyond. Starting a dialog about when they check their feet and how, may reveal that they do not check or that they cannot see the soles of their feet due to arthritis or visual impairment. Suggestions about the placement of mirrors for visual inspection of their feet and use of a magnifying apparatus may improve compliance.

Dietitians and nutritionists often are asked to teach clients with newly diagnosed diabetes about what they should eat. Most start any instruction by asking the client for a 24-hour dietary recall that can assist in assessing current eating habits that may range from good to horrible. Disregarding the need to investigate the client's prior eating habits and simply teaching from scratch is typically not productive. A person who fries everything will not be willing to avoid doing so for the rest of his or her life, even if you explain why this is important. Working with the client towards a gradual shifting away from fried foods may make it easier for the client to accept this change.

Pharmacists fill many prescriptions for diabetes medication both oral and injectible. It is important to check for drug-to-drug interactions and occasionally ask for a list of over-the-counter meds and herbal remedies. When clients pick up their medications presents an opportunity to review their meds, and how they work, when they should be taken and why, and note any side-effects they should look for. Reviewing foods that interact with drugs should be discussed as well. Giving clients written generic instructions in lieu of a face-to-face talk is often a waste of paper. Written instructions may be too long and not written for a lay person's ability to comprehend. Meeting face-to-face for a few minutes can start a personal relationship that might help a client feel comfortable enough to ask a nagging question about his or her diabetes management.

Over the years I have seen various physical and occupational therapists for treatment after trigger finger release surgery, for a partial frozen shoulder, and to increase mobility in my arthritic knees. Most therapists have asked about my diabetes control, my latest A1c, and what I do for exercise. These are great starting points to encourage someone with diabetes to be more open about his or her life with diabetes. As a physical, occupational, or speech therapist, you see your clients often over a few weeks or longer. During this time you could also discuss signs and symptoms of hypo- and hyperglycemia and how a client treats these occurrences. You might suggest better methods, such as always carrying glucose tablets or limiting carbs at a meal if a blood sugar is over 200 mg/dl or complimenting the client on a well thought out plan. Encouraging someone to test glucose levels more often may illicit a discussion about the cost of strips. A referral to a community outreach source or suggesting a cheaper strip or purchasing outlet may be in order. If you treat someone after a stroke or upper extremity injury, you should ask about any difficulties with glucose testing and suggest a more user-friendly meter for them. The American Diabetes Association lists meters and other diabetes paraphernalia every year in the Diabetes Forecast. This resource guide can be found in the January issue at http://forecast.diabetes.org/magazine/features/2011-consumer-guide.

The chapter on noncompliance is a "must read" for all healthcare professionals who deal with clients with diabetes. There are many reasons why a client appears to be "noncompliant." Don't dismiss their "failure to follow directions" as noncompliance. Ask yourself if you could or would make the changes that you are asking your client to make for the rest of your life. Ask them some of the questions that I include in this chapter to assess the reasons for their behavior. Then deal with these reasons or refer them to someone who can. This may include someone who can get them free glucose strips, to a psychologist who can help them overcome feelings of inadequacy or guilt. Using the threat of chronic complications is rarely a good strategy for improving compliance.

I hope that the chapters in this section of the book inspire healthcare practitioners in any field to use opportunities to teach clients what they desperately need and want to know about how to live with this chronic illness that affects every minute of their lives. How you respond to their questions, their silence, their sarcasm, even their noncompliance will let them know if you are the one that they can finally talk to. Maybe their dumb luck is having you as their healthcare professional.

SEVEN

The Healthcare Professional as Teacher

The roots of true achievement lie in the will to become the best that you can become.
    —Harold Taylor

Healthcare professionals wear many hats, perform many functions, and fulfill many roles. These facts contribute to our immense value and also to our greatest challenges. The most important impact nurses and other healthcare professionals can have on any client and the client's family is to teach them how to promote health and prevent illness. I believe in the old saying, "If you give a man a fish, you feed him for a day. If you teach him how to fish, you feed him for a lifetime."

The American Diabetes Association (ADA), in its 2011 *Standards of Medical Care in Diabetes—2011*, states, "Diabetes is a chronic illness that requires continuing medical care and ongoing patient self-management education and support to prevent acute complications and reduce the risk of long-term complications. Diabetes care is complex and requires that many issues, beyond glycemic control, be addressed" (ADA, 2011, p. S11). Some of these issues will be addressed in the next few chapters.

Students in all of the healthcare disciplines are taught the importance of client teaching. As busy clinicians, however, the more objective clinical skills seem to matter most. Unless there is a physician's order for "diabetic teaching," it is easy to overlook this very important aspect of client care. It is also easy for healthcare practitioners to make assumptions about what clients know based on how many years they have lived with the disease. We may reinforce behaviors when clients choose "correct" foods on the menu, state what each of their medications are used for, or give insulin appropriately. However, most nurses administer insulin and other medications that clients and/or their families give at home without conducting a full assessment about this part of their overall self-care. Many dietitians fail to ask clients who cooks or does the grocery shopping for them; obtaining this information from the client is important so the cook and food shopper can be included in the client's dietary teaching. Patients who complain, ask too many questions, or who are demanding may be labeled as "difficult" or worse. When blood sugars are too high, nurses and others in healthcare may assume clients are "cheating" or are *noncompliant*.

CLINICAL EXAMPLE: I once asked a 30-something type 1 diabetic patient, whom I had assigned to one of my clinical students, why she thought her fasting blood sugars had been so high since she had been hospitalized. She started crying and stated that she was not "cheating" or guilty of the other accusations nurses and doctors had made since her admission. After explaining that she was the recipient of a transplanted kidney, that her sight was deteriorating, and that her ultimate goal was to live long enough to experience her only child's graduation from high school, she looked at me and said, "Why would I jeopardize that by eating candy?" So I started from scratch and conducted an assessment of her insulin regimen at home. The answer to the puzzle of high fasting blood sugars became obvious when the mixed dose of regular and NPH insulins she took at home before dinner was not being carried out in the hospital where she was receiving only regular insulin prior to dinner. In addition to being a type 1 diabetic with virtually no basal insulin being produced by her own pancreas, she was taking antirejection medications, including prednisone and cyclosporine, both of which elevate blood sugar. At my urging, her nurse called the physician, who promptly added NPH to her evening dose. This interaction took me a maximum of 10 minutes. On reflection, I was upset with myself that I had not taken this professional step a few days earlier when I first learned of the problem. I allowed myself to believe the "cheating" scenario without first investigating or questioning the reporting nurses about the facts that had led them to this conclusion. Because nurses drew up the client's insulin in the medication room and administered it to her, the client never realized the error, and the nurses, including me, never questioned the inappropriate lack of a second dose of NPH with the evening meal for this patient. This was an important lesson for me about giving care without appropriate and individualized assessment data.

WHAT DO CLIENTS WITH DIABETES NEED TO KNOW?

Before healthcare practitioners can impact diabetes self-management, we need to have a clear understanding of exactly what someone with diabetes and their family need to know in order to take care of himself or herself. Redman (2004, p. 66) lists the following self-management tasks required to successfully control diabetes:

1. SMBG levels
2. Daily medications (insulin and/or oral agents)

3. Nutrition—eating regularly and controlling weight
4. Regular physical exercise
5. Recognizing early symptoms of hypo- or hyperglycemia and responding appropriately
6. Adapting medication dose and timing to account for blood sugar levels, food intake, and activity level
7. Checking feet regularly for lesions
8. Getting frequent blood pressure and cholesterol checks
9. Getting periodic eye and renal function tests

Of these tasks, the first five are crucial and should be taught with the initial diagnosis and reviewed with each client encounter. The other behaviors can be added to what is discussed with the client if time permits or at a later date if the client is seen regularly. Many clients cope with the threat to their health that a new diagnosis brings with a desire to do their own research. In their research, clients should be directed to seek information from the ADA (www.diabetes.org) and the JDRF (www.jdrf.org). When doing any Web-based research, clients as well as healthcare professionals should include the current year after the search term so the latest information is seen first.

ASSESSMENT GUIDELINES

We all should know that assessment is the first step prior to deciding what care is needed. Most acute care institutions have a multipage patient questionnaire that is completed by the admitting nurse. Many outpatient facilities, clinics, healthcare practitioners' offices, pharmacies, etc. use some form of written assessment or medical history tool. Some of the data in these forms are collected in an objective format with yes/no answers from the client and/or family. All assessment forms should require a patient list of medications with dosages and usual times of administration. Also needed are questions about who administers the drugs, the timing with regard to other meds and food, the client's knowledge of the drug's purpose, and his or her thoughts concerning the drug's effectiveness. These follow-up questions ought to be asked and charted whether or not there is a line for such responses on the questionnaire. However, even the best assessment data are only good if they are read and used by every practitioner who delivers care to this individual. If care is not individualized, then such assessment tools serve only to meet The Joint Commission (TJC) requirements and those of other accrediting agencies but do not help meet the client's or family's needs. Perhaps if this assessment form were placed in front of the patient's chart or computerized, more practitioners would read it and use the information more appropriately in their care for the client.

GOALS OF CLIENT EDUCATION

Identifying goals or expected outcomes is paramount in planning care for clients. "The overriding goal of patient education should be to support the patient's autonomous decision making, not (as it has been conceptualized) to get the patients to follow doctor's orders. . . . True patient autonomy requires creating new options to meet patient needs, not just as is now frequently the case, having the right to refuse a treatment option" (Redman, 2004, p. 7). When discussing patient autonomy and decision making, it seems imperative to use the word client rather than the word patient. In order to increase client autonomy in our pattern of healthcare delivery, we all need to view individuals and families who seek healthcare as people with options. They should be able to freely choose which healthcare providers, healthcare facilities, and healthcare management systems best suit their needs and values. This should give them the power to change providers or refuse to follow any part or all of the medical management provided. Most people would agree with this.

CLINICAL EXAMPLE: When I attempted to practice autonomous decision making a few years ago, prior to elective surgery, I met with considerable obstacles and bewilderment by healthcare providers. I insisted on interviewing the anesthesiologist who was scheduled to provide anesthesia during surgery to discuss my request for an epidural as opposed to general anesthesia. In addition, I also discussed my pain management requests with him. I then interviewed the unit manager where I would be transferred after surgery in order to discuss how her staff might handle occurrences having to do with high or low blood sugars. I requested my own vials of insulin to be kept at the bedside because I wanted to draw up and administer my own insulin unless I was unable to do so. I also stated that I would use my own glucose meter and have my own supply of 6-ounce cans of orange juice and glucose tablets at the bedside. My compromise with this unit manager was to report to her staff any insulin or orange juice administered and to use their meter along with my own as ordered and at any other appropriate times. My diabetologist provided orders for the above to ensure that my need to be in control of my diabetes was met. My surgery and the resulting care I received were as positive an experience as possible because my anxiety level and my blood sugars were under my control.

Clients who are inexperienced with healthcare might not be able to anticipate potential problems with a pending hospitalization or surgery. They also may not be as assertive as necessary to customize their care appropriately. However, the healthcare professional can ask pertinent questions about how the client and/or family envision the hospital stay or agency care to help the client articulate concerns and make them feel like they are part of the team. If the client is an adult or an adolescent, he or she should be asked before family members are involved in the assessment and teaching.

Data Gathering for Customizing Client Care

Healthcare providers should ask questions that pertain to their discipline, such as some of the following:

1. "How would you like your medications given and by whom?"

This might involve a discussion by the nurse or pharmacist about the purpose and timing of each medication and allow for the client or a family member to administer the medication under supervision to assess technique. Even if the client requests that the nurse or pharmacist gives injections, the client ought to be observed doing this at least once before leaving the setting.

2. "How do you know you are having a low blood sugar and what do you usually do about it?" If in a hospital or other inpatient facility, ask "How would you like us to handle this?"

This might involve treating a low blood sugar level first and doing a blood sugar level test after or allowing the client to treat a low blood sugar and notify us after the fact. This would decrease the anxiety the client might have concerning delayed treatment. It could also involve a discussion of signs and symptoms and possible treatments unknown to the client. The rule of 15 (15 g of carbohydrates, wait 15 minutes) should be taught to prevent overtreating a low blood sugar.

3. "How often do you usually test your blood sugar? Who do you want to do them? What are the ranges of blood sugar that you aim for fasting, premeal, and at bedtime? What do you do if the blood sugar is too high at these times?"

This might involve a discussion of when blood sugars have been ordered. They may be more or less often than the client expects. If a sliding scale insulin is ordered, the client should be informed. The client may be upset that he or she might get insulin or may be dismayed that the sliding scale only starts at a blood sugar of 200 mg/dl.

CLINICAL EXAMPLE: I shared that I was writing this book with a group of insulin pump users. Before I could ask them what they wanted me to include, they all started telling me of their most recent experiences in hospitals and/or rehabilitation agencies. Most were angry either that they had to turn off their pumps and go back to shots or that their personal range for normal was disregarded. Sliding scale insulin started too high, ordered insulin doses did not account for carbohydrates in a meal or the timing of meals. In other words, they were treated as generic patients and felt they had no autonomy in controlling their diabetes. One person stated that his recovery from cataract surgery was delayed, not because he had diabetes, but because his diabetes was poorly managed in the hospital and that he was not consulted in developing his plan of care. He was angry at the doctors and their inadequate orders and the nurses who did not listen to his needs and good sense. "They should have called the doctor when the insulin ordered did not control my blood sugars."

Nurses and all healthcare professionals should be client advocates. It is a given that most clients on insulin pumps are a special group: they test often, make multiply daily management decisions based on blood sugars, value tight control, and are very knowledgeable about how diabetes affects them. This group wanted me to encourage nurses and other healthcare professionals to ask, in addition to the above three questions, the following question:

4. "Tell me how you control your blood sugar with your insulin pump? How can I assist you in doing this?"

This might involve advocating for them with the physician, who may want to discontinue pump use. It might also involve the nurse learning more about insulin pumps in general and this client and his or her pump in particular. Letting the client explain what he or she is doing and why will serve both the practitioner and client well (Chase, 2005, p. 55).

INTERVENTIONS USING LEARNING PRINCIPLES

No matter what reason brings a client with diabetes to your outpatient or inpatient facility, you must assess and evaluate the client's understanding of diabetes self-management. In fact, if diabetes has contributed to the client's admission, this may be an opportune time to increase his or her knowledge of how to recover and prevent reoccurrence. This is what is called a *teachable moment*. You have the client's attention and can teach new information or review material he or she may have ignored in the past. Figure 7.1 outlines some learning principles that guide patient teaching. The critical ones include:

- "People learn best those things that hold particular interest for them."
- "Learning occurs most quickly if a person can see how new information will benefit him" are particularly relevant here. Clients who have had a wake-up call usually are eager to avoid a repeat of this incident. See Figure 7.1 for other learning principles that should guide any teaching.

Learning occurs only when a person is ready to learn.

Learning occurs most quickly if a person can see how new information will benefit him or her.

Adults learn best when new information builds upon preexisting knowledge.

Adults learn best when rationales are explained at their cognitive level.

People learn best those things that hold particular interest for them.

People learn best by active participation.

Learning is more likely to take place in a nonstressful and accepting environment.

Learning occurs best if rewards, not penalties, are offered.

Learning ability plateaus and time is needed to process information already learned before there is interest and motivation to learn more.

Source: Reprinted with permission from Mertig, R. G. (2003). *Teaching nursing in an associate degree program* (p. 71). New York: Springer Publishing Company.

FIGURE 7.1 Learning Principles for the Adult Learner

Anyone with diabetes who needs the care of a healthcare provider should expect to learn more about his or her body, health, nutrition, and diabetes. That means that nurses and all healthcare professionals who treat clients with diabetes need to stay current by attending workshops, reviewing professional journals, and reading books like this one and/or updating our knowledge periodically on the Internet. Some of the steps to good client-centered teaching include the following:

1. Before attempting to teach anyone, a healthcare provider must assess prior knowledge and readiness to learn. Even if the client's readiness is in doubt, do something to get that person's attention. Preparing insulin with the client watching while providing commentary on the necessary steps used and the rationale for each will, at least, peak his interest. Letting a client know that prior to leaving this setting he or she will be expected to draw up and deliver his or her own insulin will certainly give the client a reason to pay attention to what you are doing. The same goes for a review of medication by a pharmacist, compiling a diet history by a dietician, or asking about exercises performed by a physical therapist before adding new ones. Building on preexisting knowledge by asking questions about technique, injection sites, medications, food groups, etc. will demonstrate your respect for the client's knowledge and ability and increase his or her self-esteem by individualizing your approach.

Giving what I call the "canned speech" ignores the client's individuality, causes resentment, and worse, may lead to the client tuning out instructions instead of listening for "pearls" that he or she did not know. By getting clients to explain their understanding of what they have learned so far, you are evaluating their interpretation of what you have told them for correctness and completeness. It gives you an opportunity to reward the client for his or her knowledge base and attention, make adjustments and updates, and fill in where gaps in knowledge exist. This should be done whether the client has a lot of knowledge, none at all, or falls anywhere in between. The canned speech fits no one, is usually too limited, and is often done when a client is leaving, which is the worst possible time to teach. Another learning principle states: "learning plateaus and time is needed to process information already learned before there is interest and motivation to learn more"; therefore, teaching should be done from admission to discharge and at multiple intervals during all of the outpatient procedures and short hospital stays a client might experience.

Begin with a review of what the client/family already knows, move from simple to complex, encourage questions or concerns, and recognize the need for repetition. If they have some knowledge, you may also want to start with what they really want to know, where they might be confused, or what their fears for the future are. As you gain their trust, develop a positive therapeutic relationship, and, most importantly, make them feel included in developing outcomes and planning what should be taught, it is more likely that they will learn and remember what was taught. See Figure 7.2 for a questionnaire that I have used to assess a client's attitude toward diabetes, his or her knowledge base, and what he or she thinks is most important.

2. Healthcare professionals must explain everything they do or assist clients in doing, such as giving insulin or testing blood sugars, and must give rationale for these actions at the client's cognitive level using methods that he or she has identified as ways in which he or she learns best. The client may prefer to watch videos on technical skills or read about procedures with pictures depicting each step. Handouts reinforce what has been taught, increase a client's sense of self-confidence, and reduce anxiety, as the client can take written material home as reference material. Many clients prefer to watch a live demonstration several times and then redemonstrate with guidance until they feel confident that they can perform the task on their own. This cannot be done adequately when they are ready to leave.

3. Because "people learn best by active participation," involving the client in redemonstrating skills or repeating signs and symptoms of hypo- and hyperglycemia, as well as actions that should be taken when these occur, helps to solidify what has been taught. Using a client's past experiences can provide an occasion to praise the client for good problem solving when things went well or help the client to rethink his or her decisions to better resolve a similar situation in the future.

Problem solving is often one of the most difficult skills to teach, and yet it is the key to appropriate and effective self-management. Redman (2004) recounts a study of a low-income, inner-city population, comparing those

Please complete the following sentences with as many answers that apply describing your feelings and knowledge base about diabetes.

1. I have had diabetes for _____ years/months.
2. In my opinion, diabetes is a (circle as many as apply)

    challenge   opportunity   learning experience   curse   death sentence
    disaster   doable   family problem   no big deal   wake-up call

    Other_____

3. I feel that my diabetes control is

    terrible   improving   good   excellent

Please rate your knowledge about the following from 1–4.

1 = none   2 = minimal   3 = average   4 = very knowledgeable

4. My knowledge about diabetes is   1   2   3   4
5. My knowledge about a healthy diet is   1   2   3   4
6. My knowledge about exercise and diabetes is   1   2   3   4
7. My knowledge about my diabetes   1   2   3   4
    medications is (insulin and/or pills)
8. My knowledge about high and low blood sugars is   1   2   3   4
9. My knowledge about foot care is   1   2   3   4
10. My knowledge about long-term complications is   1   2   3   4
11. My knowledge about blood sugars is   1   2   3   4
12. My family's knowledge of diabetes is   1   2   3   4
13. With regard to controlling my blood sugars, I would describe myself as

    motivated   discouraged   confused   aggressive   apathetic
    compulsive   fatalistic   don't care   angry   optimistic

14. Most of my information about diabetes comes from

    _____

15. I would like to know more about

    _____

16. What would help me the most to improve my diabetes control is

    _____

17. The biggest problem I have in controlling my diabetes is

    _____

18. I would like my healthcare provider (MD, nurse practitioner, diabetes educator) to

    _____

19. I learn best with (circle as many as apply)

    discussion   written material   computer material   videos
    demonstration   hands-on   support group   audio tapes

20. I would describe my self-management of diabetes as (circle only one)

    Nonexistent   following the rules   hard work   part of living

21. What worries me the most about having diabetes is _____
22. My idea of a good blood sugar is

    _____before breakfast   _____before lunch   _____dinner   _____at bedtime

23. Diabetes has affected my life by

FIGURE 7.2 Diabetes Mellitus Client Questionnaire

with good disease control to those with poor control. They all had similar problems, complaints, and concerns about their disease state; however, "Those in good control showed good problem-solving skills, reflected a positive orientation toward diabetes SM [self-management], and a rational problem-solving process, and actively used past experience to solve current problems" (Redman, 2004, pp. 67–69).

4. Timing is everything. "Learning is more likely to take place in a non-stressful and accepting environment," so make sure the client is not in pain or worried about a test or procedure unless what you teach will decrease the client's anxiety. Simply asking if this is a good time to discuss a topic demonstrates respect and sets the stage for a positive interaction. Make sure it is truly a discussion with input from the client and/or family and not just another lecture. If it is never a good time for a certain client, then the approach might be, "Mr. Smith, we need to discuss how your medication works. Would you like to do this before or after I fill your prescription or you finish your therapy, or whatever?" This way you give the client options you can live with.

5. Ask the client what he or she would like to learn first or most. "Learning occurs most quickly if a person can see how new information will benefit him," so providing a short list and letting the client set the agenda, including questions and concerns, allows you to tailor your information to the client's specific learning needs at this time in his or her life. Giving a client some real-life scenarios to ponder will help him or her to use what he or she already knows or has just learned in new and different ways. Ask questions like, "What would you do if you realized that you were having a bad low blood sugar?" The client may have already experienced this, or you may need to help the client plan for such an event by suggesting that he or she always have a fast-acting, simple sugar with him or her. A follow-up question might be, "What if this happened when you were driving?" A question like this helps to develop problem-solving skills.

6. Another area of concern may be the financial impact of the cost of medication and supplies. If this is not expressed by the client, ask, "What would you do if you realized you were going to run out of your diabetes medication before you received your next paycheck?" It would be important for you to help the client troubleshoot this potential problem. Consequences of not taking the appropriate dose of medication due to cost need to be emphasized, and a new approach needs to be thought out, from borrowing money to getting a partial refill from the pharmacist until the client can pay for the rest. The client may also qualify for free or reduced-cost drugs from the many companies that offer such assistance. Refer the client to the Partnership for Prescription Assistance at http://pparx.org. See Chapter 4 for a list of other websites related to patient medication assistance.

7. "Learning occurs best if rewards, not penalties, are offered." Praise goes a long way in reinforcing positive behavior at any age. Evaluating a client's responses to questions and his contribution to the discussion in a positive manner will increase his or her self-esteem and sense of accomplishment. Thank the client and his family for their attention. Make an appointment with them to continue the discussion and work on other learning needs.

EVALUATING TEACHING

Teaching is never completed until learning has been evaluated to determine whether teaching efforts have been successful. Learning is best demonstrated by a change in behavior, ability, or attitude. When a client learns what has been taught, the client's behavior changes. The healthcare professional can ask questions to evaluate how a client feels about himself or herself and his or her ability to cope with chronic illness and how those feelings or coping abilities have changed as a result of teaching.

CLINICAL EXAMPLE: When I became a participant in the research group described at the beginning of Part II, I was asked how I felt about my diabetes. Some of the options included crisis, catastrophe, curse, death sentence, demoralizing, and disaster, as well as challenge, opportunity, new beginning, learning experience, wake-up call, no big deal, and doable. Although I chose "disaster" to describe how I felt about my life with diabetes that first day, I changed it to "challenge" at the end of the 6 weeks. I had learned so much about how to tell if my blood sugar was high or low that I felt I could learn to control this disease and still live the life I wanted to live. My attitude and my outlook had been changed, thanks to the knowledge I had acquired.

With short stays in an acute care facility or outpatient teaching opportunities, the behavior change that you would be able to evaluate might not be so dramatic, but getting the client to choose among some of the options listed above provides a current status of the client's feelings compared with how the client felt at the time of your first meeting. Before clients leave, ask if they feel they have a better handle on diabetes self-management. This, of course, requires a yes or no response. No matter which answer they give, ask the follow-up question "In what way?" (Asking "Why?" puts most people on the defensive because they are being asked to justify their prior response.) A positive answer might indicate growth. Other means of evaluating learning have already been discussed, such as return demonstrations of glucose monitoring or insulin injections and asking for symptoms of hypo- or hyperglycemia. Questions about when the client would call the doctor or dial 911 might evaluate his or her knowledge of what is serious as opposed to what he or she could handle. Asking questions about food choices and how the client might fit in food items important to him or her would give you both some idea of how important the client feels nutrition is to his or her overall well-being. It can be as simple as asking, "What do you intend to change about your diabetes self-care at home?" "What have you learned while you were here that might prevent your returning?" or "In what way has the information you have received changed you?" You may find that your goals and the client's goals were incompatible, not met, or only partially met. At this point it is time to reassess. Ask about what could have been done or said differently. What was missing? What needed more time or more practice? Then refer the client to diabetes websites, a diabetes educator, and/or give him or her written material, whatever is appropriate for this client. Encourage clients and their families to join the ADA. Part of the fee pays for the very informative *Diabetes Forecast,* which helps increase self-management skills, keeps clients updated on new drugs, new tests, examples of how to increase their activity level, and new dietary guidelines, and includes recipes and all sorts of appropriate information for anyone along the road to living life to the fullest despite having diabetes. Obviously, evaluation of learning is an ongoing process and is not best achieved as the client heads out the door. It is also a great way to evaluate your own skills at teaching diabetes self-management. If something works well, continue to use it with other clients and add variations to your teaching methodology so that you can adapt it to different clients. On the other hand, if something is not working after several tries with different individuals, then change it or look for a new approach. No one is perfect, and some clients really do not want to learn to take care of this disease or at least not at this time. Either way, it should always be considered a growth opportunity and should be valued.

Most of my preparation for writing this chapter consisted of reviewing materials written for advance practice nurses and diabetes educators. Yet how many clients have an opportunity to sit down with a nurse practitioner or diabetes educator for the purpose of reviewing aspects of their diabetes care? It is likely that most clients with diabetes and their families encounter nurses and other healthcare providers at the doctor's office or clinic, in acute care and long-term care facilities, or at the pharmacy or physical therapy site. How much better educated would they be if each healthcare professional were as knowledgeable as possible about diabetes care and willing to implement the steps listed above to individualize patient teaching? The immediate and long-term learning needs of clients who have to live with and make daily healthcare decisions about this chronic illness would more likely be met. Providing the tools of self-management for our clients is mandated so they can stay healthy. Working ourselves out of a job *is* our job.

REFERENCES

American Diabetes Association. (2011). Standards of medical care in diabetes—2011. *Diabetes Care, 34*, S11–S74.

Chase, P. (2005, September). Don't take my pump. *Diabetes Forecast, 58*(9), 55–58.

Mertig, R. G. (2003). *Teaching nursing in an associate degree program.* New York, NY: Springer Publishing Company.

Redman, B. K. (2004). *Advances in patient education.* New York, NY: Springer Publishing Company.

EIGHT

Teaching and Motivating Children With Diabetes and Their Parents

Parents learn a lot from their children about coping with life.
—Muriel Spark

WHAT IS IT LIKE TO HAVE A CHILD WITH DIABETES?

It was the middle of January when Kearsten started to wonder what was wrong with her 2-year-old son, Brennan. He was frequently soaking his diaper. In addition to that, he would stand at the refrigerator with his hand on the door screaming, "I'm thirsty, Mommy! I'm thirsty." It took about a week of this continuing behavior for Kearsten to suspect the worst—that Brennan had diabetes. Kearsten's ex-husband was a diabetic, and she knew that the signs of frequent urination and excessive thirst were classic symptoms. At first, she tried to ignore the signs, thinking it was just a phase her son was going through. However, over the course of the second week, Brennan seemed to be getting worse. She noticed her son's jeans were getting very loose, and his complexion was poor. Finally, she couldn't ignore the signs anymore.

Kearsten took Brennan to the doctor on a Thursday afternoon. She told the doctor of his symptoms and that Brennan had had a stomach virus right after Christmas. The doctor said he would run some tests, but he doubted Brennan had diabetes. After all, he was only 2, and that was awfully early for children to be diagnosed with diabetes. Kearsten went home, hoping she was wrong and that it was something minor. But on Saturday morning, she received a phone call from the doctor. Her worst fears had come true; Brennan's blood sugar was in the 200s, and he had diabetes. Kearsten was told he needed to go to the hospital right away. Her doctor made arrangements for the family to take Brennan to the hospital in Richmond, about an hour from her home. She called her parents, and her stepfather took Brennan's twin brother, Patrick, home. Her mother then drove Kearsten and Brennan to the hospital.

On the way there, Kearsten was in shock. She knew diabetes was something terrible. Her ex-husband hadn't taken care of himself, and he was already suffering from health problems at the age of 28. She blamed herself because she knew that the disease was genetic, and she had had children with a man who was diabetic. She had always known it was a possibility, but she was hoping it wouldn't happen to either of her babies. Kearsten kept thinking, "How could God do this to my beautiful baby? How will I be able to cope with taking care of a diabetic?"

Brennan was checked into the hospital, where he was immediately given a shot of insulin. Because he was so young, he stayed in a tall crib with bars that reminded Kearsten of a jail cell. Sometimes she lowered the side rail and crawled into the crib just to hold him and stay close to him. She stayed with him that night and every night for 4 days. It was hard to accept that he had this diagnosis when he seemed okay. During his stay, he flirted with the nurses and had the run of the halls. But Kearsten roamed those same halls and saw the really sick babies, and she accepted the truth.

On the second day, Kearsten gave Brennan his shot. The nurses kept saying the shot would go in very easily, but it was one of the hardest things his mother had ever done, and she knew eventually he would have to do it every day, and for the rest of his life. While in the hospital, Kearsten met with dieticians, nurses, and doctors. She learned Brennan's eating habits would not have to change too much, as she had always tried to serve nutritious meals. She also learned how to test Brennan's blood, where to give him shots, and what to do if his blood sugars went too high or too low. Brennan's father and his family also came to visit Brennan in the hospital. His father cried, as he also blamed himself for Brennan having diabetes. Even though Kearsten knew it was really no one's fault, it was still hard to be kind to him because she was so angry.

After the 4 days in the hospital Kearsten's family came to get her and Brennan. They were making the trip home, and Brennan's blood sugar was better, but Kearsten knew this was only the beginning of a very long, difficult journey. She kept thinking of what her ex-husband's mother had once told her. She said, "It's so hard to know your child may die before you." Now Kearsten had those same thoughts about her own precious son. How was she going to handle the day-to-day challenges of having a child with diabetes? Kearsten also had a special challenge; how was she going deal with her son as a twin? Brennan had diabetes, but Patrick did not. How was she going to be fair while still accepting the fact that her two children had very different needs?

The day parents discover their child has diabetes is one of the worst days of their lives. All sorts of question, fears, and doubts come to mind. Will he or she be okay? Will I be able to give shots? How much does it hurt to test blood? What changes do I have to make to his or her diet? Will my child be able to enjoy holidays like Halloween and Easter? What will

I even do about birthday cakes? And HOW WILL I MANAGE IT ALL? Being a parent of diabetic child is a challenge at any age, but each stage has special needs that parents must understand.

AGES AND STAGES

Baby/Toddler Years

Parents of very young children with diabetes deal with one of the most difficult challenges. Healthcare professionals need to alert parents that young children lack the ability to communicate how they feel. For example, sometimes it is even difficult to be aware the child is showing symptoms of diabetes. A parent may not be aware his or her child's overly wet diaper or constant drinking is a sign of diabetes, unless that parent is already familiar with the signs. Frequently, a baby or toddler must be pretty sick in order for the parent to take the child to the doctor.

Once diagnosed and sent home from the hospital, parents not only must learn how to initially treat the disease but also must become *detectives* when trying to determine how the child is feeling. "Is my child showing signs of low blood sugar? Is he or she acting 'high'?" It is very difficult to figure this out when the child is unable to use words to communicate with his or her parent. Many parents of babies, toddlers, and preschoolers are in constant contact with their nurses and physicians, simply because they can't tell. Parents should keep a log of questions they have and call the nurse weekly for answers and clarification.

Nurses should remind parents that they know their child better than anyone. For example, one child may cry uncontrollably over something he or she would never cry about, and this could mean the child is "low."

Other children may become sleepy or cranky or even angry. Still others will show signs of low blood sugar physically rather than emotionally. They may appear shaky or unstable. Maybe it's a look in the child's eyes that only the parents understand. Parents must have more faith in their ability to know that something is wrong and use these clues to figure out what it is. This is difficult because their child was just diagnosed with something new and scary. To parents, it feels like they are bringing home that tiny newborn baby all over again.

At the point a child is diagnosed, it is important for nurses to assess parent expectations of their healthcare professional. Get to know their personality. Some parents may want exact instructions, whereas others may need the freedom to experiment with what works for their child. Attention to these details will put parents more at ease, making the transition to diabetes management easier for the patient, the child's parents, and the whole family.

Parents must become familiar with the signs of low and high blood sugars in general and then determine what applies specifically to their child. See Table 8.1 for signs and symptoms of hypo- and hyperglycemia in a young child.

The School-Age Child

In this stage, it is very important for all parents to remember they have rights within the school system. Whether entering school with a child who has been previously diagnosed with diabetes or whether a child who has been in school has been recently diagnosed, schools are responsible for the care of the child enrolled. This is the law!

TABLE 8.1

Signs and Symptoms of Hypoglycemia and Hyperglycemia in Children

HYPOGLYCEMIA	YOUNG CHILD	HYPERGLYCEMIA	YOUNG CHILD
Tremors, shakiness, jerky movements	Same	Excessive urination	Soaked diapers or accidents if potty trained
Dizziness, feeling faint, headache	Lethargic, unable to sit up	Excessive thirst	Crying for more fluids
		Excessive hunger	Craving sweets
Sweating, pale moist skin	Same	Headache	Crying more than usual
Excessive hunger	Craving sweets	Sleepiness	Sleeping longer than usual
Mood swings or erratic behavior	Irritability	Difficulty concentrating	Not able to do usual tasks
Tingling or numbness	Difficult to assess	Visual disturbances	Difficulty focusing
Difficulty paying attention, confusion	Same	Dry or flushed skin	Same
Visual disturbances, dilated pupils	Dilated pupils	General malaise	Crying without relief, irritable
Increased heart and respiratory rates	Same	Weight loss	Same
		Fruity breath	Same, sweet odor to urine
Seizures and coma	Same	Coma	Same

For those children entering school with diabetes, it is imperative for parents to inform the school beforehand and meet with the professionals in charge of the child's care. This includes the school nurse, the regular education teacher, the physical education teacher, and any other educational professional deemed necessary by the parents and school. At this time, a plan will be devised to most effectively manage the child's diabetes (ADA, 2010). There are three basic types of plans within the schools.

It is currently the position of the JDRF that all type 1 diabetic students, from elementary school to highschool, obtain a 504 Plan. A 504 Plan is a legal agreement between the student and a school to ensure the child will be able to participate in all activities while having his or her diabetic needs met (JDRF, 2011). Even if the child's school is currently meeting the student's needs, it is advised to have one in place in case a problem arises in the future. The 504 Plan ensures the child's medical and educational needs are met. For example, a child who is not allowed to eat a snack in the classroom may miss valuable class time leaving to eat, and consequently, the child's grades may suffer. A 504 Plan would suggest the child eat the snack in class so as not to miss valuable instructional time. This plan can be accessed at www.diabetes.org/living-with-diabetes/parents-and-kids/diabetes-care-at-school/written-care-plans. In addition another useful resource for issues related to school-aged children with diabetes is Lawlor and Pasquarello's "School Planning 101", which can be accessed at www.diabetesself management.com/articles/kids-and-diabetes/school_planning_101/4/.

Section 504 of the Rehabilitation Act of 1973 is a civil rights law that prohibits disability-based discrimination in all programs that receive or benefit from federal financial assistance. If a parent wishes for a 504 Plan to be put in place, the parents first contact the guidance department of their child's school. At that time, a team will meet to determine if a 504 Plan is necessary. The team usually consists of the parent(s), guidance counselor, regular education teacher, school nurse, and other necessary school personnel. It is important for parents to remember they have the right to a 504 Plan if they feel it is necessary to avoid any discrimination due to diabetes. A 504 Plan may include many of the guidelines put in place by the Diabetes Medical Management Plan (DMMP); however, a 504 Plan is a legal document, and the school must comply with it by law (ADA, 2009). In addition, the 504 Plan can be used in most colleges and universities; however, the procedures may change. Typically, it is the student's responsibility to inform the school that a 504 Plan exists. Colleges and universities expect diabetic students at this age to be their own advocates.

Diabetes Medical Management Plan

The DMMP is a plan that includes information on who is responsible for diabetes management, instructions on how to handle emergency situations, specific instructions for how to deal with levels of high and low blood sugars, and basic "rules of thumb" on how to deal with the child's needs. For example, one parent might wish to be called if the blood sugar is lower than 70. However, another child's DMMP may state to simply give the child a snack and check blood sugar in 15 minutes. The DMMP is usually included with a 504 Plan as it contains pertinent information from the child's healthcare team. See Table 8.2 for content that should be on a DMMP. A parent who is interested in obtaining a DMMP should call the ADA at 1-800-DIABETES (342-3837) or go to www.diabetes.org/living-with-diabetes/parents-and-kids/diabetes-care-at-school/written-care-plans/diabetes-medical-management.html to download the form.

Individualized Education Plan

An Individualized Education Plan (IEP) is for those diabetic students who have special educational needs that affect the child's academic performance. Many children with diabetes who have an IEP are labeled as Other

TABLE 8.2
What Should Be Included in a DMMP

DIABETES MANAGEMENT	INSULIN	MEAL PLANNING
What type of meter is used?	What type(s) of insulin does the student take?	What time does the student eat lunch?
Where is the meter stored and used?	Where is the insulin stored?	Does he or she eat a school lunch or bring lunch from home?
Who writes down monitoring results and where?	How is the insulin stored?	Is there a plan if the student refuses to eat lunch?
How should parents be informed of blood glucose results and treatments?	How is the insulin dose determined?	Who is responsible for making sure the student eats a snack?
What are the blood glucose target ranges?	When is insulin administered?	Does the school restrict where food can be eaten?
What action is to be taken if the blood glucose level is outside the target range?	Who administers insulin?	Can snacks be eaten in the classroom? If the whole class has a snack, how will the student with diabetes be accommodated?
Are ketones to be checked?		Are there classroom parties or special projects that involve food?
At what blood glucose level should ketones be checked?		If so, what are the guidelines and accommodations for the student with diabetes?
By whom should they be checked?		
What should be done with information on ketones?		

Health Impaired (OHI). This means that diabetic-related complications significantly affect the child's ability to learn. For example, a child with extremely fluctuating blood sugars may have difficulty paying attention in class, which in turn would affect his or her ability to learn. With an IEP, accommodations such as extra time on assignments or repeating of directions will be put into place to help improve the child's performance.

Putting an IEP into place is a process that takes some time. Usually, a child must be referred for an initial meeting. Those present usually include the same team as that needed for a 504 Plan, in addition to a school social worker and a school psychologist. Several components are then needed to determine if the child is eligible for an IEP. These may include a medical history and exam, interview of the family by the school social worker, teacher evaluations, classroom observations, and various diagnostic tests given by the school psychologist. The team will then reconvene to determine the significance of the data. If a significant discrepancy is found between learning ability and achievement, then the child will qualify for an IEP.

The IEP will include goals to improve the child's educational performance. Within these goals accommodations will be created. The DMMP serves as a good basis for the goals. An IEP is a legal document that must be reviewed once a year. The parents also have the right to review the goals and make changes at any time if they are not pleased with their child's performance or the plan is not meeting the child's needs. An example of an IEP can be retrieved from www.diabetes.org/living-with-diabetes/parents-and-kids/diabetes-care-at-school/written-care-plans/.

The DMMP, 504 Plan, and IEP are all plans designed to ensure the best care for a child with diabetes. It is the right of the parents to decide which plan(s) is (are) the best for their child.

The Prepubescent Child

As if diabetes were not enough of a challenge itself, children between the ages of 9 and 12 have a whole new set of challenges. After all, they are about to become teenagers!

For those children aged 9 to 12 years who have been diabetic for some time, parents are frequently lulled into thinking their child is capable of taking on his or her own diabetic care. The healthcare professional should remind parents that while most children are capable of performing the daily medical tasks, they are not emotionally ready to assume all the responsibility for their care. For example, almost all diabetic children at this age are able to test their own blood and even give themselves an injection. However, a 9-year-old probably will not be able to correctly measure the insulin for the syringe, especially if half units are necessary. Children in this age group are also not able to comprehend how serious it is to measure the appropriate amount and the consequences of giving themselves too much or too little insulin.

The prepubescent child is also prone to "cheating" or "sneaking," as it is sometimes called. This is the age of peer pressure, and many children want to be "normal" and eat junk and sugary foods. Parents must be mindful of cheating, and healthcare professionals should advise them to keep a close eye on their child's blood sugar levels, but it must be handled while still respecting the growing independence of their child. Some parents allow their child to test his or her blood, but the parents record the readings. By doing this, parents can see if there are highs at certain times. If so, then the child should be asked what might have caused the high reading. If high blood sugars become a pattern, then parents must work to find the underlying cause (Schmidt, 2003).

For example, a child consistently has high blood sugar readings at dinner. After some discussion, the parents find that their child walks home with a group of children who like to buy extra pies and candy at lunch in order to have something to eat on the way home from school. When offered the snacks, she eats them because she is too embarrassed to tell her friends she is diabetic and can't eat them. This results in an extremely high blood sugar at dinner.

What should a parent do in this situation? First, parents must remember their child is human, and all people, including parents themselves, eat food they should not. No one is perfect at all times, and children are desperate to fit in with their peers. It is important not to blame the child. Once the child is caught, he or she usually feels badly enough without adding on extra guilt. The best approach is to sit down with the child and talk about why the child cheated. Find out the underlying cause of the cheating and acknowledge it. If it is due to peer pressure, parents must be empathetic and explain that they understand the importance of fitting in with friends. In the case of peer pressure, parents must continually remind their child of the importance of keeping blood sugars under control in order to best take care of his or her body. Perhaps the child is going through a growth spurt and is seriously hungry at that time of day. If so, then parents should work with the child to incorporate an appropriate snack into his or her meal plan so that cheating is no longer necessary.

Sometimes children at this age are starting to rebel against the fact that they have diabetes. They become angry with their situation and decide to ignore the consequences of not taking care of themselves properly. Parents may need to enlist the support of someone outside the family, such as a teacher, nurse, guidance counselor, or coach, to provide positive support to the child. These people may be able to gently steer the child back on to a more rigorous management plan for his or her diabetes. It is important for parents to remember that these behaviors are normal for their child's age and that diabetes is simply another area that will involve the normal growing pains of independence and questioning of authority.

Another Child in the Family Is Diagnosed With Diabetes

It was the summer of 2006, and Patrick and Brennan were turning 10. Ever since Brennan had been diagnosed with type 1 diabetes in January 1999, the possibility of his twin brother Patrick developing it loomed in the back of Kearsten's mind. Every time Patrick seemed to be drinking or urinating more than usual, she would pull out Brennan's test kit, and it was always normal. Waiting for the result to appear on the screen would be an anxiety-filled 5 seconds, followed by a rush of relief. Kearsten did this frequently for the first couple of years after Brennan's diagnoses, but as time wore on she became complacent in her concern. His father's family had several people with diabetes, but Patrick and Brennan were not identical twins, and the chances of Patrick developing diabetes were only approximately 5%. She kept telling herself there was a 95% chance he wouldn't develop diabetes, and those were very good odds!

Kearsten had noticed throughout the summer that Patrick was drinking more than usual, but it was extremely hot with many days over 100°, so she told herself he was justifiably thirsty and nothing was wrong. The family continued enjoying their summer: playing at the pool, attending swim meets, and planning the boys' 10th birthday celebration. Ever since the boys were 6, the family had been visiting local theme parks instead of having birthday parties, and this year was no different. On July 23, just 2 days before their birthday, they spent the entire day at King's Dominion. All day long the boys enjoyed rides, splashed at the water park, and ate all sorts of junk food. The family had pizza, fries, drinks, ice cream, snow cones, and anything else their hearts desired. Throughout the day Kearsten managed Brennan's diabetes, giving him the extra insulin he needed to enjoy his special day. The family arrived home late that night after a wonderful day, and everyone fell into their beds completely exhausted.

The next morning was sunny, and Kearsten woke up fairly early. She wanted to enjoy some alone time before the boys woke up. However when she walked into the living room she was surprised to find Patrick asleep on the sofa. Kearsten woke him and asked why he was sleeping downstairs. Afraid his mother would be angry, he sheepishly said, "Mommy, I kept having to wake up all night to pee, and I finally peed in the bed." Immediately, Kearsten's mind flew to diabetes. She was terrified to test him, but she had to know the truth. Kearsten pulled Brennan's test kit out of the kitchen drawer and told Patrick she wanted to test his blood. He sat up, put out his finger, and patiently waited for his mother to prick his finger. Kearsten could see the worry on Patrick's face, but he didn't say a word. Waiting for the numbers to appear was awful, but it was nothing compared to actually seeing them. His blood sugar was over 300. Kearsten's world fell apart; Patrick most certainly had diabetes. Patrick said, "What is it?" She looked at him and spoke the words she never wanted to utter, "Patrick, honey, you have diabetes."

Kearsten looked at him, and the tears started for both of them. She hugged him, and he sobbed. He told his mother he had always told his Nana that the one thing he never wanted was diabetes. As for Kearsten, she was in shock. She couldn't believe it was happening again to her other sweet child. Wasn't one child with diabetes enough? Why was God doing this to her family? She was angry and so incredibly sad for her baby.

Kearsten immediately called her mom and the boys' father to tell them the news, and then she called Patrick's pediatrician. As soon as family arrived to take care of Brennan, Kearsten drove Patrick to the doctor. She kept hoping that maybe she was wrong, maybe Brennan's meter wasn't calibrated, maybe he had something on his hands to cause the high blood sugar, but unfortunately the pediatrician confirmed the mother's finding. The pediatrician called Brennan's doctor for the family, and they left for Patrick's first appointment with a diabetic specialist.

Patrick, his father, and Kearsten spent over 6 hours with the specialist that day. She was pleased to find out Patrick wouldn't have to spend the night in the hospital. Kearsten already knew how to take care of a diabetic, and Patrick was very familiar with the routine. Kearsten admits to being a complete wreck though. She was in a daze of denial and spent much of the day in tears or in a fog. At some point her mother told her she had to pull herself together for Patrick and get over it. That day she couldn't bring herself to do it, and she felt like a terrible mother. Kearsten was the one who was supposed to be a rock for him, and she didn't have the strength.

Patrick, on the other hand, was amazing. He cried and was angry, but he handled it well. The day after his diagnosis Patrick began injecting himself, and Kearsten has not given him a shot since. It's almost 5 years later, and he still refuses a pump, stating that he "doesn't want a machine to control his body." He is shaving now, active in sports, a good student, and rarely ever misses school. Patrick is a great kid. Sure, he still gets angry, forgets to record his blood sugars, and thinks having diabetes is unfair, but he lives with it and doesn't let it control him.

The family's life is good, but it's hard. Kearsten's stepbrother once told her it was normal to be angry and question God after what her family had been through. After that first day of Patrick's diagnosis she was able to move on and be the parent her son needed. The boys have two different regimens, and it's difficult to keep track of them. Kearsten certainly wouldn't call herself the best mom of a diabetic. The family does their best, and that is all the family can ask. Kearsten only hopes she has raised them to be responsible with their diabetes as adults because she wants to enjoy her sons for a long, long time.

Diabetes and the High School–Aged Child

Dear Jane,

This is Oliver! I no longer live in Hawaii but I got your letter and I will still talk to you about how I feel about being a dietbetic. It is probably the most stressful medical problem a 14 year old could have. Because everybody will always be on your tail so that you will do what is proper. One way I think will make a dietbetic's life easier is for a cure, but it won't happen soon. But to me the best treatment for dietbetes is having friends, parents, doctors, and even strangers supporting you, helping and always being there for every little thing. But this disease has brought frustration, stress, anger, and lots of problems for me. It is like having a parol officer on your tail. You know what I mean checking in at a certain time just to put a shot on, check your blood sugar, and trying not to cheat on your diet by eating delicious looking foods. And another way people can help make a dietbetics life easier is by making more sugar free selections that taste good and don't cost a fortune. And put more organizations for kids, teens, and adults in more states. Well, hope you have a successful career. And don't forget these are my opinions only. I only talk for myself not others, Bye!

Your Friend,

Oliver

This letter from Oliver to Dr. Kadohiro (2000, p. 81), in her journal article "Diabetes and Adolescents: From Research to Reality," states what almost every teen with diabetes feels. Above all, teens want to fit in with their peers, assert their independence, and obtain flexibility in their daily activities. Unfortunately, these goals run contrary to the goals of tight blood sugar control; thus teens begin to rebel and become lax in their diabetes management. And honestly, what teen wouldn't rebel? As Oliver said, "It is like having a parol(e) officer on your tail." Parents and healthcare professionals must recognize and remember the difficulties of simply being a teen, let alone a teen with diabetes. Healthcare professionals need to assist parents in the transitioning relationship of primary care giver to helpful coach of their diabetic children.

In addition parents need to recognize teens with diabetes will change in their attitudes. Those children who were comfortable with people knowing about their diabetes may want to keep that information hidden from their peers. As stated in Attitude Changes by McCarthy and Kushner (2007), "The girl who once simply clipped her pump to her belt and let it hang out there now painstakingly finds way to hide it. The boy who whipped out his meter on the sidelines at Little League now wants to check only in the car and not bring his meter with him." All of the normal challenges discovered in raising a teenager can be applied to diabetes as well.

Parental Missteps

All parents ultimately want their child to be happy and healthy; however, many parents have no idea how to achieve this. Do any of these parents sound familiar?

The *overanxious* parent does everything for the child. He or she is in complete control of the diabetic child. This creates an overanxious child who becomes dependent on the parent and is not capable of managing his own her own diabetes (Rossini and Lundstrom, 2010, p. 5). For example, the overanxious parent may make all meals, including packing the child's lunch and preparing the daily injections for the child and bringing it to the dinner table. He or she will then write down all blood sugars to ensure accurate records are being kept. The diabetic child of the overanxious parent is frequently also overanxious and often does not learn self-care management because the parent has done everything for the child.

The *overindulgent* parent feels sorry for the child with diabetes and feels that injections and dietary restrictions are too difficult for the child to handle. The children of overindulgent parents feel ill equipped to cope with their diabetes and feel inadequate (Rossini and Lundstrom, 2010, p. 5). They frequently are not able to understand the consequences of their actions.

The *perfectionist* parent is overly concerned with diabetes management. When the child is young, parents may obtain success with discipline. As the child of a perfectionist parent grows into a teenager, the child may rebel against the parent and his or her diabetic regimen. Also, the child may feel guilty about high and low blood sugars and begin lying to the parent about food or blood sugar testing (Rossini and Lundstrom, 2010, p. 5). For example, a parent may notice his or her child is not recording blood sugars. In an effort to improve recording, the parent tells the child he or she will be grounded if blood sugars are not recorded, so the child complies. At the child's next appointment, it is discovered the child's HbA1c is very high. The doctor notices the recorded numbers appear to be in the normal range, so he downloads them from the child's meter and sees that the numbers don't match. The child did not properly record high readings and made up numbers when forgetting to test in order to avoid punishment from the perfectionist parent.

The *indifferent* parent is not an active participant in the child's diabetic regimen. He or she gives too much control to the child for a number of reasons, perhaps frustration on the parent's part or the feeling of being overwhelmed. Children of these parents may become depressed or seek attention by skipping insulin injections or not following the diet. Also children of indifferent parents have a higher occurrence of hospitalization.

How can parents avoid these traps? Research shows that the more open and caring the parent is with the child, the better the child's management of his or her diabetes. Parents need to work together with their child, the school, and healthcare professionals to create a team in which the child is able to successfully transition to the lead role in his or her own diabetes management. Dr. Wysocki (2002, p. 2), chief of the Division of Psychology and Psychiatry at Nemours Children's Clinic in Jacksonville, Florida states, "Parents who actively supervise the diabetes management skills of their younger teens, who praise and encourage success and proficiency while offering gentle remedial instruction when needed, and who solve diabetes problems with, rather than for, their adolescents are more likely to find these transitions to be smooth."

However, this is easier said than done for parents who are in the middle of experiencing the teenager who exhibits poor control over blood sugars. It is easy to understand why parents may scold or negatively question the child in regards to testing and blood sugars. Parents worry about their children and want what is best for them, so they are understandably concerned when their children do things that could hurt themselves, such as skipping insulin doses or forgetting to test blood sugars. As healthcare professionals, it is important to be supportive of the parents as well as the patient. Remind parents to be positive and open with their child, but tell them no one can be perfect. Reinforce to parents that more children have positive outcomes if they grow up in a family who has the following characteristics:

- Diabetes management is seen as a vehicle to accomplish broad life goals, rather than being defined more narrowly.
- Loved ones' concerns are expressed through warmth and empathy, and the adolescents become comfortable with relying on the support of others. There is more praise and admiration for self-care success and effort than there is criticism and punishment for self-care failures.
- Diabetes responsibilities are transferred actively to the adolescents for the right reasons rather than as a result of parental burnout.
- Parent-adolescent communication is frequent, mutually respectful, and constructive rather than conflictual and destructive. (Wysocki, 2002, p. 3)

High School Sports and Diabetes

Today, many athletes with diabetes are able to compete at the top level of their sports. Professional football quarterback Jay Cutler, pro basketball player Adam Morrison, and Olympic gold medalist swimmer Gary Hall, Jr. are just a few of the growing number of diabetic athletes (Black, 2009). While exercise is important to the health of a diabetic, there are special concerns that the high school athlete with diabetes, the coach, school nurse, parents, and diabetic's team must address in order to ensure a safe and successful season.

Responsibilities of the Student Athlete With Diabetes

In high school, the student with diabetes plays a more active role in his or her diabetes management. Students at this age should be a part of the healthcare team that creates and revises the DMMP. It is especially important to communicate with the coach by telling him or her about diabetes, the symptoms of hypoglycemia and hyperglycemia, and when the student is feeling high or low blood sugars. Students should also wear medical alert bracelets and keep fast acting glucose close in case of a low blood sugar. In addition, the athletes should also carry their insulin and necessary supplies with them at all times. Most athletes have a bag to carry their equipment; and diabetic athletes should pack their glucose meters, insulin and supplies, and easy-to-carry snacks such as crackers, glucose tablets, and juice boxes. They need to remember to restock these supplies as they are used and check their bags regularly, especially when they travel for games and events. Healthcare professionals need to discuss these responsibilities with their patients and provide tips on how to self-monitor variations in blood sugar when exercising (National Diabetes Education Program, 2010, p. 95).

Responsibilities of the Parent or Guardian

Parents and guardians of diabetic athletes need to remain in contact with the coach and other healthcare team members, especially if their child is participating in sports. Initially, they should talk to the coach and inform him or her about their child's condition. They should ensure the school nurse provides the coach a copy of the DMMP and includes symptoms and care for high and low blood sugars. Parents can also create a portable "snack box" for the coach to keep on hand, both at practice and during sporting events, in case the athlete has a low blood sugar. Finally, parents need to notify the coach if there are any changes to the student's diabetes management (National Diabetes Education Program, 2010, pp. 93–94).

Responsibilities of the Coach of a Diabetic Athlete

When coaches first discover they have a diabetic athlete, they may initially be nervous in regards to the student's care. Coaches should initially visit the school nurse for a copy of the DMMP and discover the amount of care they may be expected to provide and receive the proper training for that care. They must also be aware of the signs of hypoglycemia and hyperglycemia and be able to treat it immediately; therefore, appropriate supplies should always be carried in the first aid kit. In addition, it is the responsibility of the coach to treat students with diabetes the same as any other student, except in regard to their medical needs. Diabetic athletes need to have permission to monitor their blood sugars and give themselves insulin as directed in their DMMP. As coaches develop a relationship with their athletes, they may notice changes in behavior that could be indicative of blood sugar changes in diabetics. Coaches need to watch for these signs and ask the students to check their blood sugar. Finally, coaches need to be aware that low blood sugars frequently occur during exercise, so they need to keep an eye out for signs of hypoglycemia in the diabetic athlete (National Diabetes Education Program, 2010, pp. 83–84).

Responsibilities of the School Nurse

The school nurse acts as the ultimate link between parents, the student, and the coach. He or she is responsible for providing the diabetic care guidelines created by the personal healthcare team and the school health team. The school nurse should meet with the coach to review the student's plan for an emergency situation, train the coach in how to treat medical emergencies, and recognize symptoms for which the coach should watch during practices and sporting events. The school nurse should also verify the coach has the proper diabetic supplies for the student, both at school and for times when the student is off campus. At school the nurse is the chief advocate for the student and needs to keep the lines of communication open between the student, his or her parents and health providers, and the teachers and coaches with whom the student comes in contact (National Diabetes Education Program, 2010, p. 75).

Responsibilities of the Healthcare Professional of a Diabetic Athlete

Healthcare professionals play an important role in the care of the diabetic athlete in high school. They should be available to speak to the school nurse as the school's main advocate for the child. In addition, the healthcare professional must remind the athlete and parents that special care needs to be taken to watch for signs of blood sugar changes, especially hypoglycemia, during exercise. Sports such as football and swimming can affect a diabetic differently, and the healthcare professional should provide various kinds of plans for the differing levels of physical activity. Ultimately, it is the responsibility of the healthcare professional to ensure both diabetic athletes and their parents or guardians that not only can diabetics participate in athletic activities, but they can excel in them. If the proper precautions are taken by diabetic athletes, their parents, and their school; students can compete at the top level in their sport, maintain proper health, and enjoy the same physical activities as their peers (National Diabetes Education Program, 2010, p. 21).

There are many resources for teachers, child care providers, parents, and health professionals. For a comprehensive list and directions for obtaining copies, call the ADA at 1-800-DIABETES (342-3837) or visit the ADA's website for Diabetes Care at School at http://www.diabetes.org/living-with-diabetes/parents-and-kids/diabetes-care-at-school/.

AN APPOINTMENT AT THE PEDIATRIC ENDOCRINOLOGIST

Kearsten left the pediatric endocrinologist appointment with her boys yesterday, determined not to cry this time. After sitting in the small office for over 3 hours with her two teenage sons, she felt disheartened and thought she was a terrible mother. Yet again, the boys' HbA1c levels were not where they should be; Patrick's was at 8.2, up 0.2 from the last appointment, and

Brennan's was 8.0, down 1.0 from the last appointment. Kearsten felt most of the appointment was negative and overly critical of herself and her sons.

First, the diabetes educator came in to talk to them. She delivered the news of the HbA1c levels with much criticism and no positive interaction. She continued by reminding Patrick and Brennan of the threat of not being able to get their license if they were unable to get their levels under control. When it was time to check Brennan's numbers and noticed his basal levels were not complete, she immediately told him he had to fill in the numbers himself and hastily handed him the paper. Brennan, with a shocked look on his face, told the educator that he was told they could be filled out during the appointment if he didn't have the time to do it himself. She told him, "Nope, nope, nope," and even handed him the paper back when he had missed a line. Kearsten understood the educator was trying to teach Brennan how to do these things himself, but the educator could have done this in a more positive manner. Kearsten was also thinking that clearly the educator had no understanding of Brennan's learning disability in writing.

About 30 minutes later the doctor arrived. Both Patrick and Brennan love their doctor because he is the first doctor they have seen who has diabetes himself. He wears a pump and understands all the frustration of being diabetic. As usual the doctor was firm but kind with Brennan and Patrick. He explained the advantages they have over his other patients because they are athletes, and he wanted them to use their swimming to their diabetic advantage to get their HbA1c levels down to more acceptable numbers.

After Kearsten and her sons had been in the examining room for well over 2 hours, the final doctor came in to exam them. She was kind, but she was clearly criticizing both Kearsten and her sons in regards to their diabetes management. Kearsten was asked why she wasn't more involved in her sons' diabetes as she seemed to be more involved several years ago. Immediately, Kearsten was put on the defensive and explained that she felt overwhelmed when Patrick was diagnosed and chose a different regimen than his brother. Then she remarried, had a daughter, and was currently extremely busy trying to raise two teenage sons and a toddler while working full time. The doctor told Kearsten she needed to take a more active role in her children's diabetes, and she needed to sit down with them every 2 to 3 days to discuss the trends and patterns in her sons' blood sugar after she put her daughter to bed. She was also told her sons must wake up in the middle of the night to test their blood at 12:00 midnight and 2:00 a.m. Again, Kearsten was wondering how she was going to do this. She was already so tired, and she only had one alarm on her clock and didn't want to wake her husband by turning on the light.

The doctor was more positive with Patrick and Brennan. She told them it had been her experience that athletes with diabetes performed much better when their blood sugars were under excellent control. She charged the boys with testing her theory by improving their control and thus swimming faster times. Kearsten was hopeful this challenge would do the trick. For the first time in years, Patrick and Brennan seemed truly interested in an idea regarding their diabetes. Kearsten felt like she had tried everything she knew with her sons, and maybe this would be the tactic that would finally work with them to manage their diabetes better.

After the appointment, Kearsten rode down the elevator with another mom whose child was about 4 years old and had just been diagnosed with diabetes. She was frantic because the appointment had taken so long, and now her son wouldn't have dinner at the precise time and his blood sugar would be high. Kearsten told the mother not to worry too much. There was this thing called life that would get in the way of managing her son's diabetes perfectly, especially as he got older. Kearsten told the mother not to expect perfection, but to remember she could only do the best she could do. The mother thanked her, and Kearsten could tell the woman was happy to have someone to talk to who could understand.

Kearsten went home that night and cried after the boys went to bed. She felt like such a terrible mother because she knew there were things she should be doing better regarding her sons' diabetes, but she didn't know how to implement them. She felt so alone and inadequate, but she was going to do her best to improve.

A REQUEST TO HEALTHCARE PROVIDERS FROM A PARENT OF A DIABETIC

Parents worry about their children all the time; it is their job. Parents of children with diabetes worry about their children a great deal more on a daily basis. Additionally, many parents of diabetics feel anxiety as the time approaches for their child's appointment with their pediatric endocrinologist. Parents are under a great deal stress as they wait for that elusive HbA1c number, and they fear the repercussions from the healthcare provider if that number is higher than it should be. Nurses, doctors, and educators need to remember that being a diabetic is really hard, but it is also hard being the parent of a diabetic. They need to remember empathy and to be supportive and positive while still being honest with consequences and care. Many parents feel alone and would appreciate information on support groups for parents of juvenile diabetics. Remember to give them and their children compassion no matter how well or poorly their child's diabetes is managed.

REFERENCES

American Diabetes Association. (2009, December 30). *Diabetes care in the school and daycare setting*. Retrieved April 18, 2011, from http://care.diabetesjournals.org/content/33/Supplement_1/S70.full?ijkey=f013bb43f4c1f54a97a307e4b024a1117a218d9b&keytype2=tf_ipsecsha

American Diabetes Association. (2010). *Your school and your rights*. Retrieved May 18, 2011, from www.diabetes.org/assets/pdfs/schools/your-school-your-right-2010.pdf

Black, R. (2009, December 28) Juvenile diabetes and sports. In *Quality health*. Retrieved April 1, 2011, from. http://www.qualityhealth.com/diabetes-articles/juvenile-diabetes-sports

JDRF. (2011). *JDRF position statement*. Retrieved April 20, 2011, from http://www.jdrf.org/index.cfm?page_id=107280

Kadohiro, J. (2000). Diabetes and adolescents: From research to reality. *Diabetes Spectrum, 13*(2), 81–82. Retrieved April 1, 2011, from http://journal.diabetes.org/diabetesspectrum/00v13n2/pg81.htm

Lawlor, M. T., & Pasquarello, C. (2004). School planning 101. *Diabetes Self-Management, 21*(3), 69–74.

Managing diabetes in young athletes. (2009, August 10). In *UW Health*. Retrieved April 20, 2011, from http://www.uwhealth.org/news/managing-diabetes-in-young-athletes/20715

McCarthy, M., & Kushner, J. (2007). Attitude changes. In *Netplaces*. Retrieved March 30, 2011, from http://www.netplaces.com/type-1-diabetes/teen-issues/attitude-changes.htm

National Diabetes Education Program. (2010). *Helping the student with diabetes succeed: A guide for school personnel*. Retrieved April 1, 2011, from U.S. Department of Health and Human Services. http://www.ndep.nih.gov/media/Youth_NDEPSchoolGuide.pdf

Rossini, A. A., & Lundstrom, R. (2010). *The healing handbook for persons with diabetes*. Worcester, MA: University of Massachusetts Medical School. Retrieved April 20, 2011, from http://www.umassmed.edu/healinghandbook/chapter13/index.aspx

Schmidt, C. (2003). Mothers' perceptions of self-care in school-age children with diabetes. *MCN: The American Journal of Maternal/Child Nursing, 28*(6), 363–370.

Wysocki, T. (2002, January). Parents, teens, and diabetes. *Diabetes Spectrum, 15*(1), 6–8. Retrieved April 1, 2011, from http://spectrum.diabetesjournals.org/content/15/1/6.full

NINE

Teaching and Motivating Adolescents and Their Parents

Nobody can make you feel inferior without your consent.
—Eleanor Roosevelt

In the United States, about 215,000 individuals under age 20 are living with diabetes, primarily type 1, although type 2 cases are increasing yearly (American Diabetes Association [ADA], 2011). The expected developmental struggles and transitions of adolescent life are complicated by the necessity of managing diabetes. New issues may arise when adolescents who are accustomed to living with the disease begin to assert their independence and seek more autonomy in self-management. New onset diabetes can present even more complex challenges. Recent landmark studies have emphasized that maintaining glycemic control during adolescence is critical in preventing and delaying long-term complications of diabetes (Anderson, Svoren, & Laffel, 2007). Adolescents and their families need guidance and support to adjust to new or evolving health concerns.

Adolescence is a time of rapid physiological, cognitive, psychological, and social changes that also requires adaptation within the family system. Physiologically, the onset of puberty is accompanied by dramatic hormonal shifts that drive the obvious physical changes, as well as the often intense and unpredictable fluctuations in mood that characterize the teen years. Cognitively, adolescents begin to develop new problem-solving skills, think more abstractly, and test previous assumptions about the world. They begin to develop a personal sense of morality and values and attempt to define and express their identity as individuals. Although they can visualize and plan for the future, many adolescents tend to be quite present-oriented, with little consideration for long-term consequences of their behaviors. Impulsivity and a sense of invulnerability may contribute to a willingness to take risks. Increasing importance is placed on self-image, sexuality, and peer acceptance. Family relationships are being redefined and boundaries renegotiated. If family relationships are dysfunctional prior to adolescence, the problem is compounded. Previously stable relationships may become more unpredictable.

What do these changes mean in terms of diabetes management? First, the physiological changes associated with adolescence are believed by many clinicians to contribute to blood glucose fluctuations and insulin resistance, making consistent glycemic control in this population more difficult to achieve (Rosenberg & Shields, 2009). This is important to keep in mind because diabetes management involves such a focus on adherence. Parent and adolescent education that includes information about these responses can prevent erroneous assumptions by parents that adolescents are being irresponsible with self-care, and feelings of incompetence on the part of the adolescent.

Unfortunately, other manifestations of adolescent development more typically complicate matters. The desire to be spontaneous, conform to social norms, and avoid appearing different can lead some adolescents to take risks with their health. The normative developmental movement toward independence and individuality that contributes to parent–teen conflicts in general may be enacted in various aspects of diabetes management. Even teenagers with type 1 diabetes who are knowledgeable about their condition and have been compliant with treatment regimens may exhibit sudden shifts in attitude and behavior that are a cause of alarm to parents and healthcare providers. Teenagers may want increased responsibility and control in managing their condition and resent the degree of dependence on parents and healthcare providers that is necessary to help ensure their ongoing wellness (Anderson et al., 2007). The response to perceived interference may be rebellion against regimented treatment protocols. However, allowing adolescents to assume full responsibility for their diabetes management too soon can be risky. To achieve optimal outcomes, healthcare providers must foster a genuine collaboration with adolescents and their families to plan for the transition to increased adolescent autonomy (Paterson & Brewer, 2009). This collaboration serves several purposes: to prepare the adolescent to assume total responsibility for self-care as an adult; to reassure parents that the adolescent has the resources and competence to make appropriate decisions; and to increase the likelihood that adolescents will adhere to treatment regimens.

THE TRANSITION TO SELF-CARE

The ADA recommends a gradual transfer of responsibility for carrying out tasks related to the management of diabetes, progressing through middle and high school, with continued parental involvement throughout the process (ADA, 2005). Some adolescents are quite enthusiastic about increasing their self-care roles, whereas others may be less confident, especially those who are newly diagnosed. The changing roles can be anxiety-producing for everyone, even if the transition is mutually viewed as necessary and desirable. Parents who have been helping their child to manage their diabetes for many years may need help determining how much control to relinquish and when the adolescent is developmentally ready to assume more autonomy (Paterson & Brewer, 2009). This readiness differences by individual, and involves both cognitive ability and psychological motivation. Does the adolescent express a desire to take on more responsibility? Is understanding and competence in following the prescribed treatment regimen clearly demonstrated? Does the adolescent behave responsibly in other aspects of life? Are there intellectual or emotional situations that could impair the adolescent's ability to assume an increased role in self-care?

What is very clear is that adolescents with diabetes are healthier when parents remain involved in their care (Greening, Stoppelbein, & Reeves, 2006; Hoey, 2009). In fact, the decreased glycemic control often seen in older adolescents might in part be attributable to diminishing parental oversight. However, high levels of family involvement at a time when adolescents are increasing activities outside of the home, forming close relationships with peers, and separating from parents to assert their individuality, complicates the normal course of adolescent development. The challenge is to find the line between too much involvement and too little—not an easy task, and one that requires ongoing assessment and adjustment as the adolescent matures or healthcare needs change. Additionally, cultural norms and values surrounding parent–child relationships have to be taken into account and respected when assisting adolescents and their families to integrate diabetes management into the broader tasks of moving towards adulthood.

CLINICAL EXAMPLE: Western norms stress authoritative parenting, which emphasizes support and moderate control, whereas Chinese American parents tend to be stricter and less verbally demonstrative. Control is seen as a way of protecting children and emotional expression is considered unhealthy, so is discouraged. Consequently, their children may be more conscientious about self-care, but less likely to ask questions or express a desire to make independent decisions (Van Kampen & Russell, 2010).

Adolescent and parental perspectives may be quite different, requiring the provider to communicate and work closely with both to foster a healthy balance between autonomy and appropriate parental involvement. Part of this process is clarifying adolescent and parental roles and expectations of each other, and planning for regular review and reassessment as the adolescent matures or circumstances warrant. As responsible behavior is demonstrated, oversight can be reduced.

BALANCING PARENTAL INVOLVEMENT

Ideally, parental roles in diabetes management involve helping the adolescent stay motivated, helping with self-care tasks when necessary, providing support, and assisting the adolescent to problem-solve around issues that may arise as responsibilities for the self-care regimen are gradually relinquished to the adolescent (Greening et al., 2006). Just as adolescents who perceive relationships with parents to be warm, accepting, and supportive of their independence tend to achieve better health outcomes, poorer metabolic control is associated with adolescent perceptions of parental over-involvement and controlling behaviors (Hoey, 2009).

Coping with an adolescent is challenging for parents; coping with an adolescent with diabetes can be much more challenging. Parents of newly diagnosed adolescents will need education concerning their child's condition and its management (Paterson & Brewer, 2009). They may need reassurance that both they and their child are capable of coping with this new reality. Parents may need help determining how to incorporate the elevated needs of the adolescent with diabetes into the family structure and avoid treating the adolescent as "different" from siblings, which can lead to sibling conflicts. This is a good opportunity for healthcare providers to help foster an atmosphere of cooperation and closeness between parents and adolescents as they face the new situation together.

Similarly, it is important for the provider not to assume that parents experienced with diabetes management will require little support or education (Paterson & Brewer, 2009). Parents who have previously taken charge of their younger child's healthcare regimen may be anxious about relinquishing control—after all, their diligence is their way of showing love and caring for their child. As parent–adolescent relationships naturally become less cohesive, the degree of control that was successful in childhood is more likely to be counterproductive in adolescence, leaving parents frustrated and confused about how to respond. When there is an ongoing provider–family relationship, it can be helpful for the healthcare provider to broach the topic of shifting responsibilities at the preadolescent stage so that individuals and their families can anticipate the changes that adolescence will bring and be better prepared for what lies ahead. Including both parents in conversations, listening to them, and encouraging them to speak openly and strategize together can help avoid parental disagreements about the appropriate level of involvement with their adolescent's care, which can lead to conflict in the couple if their concerns, fears, or parenting approaches differ.

Assessing parents' feelings and perceptions about diabetes and the adolescent's competence to manage care can guide the healthcare provider's priorities for intervention. For some parents, close monitoring fills a need for some degree of control over a frightening circumstance. Fears about the implications of the illness and the often valid concerns that adolescents take these implications less seriously may make parents reluctant to share responsibility for care. Other parents may feel so badly for their child, or even harbor guilt about the genetic component of diabetes, that they hesitate to maintain expectations about behaviors aside from diabetes management, which may give tacit permission for limit testing in diabetes management also (Dahan & McAfee, 2009). Many years ago, Coyne, Wortman, and Lehman (1988) used the term "miscarried helping" for excessive parental attempts to provide care that undermined healthy adolescent development. Parents who are too attentive or overprotective concerning their child's illness can unknowingly reinforce excessively dependent behaviors. Alternately, some adolescents respond with resentment and sabotage their own care. Providers should take care that, while supporting the adolescent's autonomy, parents are not excluded from healthcare conversations, because feeling uncertain and inadequately informed can lead to anxiety and overly vigilant behaviors (Paterson & Brewer, 2009).

On the other hand, parental expectations that the adolescent will assume too much responsibility too quickly also result in poor outcomes. Most of the literature assumes that parents are willing and able to be collaborative partners in their adolescent's care. Circumstances such as single parenthood can make some parents less readily available, and parents who themselves have psychological problems or chronic illnesses may need additional support (Wysocki & Greco, 2006). Extended family members can sometimes become supportive allies.

In other situations, dysfunctional family dynamics prevent parents from offering adequate support. Family conflict, whether or not it involves diabetes-related issues, is associated with poor adherence and poor glycemic control (Anderson et al., 2007). Stress hormones triggered by family conflict can interfere with glycemic control, and conflict can directly interfere with performance of self-care activities. Referrals for counseling may be indicated for these families, or if they are unwilling to participate, the adolescent may need help developing additional support systems. In addition to extended family members, diabetes camps, teen support groups, or online forums with peer and professional participation (e.g., *www.diabetescommunity.dlife.com* or *juvenation.org*, a site sponsored by JDRF) can be useful resources to provide support and prevent a sense of isolation.

TEACHING AND PROMOTING ADOLESCENT ADHERENCE

Working individually with adolescents, in addition to working with them within the family setting, helps build trust and demonstrates respect for the teenager's desire for independence. If adolescents were diagnosed in early childhood, most of the education efforts have probably focused on their parents, so adolescents will need information and practice in learning the practical aspects of their diabetes management. Teaching coping skills related to managing stress, setting priorities, and problem solving in potentially awkward social situations will also help prepare teenagers to assume greater responsibility in their self-care (Greening et al., 2006).

Many new situations can arise during adolescence. Anticipating and developing problem-solving strategies ahead of time can be reassuring to both adolescents and their parents as new roles are being negotiated. Teens will be dating, going to social events, learning to drive, participating in sports, visiting friends' homes, and traveling—all can be enjoyed safely but may require planning and adjustments. Throughout adolescence, teens will also encounter peer pressure to participate in high-risk behaviors. It is important to discuss issues such as smoking and alcohol and substance use with all teens, but especially those with diabetes, as these behaviors have even more serious consequences for them. Choices about sexual activity is another topic of critical importance during this developmental stage. Like all adolescents, those with diabetes need access to sound information about birth control and risks of unprotected sex in terms of unplanned pregnancy and STDs, as well as the implications of diabetes and pregnancy (see Chapter 10 for more about pregnancy and diabetes).

Although you must tailor your interactions and teaching to each individual's cognitive level, avoid talking down to adolescents, and treat them as individuals who are separate from their illness and who are capable of making healthy choices (Gelder, 2009). These approaches will help counteract the tendency for adolescents to rebel in order to assert their own identity. Working collaboratively will permit a sense of control and increase your credibility. When teaching, use instructional methods that will stimulate and hold the adolescent's interest. Most teenagers are frequent and competent users of the Internet. You can direct them to websites where they will find accurate information about their illness (see the list at the end of this chapter). Online discussion groups can be a means of both information and peer support. Parents may find the Internet a valuable resource as well.

The importance of peers during adolescence means that group interventions may be particularly appropriate for teenagers (Plante & Lobato, 2008). Group interventions have been successful at addressing psychological adjustment and adherence, more so than consistently achieving glycemic control, but the enhanced well-being and positive habits that they promote may have implications for the future that have not yet been documented (Anderson et al., 2007). Support groups and camps can provide practical information, enhance motivation, and opportunities to interact with peers who share their health challenges. An additional benefit of camps is that they are usually held in the summer, a time when most adolescents' days are less structured and they may eat less regularly or become more sedentary (Wang, Stuart, Tuli, & White, 2008). Other adolescents and their families benefit from more structured group interventions focused on communication, stress management, teamwork, and conflict management (Anderson et al., 2007). Check local hospitals, clinics, pediatricians' offices, or newspapers to find resources in your area for children with diabetes and their families. Some resources are listed at the end of this chapter.

Unfortunately, an ongoing challenge among healthcare providers is how to target low income adolescents who lack access to comprehensive healthcare and may not have an ongoing relationship with a provider or appropriate parental involvement. Adolescents with type 2 diabetes who often have co-occurring conditions, such as hyperlipidemia and hypertension, but may not be experiencing immediate bothersome symptoms, frequently fall into this category. In such situations, it is imperative to be sure that adolescents and their families fully understand the risks associated with their illness and the need for ongoing monitoring (Reinehr, Schober, Roth, Weigand, & Holl, 2008). There are federal and state programs available to assist with funding medical care for minors, and families may need assistance completing required paperwork. Other philanthropic resources can be helpful in obtaining free diabetic supplies.

ADDRESSING NONADHERENCE

It is frightening, but normal, for adolescents to occasionally use poor judgment. When this occurs, it is best to remain calm and avoid responding harshly. This approach will foster an environment in which the adolescent is more likely to be honest, and will provide opportunities to talk about mistakes and discuss strategies for improvement. But what if, despite education and appropriate parental support, the adolescent is consistently making poor choices? Because teenagers are at different points in their development of abstract thinking skills, they may genuinely not comprehend the long-term consequences of nonadherence. Certainly it can be beneficial to reinforce the reasons for adhering to the treatment regimen, but every healthcare provider knows that education without motivation has very little impact.

The first step toward intervening in teenage nonadherence is understanding what concerns drive the teenager's behavior. Most often, nonadherence is a behavioral response associated with adolescent development. It is especially important to foster a trusting relationship with adolescents who have diabetes. Being empathetic to their concerns, taking time to listen, maintaining confidentiality, providing positive reinforcement for healthy behaviors, and including them as collaborators in their treatment planning will help achieve this goal (Gelder, 2009). Muscari (1998) suggests working with your adolescent client to create a formal contract. The written contract should outline the desired outcome and the interventions required to achieve it. Because adolescents live in the present, setting short-term, realistic goals will be more effective than focusing on long-term consequences.

Most adolescents lead busy lives and have full schedules. If some adolescents perceive diabetes self-management to be too time-consuming or inconvenient, you can work with them to help incorporate their therapeutic regimens into their daily routines, making interventions less disruptive. Teenagers value flexibility and spontaneity. Attempts to ban specific foods or strictly regulate activities are likely to be unsuccessful. Instead, teach teenagers how to make reasonable food choices and adjust their medication to accommodate what they eat. It may be time to think about modifying the adolescent's medication or consider use of a pump.

When adolescents neglect their dietary or insulin regimens in the presence of peers, the behavior reflects not a lack of knowledge, but a desire to avoid appearing different or fears that self-care behaviors will jeopardize their inclusion in activities (Greening et al., 2006). Talking honestly about these concerns and pointing out alternative scenarios can be beneficial. Adolescents who do not have supportive relationships with their parents and other adults are more susceptible to negative peer influence (Drew, Berg, & Weibe, 2010). However, friends can be a unique source of social support that complements the support offered by parents and healthcare providers. Many adolescents genuinely want to be helpful and supportive. Most have at least some awareness of diabetes and its implications, or have family members with diabetes. Nurturing positive relationships and developing a social network in which at least some peers are aware of the adolescent's condition can help motivate adolescents to adhere to their regimens. Additionally, peers can be of assistance if complications such as hypoglycemia occur. Another useful strategy is to plan for specific events or circumstances in advance, possibly even enlisting the assistance of friends.

Adolescents may be particularly concerned about dating, when and how to disclose their condition to their date, how to deal with dining out, and how to check glucose levels and administer insulin discreetly. This is a time when talking with peers who have had similar experiences can be helpful.

A collaborative, validating approach, creativity and flexibility in care planning, and acknowledgment of the adolescent's need for support are strategies that can potentially decrease the problem of nonadherence in adolescents with diabetes. Above all, genuinely attempt to achieve an understanding of the adolescent's perspective on his or her illness. Adolescents might be inspired and gratified to learn that some of their role models—athletes, musicians, and actors—are successfully coping with diabetes (e.g., Nick Jonas, of the Jonas Brothers singing group). An interesting list of celebrities, literary figures, politicians, scientists, and other famous people can be found at *www.dlife.com/diabetes/famous_people*.

What does having diabetes mean to adolescents? What do they believe about long-term consequences? How do they think having diabetes affects them personally and socially? What are their priorities in life? What problems do they anticipate in managing their diabetes? Stepping into the adolescent's world will help you, the healthcare professional, to be viewed as a partner, rather than an adversary, in helping the adolescent to achieve optimal wellness.

SPECIAL CONCERNS

Occasionally, situations arise that defy the usually effective solutions. Adolescents with diabetes share risks for behavioral and emotional problems with other teens, although these issues may have even more serious consequences. When a collaborative plan has been made and the adolescent persistently seems unable or unwilling to follow through, underlying problems such as depression, eating disorders, or substance abuse may be in play.

Depression

Depression is a common problem during adolescence, affecting not only mood but also motivation, cognition, and behavior. The additional stressor of coping with a chronic illness can heighten a preexisting risk. As with adults, higher rates of depression have been found in adolescents with diabetes than those without, and the presence of depression is associated with poorer glycemic control (Dahan & McAfee, 2009). The risk, estimated at up to 20% of adolescents with type 1 diabetes (Grey, Whittemore, & Tamborlane, 2002), warrants the inclusion of depression screening into routine care, annually or if depression is suspected. Because adolescence is a time when moodiness and behavioral fluctuations are often considered the norm, symptoms of depression can be easily overlooked. If you or the adolescent's parents note changes in baseline behavior, investigate. In addition to typical symptoms (i.e., sad mood, crying, isolation, sleep disturbance, appetite disturbance, poor concentration, low energy, neglect of hygiene and self-care, loss of interest in activities), adolescents who are depressed may exhibit irritability, decreased grades, and behavioral problems (Berger, 2010). (Please see Chapter 11 for a more thorough discussion of depression and diabetes.) Anxiety is also frequently associated with depression, or may present as a primary condition that impedes functioning. If anxiety is persistent and severe enough to interfere with the adolescent's ability to learn and carry out self-care protocols, more intensive therapy is required.

Insulin Omission and Eating Disorders

Body image is important to adolescents. Although eating disorders can occur at any time in life, because of adolescent preoccupation with appearance and susceptibility to media ideals, adolescence is the most frequent stage at which they develop, with females being most vulnerable. Adequate glycemic control is associated with a trend towards high-normal BMI for adolescents with type 1 diabetes, which the adolescent might find unacceptable (Dahan & McAfee, 2009). Also, the medical necessity of calculating and monitoring intake and exercise can feed into the behaviors associated with abnormal eating. Excess weight is associated with having type 2 diabetes, and weight reduction is likely to be a part of regimens designed to treat this type of diabetes (Reinehr et al., 2008). Eating disorders are associated with poorer glycemic control and with long-term complications (Dahan & McAfee, 2009). Binging and purging can cause dangerous fluctuations in blood glucose, and vomiting after binging can lead to ketoacidosis.

While not always indicating a full-blown eating disorder, an alarming behavior specific to adolescents with diabetes is the manipulation of insulin for weight control, termed *diabulemia* in some circles (Dahan & McAfee, 2009). Adolescents may do this without awareness of or concern for long-term consequences. One recent study found that although adolescents with type 1 diabetes overall were more likely to report regular meal consumption and less likely to use unhealthy eating behaviors for weight control than teens in the general population, a significant number of them (10.3% of females and 1.4% of males) reported reducing or omitting their insulin as a means of weight control (Ackard et al., 2008). These statistics increase among adolescents who have co-occurring eating disorders, with insulin manipulation being the preferred weight control strategy over the more typical behaviors of purging, laxative use, and excessive exercise. While the immediate threat to health is apparent, there is also evidence that the damage is cumulative, leading to microvascular complications in young adulthood (Peveler, Bryden, & Neil, 2005). Serious issues such as the risk of ketoacidosis related to insulin omission require heightened parental involvement. If such behaviors continue after the adolescent is counseled, increased oversight and assessment for an eating disorder is indicated.

Substance Use/Abuse

It is almost inevitable that adolescents will at some point encounter peer pressure to smoke, drink alcohol, or even use illicit drugs. Speak frankly about these topics, and avoid lecturing. Acknowledge that choices may sometimes be difficult and you want the adolescents to have the information they need to make informed decisions. Although rates of teen smoking have decreased in recent years, it is still not an uncommon behavior. Most school curriculums include antismoking education, so most adolescents are well aware of the health hazards associated with smoking. They may not know, however, that nicotine can decrease insulin absorption and is a potent vasoconstrictor, which can exacerbate cardiovascular and neurological complications of diabetes.

Adolescents are even more likely to be faced with choices about alcohol use. The unfortunate reality is that experimentation with substances is not uncommon in adolescence, and adolescents with diabetes are no exception. Teens need to understand how substances will affect diabetes. These consequences can be particularly serious for individuals who are experimenting and do not know their tolerance.

Adolescents also need to learn what precautions to take if experimentation does occur. Providing information about precautions is not the same as condoning behaviors. You, as well as the teen's parents, can make it clear that you do not approve of experimentation. Because adolescents make bad decisions at times, withholding information can result in life-threatening situations. Adolescents should be specifically warned about the dangers of using alcohol or any other substance while alone or without someone present who is able to seek assistance if needed. Wearing a medical ID or carrying information about their illnesses can help save their lives if they become unconscious and require treatment.

For some adolescents, substance use does not end with experimentation. Substance abuse can stand alone or be a symptom of depression and other emotional disorders. Alcohol and drugs can affect the management of diabetes through their physiological effects and impact on adherence and self-care behaviors. Surveys indicate that about 75% of high school students have tried alcohol, and almost 25% report having been drunk within the previous 30 days (Centers for Disease Control and Prevention [CDC], 2010). Alcohol is particularly dangerous for individuals with diabetes because it inhibits the liver's ability to produce glycogen, and its effects on blood glucose can be lingering. Alcohol can lead to potentially dangerous hypoglycemia, even hours after consumption (Dahan & McAfee, 2009). Further, symptoms of hypoglycemia can be misinterpreted as intoxication.

Stimulant use is associated with decreased appetite and increased metabolism (Sheldon & Quinn, 2005). Stimulants such as cocaine activate hormones that increase blood glucose levels and alter carbohydrate metabolism, leading to hyperglycemia. The physiological risk, and the tendency to omit insulin, make cocaine a serious risk factor for diabetic ketoacidosis. So-called designer drugs, such as Ecstasy, popular in "rave" dance cultures, also have documented risks (Lee, Greenfield, & Campbell, 2009). Ecstasy increases heat production and causes dehydration, so users increase their fluid intake. Excessive water intake, when combined with prolonged exercise, increases the risk of ketoacidosis and hyponatremia. Stimulants may also cause an intense "crash" and long periods of sleep, during which insulin doses can be missed. [Note: Parents may be concerned about stimulant medications prescribed for attention deficit disorder (ADD) or attention deficit hyperactivity disorder (ADHD). Adolescents with diabetes who have co-occurring ADD or ADHD can safely take medications for these conditions, but should be closely monitored for changes in appetite that could affect intake, weight, and insulin requirements, and should be cautioned not to self-adjust their medication doses.] Opiates such as heroin are associated with hyperglycemia, and with glucose and insulin abnormalities similar to those seen in type 2 diabetes even in individuals without the disease (George, Murali, & Pullikal, 2005). Insulin syringes are popular among IV drug users, so adolescents should be cautioned not to provide syringes to others.

Although the physiological impact is minimal, the use of marijuana can cause impaired judgment and is associated with increased appetite and binging, which can increase risks of hyperglycemia (Ng, Darko, & Hillson, 2004). Substance abuse is a high-risk behavior on multiple levels, but the risk is compounded for adolescents with diabetes. It is always prudent to seek assistance from professionals who are familiar with the assessment and treatment of substance abuse if you are concerned that an adolescent in your care is developing a substance abuse problem of any kind, before a crisis occurs.

Routine care should include education about behavioral risks and screening for emotional and behavioral problems common in adolescence. If you suspect a problem or even if you are unsure, approach the topic compassionately and nonjudgmentally, and refer the adolescent to a mental health professional for assessment and counseling. Outcomes improve with early intervention. The inclusion of mental health professionals in the collaborative adolescent-parent-provider alliance will help ensure that the adolescent receives comprehensive care that addresses psychological and physiological needs.

SUMMARY

The psychosocial and hormonal changes that accompany the onset of puberty bring challenges to the achievement of optimal metabolic control in adolescent clients. Adolescents desire more autonomy in decision-making and management of their condition, while the normal developmental changes associated with adolescence can adversely affect adherence to self-care regimens. Both adolescents and their parents require education, support, and guidance to successfully negotiate the transition of primary diabetes management responsibility from parent to adolescent, while maintaining the degree of parent involvement necessary to promote favorable outcomes. Using a collaborative approach, the healthcare provider is in a position to advocate for adolescents and their families in the quest to achieve optimal wellness and prepare for lifelong management of diabetes.

REFERENCES

Ackard, D. M., Vik, N., Neumark-Sztainer, D., Schmitz, K. H., Hannan, P., & Jacobs, D. R. (2008). Disordered eating and body dissatisfaction in adolescents with type 1 diabetes and a population-based comparison sample: Comparative prevalence and clinical implications. *Pediatric Diabetes, 9,* 312–319.

American Diabetes Association. (2005). Care of children and adolescents with type 1 diabetes. *Diabetes Care, 28,* 186–212.

American Diabetes Association. (2011). *Data from the 2011 Diabetes Fact Sheet.* Retrieved April 11, 2011, from http://www.diabetes.org/diabetes-basics/diabetes-statistics/

Anderson, B. J., Svoren, B., & Laffel, L. M. B. (2007). Initiatives to promote effective self-care skills in children and adolescents with diabetes mellitus. *Disease Management and Health Outcomes, 15*(2), 101–108.

Berger, F. K. (2010). *MedlinePlus: Adolescent depression.* Retrieved April 12, 2011, from http://www.nlm.nih.gov/medlineplus/ency/article/001518.htm

Centers for Disease Control and Prevention. (2010). Youth risk behavior surveillance—United States, 2009 [pdf 3.5M]. *Morbidity and Mortality Weekly Report, 59*(SS-5), 1–142.

Coyne, J., Wortman, C., & Lehman, D. (1988). The other side of support: Emotional overinvolvement and miscarried helping. In B. Botlieb (Ed.), *Social support: Formats, processes, and effects* (pp. 305–333). New York: Sage.

Dahan, A., & McAfee, S. G. (2009). A proposed role for the psychiatrist in the treatment of adolescents with type 1 diabetes. *Psychiatric Quarterly, 80,* 75–85.

Drew, L. M., Berg, C., & Weibe, D. J. (2010). The mediating role of extreme peer orientation in the relationships between adolescent-parent relationship and diabetes management. *Journal of Family Psychology, 24*(3), 299–306.

Gelder, C. (2009). Care of adolescents in transition. *Practice Nursing, 20*(9), 444–448.

George, S., Murali, V., & Pullickal, R. (2005). Review of neuroendocrine correlates of chronic opiate misuse: Dysfunctions and pathophysiological mechanisms. *Addictive Disorders and Their Treatment, 4*(3), 99–109.

Greening, L., Stoppelbein, L., & Reeves, C.B. (2006). A model for promoting adolescents' adherence to treatment for type 1 diabetes mellitus. *Children's Health Care, 35*(3), 247–267.

Grey, M., Whittemore, R., & Tamborlane, W. (2002). Depression in type 1 diabetes in children: Natural history and correlates. *Journal of Psychosomatic Research, 53,* 907–911.

Hoey, H. (2009). Psychosocial factors are associated with metabolic control in adolescents: Research from the Hvidoere Study Group on Childhood Diabetes. *Pediatric Diabetes, 10,* 9–14.

Lee, P., Greenfield, J. R., & Campbell, L. V. (2009). Managing young people with type 1 diabetes in a "rave" new world: Metabolic complications of substance abuse in type 1 diabetes. *Diabetic Medicine, 26*(4), 328–333.

Muscari, M. E. (1998). Rebels with a cause: When adolescents won't follow medical advice. *American Journal of Nursing, 98,* 26–30.

Ng, R. S., Darko, D. A., & Hillson, R. M. (2004). Street drug use among young patients with type 1 diabetes in the U.K. *Diabetic Medicine, 21,* 295–296.

Paterson, B., & Brewer, J. (2009). Needs for social support among parents of adolescents with diabetes. *Journal of Nursing and Healthcare of Chronic Illness, 1,* 177–185.

Peveler, R. C., Bryden, K. S., Neil, H. A., Fairburn, C. G., Mayou, R. A., Dunger, D. B., & Turner, H. M. (2005). The relationship of disordered eating habits and attitudes to clinical outcomes in young adult females with type 1 diabetes. *Diabetes Care, 28,* 84–88.

Plante, W. A., & Lobato, D. J. (2008). Psychosocial group interventions for children and adolescents with type 1 diabetes: The state of the literature. *Children's Health Care, 37*, 93–111.

Reinehr, T., Schober, E., Roth, C. L., Weigand, S., & Holl, R. (2008). Type 2 diabetes in children and adolescents in a 2-year follow-up: Insufficient adherence to diabetes centers. *Hormone Research, 69*, 107–113.

Rosenberg, T., & Shields, C. G. (2009). The role of parent-adolescent attachment in the glycemic control of adolescents with type 1 diabetes: A pilot study. *Families, Systems, and Health, 27*(3), 237–248.

Sheldon, B. H., & Quinn, J. D. (2005). Diabetes and illicit drug use. *Practical Diabetes International, 22*(6), 222–224.

Van Campen, K. S., & Russell, S. T. (2010). *Cultural differences in parenting practices: What Asian American families can teach us.* Frances McClelland Institute for Children, Youth, and Families ResearchLink, Vol. 2, No. 1. Tucson, AZ: The University of Arizona. Retrieved April 17, 2011, from http://mcclellandinstitute.arizona.edu/PDFs/Publications/Research%20Link/ResearchLink2_1.pdf

Wang, Y. A., Stuart, S., Tuli, E., & White, P. (2008). Improved glycemic control in adolescents with type 1 diabetes mellitus who attend diabetes camp. *Pediatric Diabetes, 9*, 29–34.

Wysocki, T., & Greco, P. (2006). Social support and diabetes management in childhood and adolescence: Influence of parents and friends. *Current Diabetes Reports, 6*(2), 117–122.

TEN

Teaching and Motivating Adults

There is only one way . . . to get anybody to do anything. And that is by making the other person want to do it.
—Dale Carnegie

Most of Chapter 7, "The Healthcare Professional as Teacher," could apply to many adult clients, but there are two groups of adults with diabetes who are particularly vulnerable to accelerating tissue damage and, perhaps, more amenable to intervention. In my view, these include pregnant women and the aging population. This chapter also covers how diabetes may impact adults of all ages in areas such as family life, employment, health insurance, and self-esteem and discusses options to use for motivating these adults to achieve more optimal diabetes control.

DIABETES AND PREGNANCY

Pregestational Diabetes

Many women often wonder about the effects of pregnancy on their body, but women with preexisting diabetes have good reason to be concerned.

Type 1 Diabetes

Years ago women with type 1 diabetes diagnosed as children were discouraged from getting pregnant. Prior to the development of insulin in 1922, children with diabetes did not live long enough to procreate. Anyone who remembers seeing the 1989 film *Steel Magnolias* is aware that pregnancy can cause damage to glucose-sensitive organs in women with type 1 diabetes. In the film, Julia Roberts plays a type 1 childhood-onset diabetic. She is warned not to attempt pregnancy by her physician and her mother. She does so anyway, has a difficult time with the pregnancy and delivery, and ends up dying of renal failure a year after the birth of her son. Even though there have been many advances made in the care of pregnant women in general, and those with diabetes in particular, many parents of young diabetic women may still consider pregnancy a death sentence for their daughters. More sophisticated glucose meters, rapid-acting insulin, insulin pumps, and research have greatly impacted the safety of pregnancy for women with diabetes. More women with long-standing disease have fewer complications today due to better glycemic control before and during pregnancy, decreasing potential complications.

Pregnancy for anyone is considered a complex metabolic state, causing dramatic shifts in glucose, fat, and protein utilization. During the first trimester, the body is insulin sensitive and burns more fat for energy than usual, thus decreasing insulin demands. By the end of the first trimester, insulin requirements may have dropped by 10% to 20% of the dosage taken before pregnancy and nocturnal hypoglycemia is especially common (Jovanovic, 2009). Many women are also nauseated, and normal weight gain is typically less than 4 pounds during this time. Some women actually lose weight due to nausea and vomiting. As the placenta becomes fully functional during the second trimester, it produces an increasing amount of hormones (human placental growth hormone, human placental lactogen, and progesterone) that cause insulin resistance. By the third trimester, the pancreas must produce up to three times the amount of insulin for the body to remain normoglycemic. In addition, the basal metabolic rate increases tremendously, and both the woman's demands for glucose and that of her fetus are considerable (Jovanovic, 2009). Normally, weight gain during the second and third trimester equals up to a pound per week, with a total weight gain of 25 to 35 pounds. During normal pregnancy, women have a lower fasting glucose and are hyperinsulinemic due to insulin resistance from placental hormones. This increase in insulin secretions from the pancreas facilitates the increase in glucose uptake by the fetoplacental unit and by the cells of their own bodies. With a normal pancreas, the added insulin needs are fulfilled automatically. When an actual diabetic state is added to the normal changes in pregnancy, glycemic control is further challenged. The consequences of not controlling blood sugars to the pregnant woman can include a worsening of any preexisting chronic complications, such as retinopathy, nephropathy, neuropathy, hypertension, and cardiovascular disease. Even without preexisting diabetic complications, these women are at increased risk for pregnancy-inducted hypertension (PIH), miscarriage, and DKA, as well as the beginning of chronic long-term complications, if glycemic control is not achieved. Therefore, preconception care for women with diabetes focuses on achieving optimal blood sugar control. Poorly controlled diabetes prior to pregnancy and during the first trimester increases the risk of spontaneous abortion by 15% to 20% and causes major congenital anomalies in 5% to 10% of pregnancies (Centers for Disease Control and Prevention [CDC], 2011). Maternal hyperglycemia can be teratogenic in the first few weeks of gestation when organogenesis is taking place. This may be occurring before a woman even suspects she is pregnant. The resulting birth defects most often include neural tube defects and cardiac anomalies, as well as those of skeletal, renal, genitourinary, and gastrointestinal systems, and chromosomal anomalies (Correa et al., 2008). With uncontrolled glucose levels later on in pregnancy, the fetus grows larger than normal (macrosomia), making vaginal birth difficult or impossible. This increases the likelihood of shoulder dystocia, fractured clavicle, and/or the need for a cesarean delivery. Hyperglycemia also increases the incidence of stillbirth and perinatal mortality rates. The infant of a diabetic mother with uncontrolled blood sugars is at risk for jaundice, respiratory distress syndrome (especially if macrosomic), prematurity, and hypoglycemia during the first 4 hours of life. During gestation, fetuses fed high levels of glucose via the placenta compensate by producing more and more insulin. This not only produces fatter babies at birth but also puts them at risk for hypoglycemia when their sugar supply is curtained with the cutting of the umbilical cord. Hypoglycemia can cause seizures and brain damage, depending on how low the blood glucose level goes before their pancreas can cut back on insulin production. Newborns of mothers with diabetes are fed early (within 1 to 4 hours) or given an IV of 10% glucose and water if the infant is too lethargic or premature to suck. Macrosomic babies usually have more fat cells than normal and are at risk for obesity and type 2 diabetes during their lifetime. Conversely, infants of diabetic mothers may be small-for-gestational age whether they are born at term or are preterm. This puts these babies at risk for obesity and diabetes later on in life (Morgan et al., 2010). Risk for diabetes is also slightly increase by being born before the 38th week of gestation, according to a study done in Sweden and reported by Crump, Winkleby, Sundquist, and Sundquist (2011).

Pregnant women with type 1 diabetes need to follow blood sugar levels very carefully because insulin needs may be lower during the first trimester and higher than prepregnant amounts at or around 20 weeks. Insulin needs increase as the pregnancy advances and by the end of pregnancy could be as much as three times more than before pregnancy. Because pregnancy can increase the likelihood of chronic diabetic complications, women should have a comprehensive eye exam via dilated pupils to document any retinopathy present at the beginning of the pregnancy and follow any further development as the pregnancy progresses and for at least 1 year postpartum (American Diabetes Association [ADA], 2011a). Blood work documenting renal function (see Chapter 6) should also be followed at the beginning and during pregnancy and compared with prepregnancy levels.

Type 2 Diabetes

Women with pregestational type 2 diabetes are often overweight and may have hypertension. It is as important for these women to prepare for pregnancy as it is for women with type 1 diabetes. A study conducted by Clausen et al. (2005), comparing pregnant women with type 2 diabetes to women with type 1 diabetes and those without diabetes, concluded that perinatal mortality increased by four to nine times and major congenital anomalies were more than doubled in women with type 2 diabetes. Type 2 diabetes is a lot more than just "a touch of sugar." The women in this study were older, overweight, had more children, were often non-White, with a shorter duration of time since diagnosis but had A1c levels during pregnancy that were lower than women with type 1 diabetes. This seems to be counterintuitive. However, most clients with type 1 diabetes in this study were in better glycemic control before pregnancy, planned the pregnancy, sought prenatal care earlier, were of normal weight, and were younger with fewer pregnancies than those participants with type 2 diabetes. Many of the women with type 2 diabetes had metabolic syndrome and were insulin resistant prior to pregnancy. This study points out the importance of having women with type 2 diabetes prepare their bodies for pregnancy by losing weight, controlling blood pressure with medication, if necessary, and controlling blood sugars, often with insulin, because most oral agents are teratogenic in the first trimester (Clausen et al., 2005). Glyburide, a sulfonylurea, has been given after 24 weeks of gestation and shown not to cross the placenta or cause any fetal problems (Moore, 2007). This might be a good choice for treatment of gestational diabetes, which develops about this time.

Metformin (Glucophage) can be used in the first trimester for women with polycystic ovarian syndrome (PCOS) to normalize glucose levels, reverse infertility, and prevent early miscarriage. For more information on PCOS see the American Diabetes Association (ADA)'s website on the subject at www.diabetes.org/Living-with-diabetes/complications/women/polycystic-ovarian-syndrome.html. Metformin has also been shown to be safe if taken throughout the pregnancy (Refuerzo, 2011).

For women with preexisting type 1 or type 2 diabetes, the ADA (2011a) recommends the following optimal glycemic goals, which are 20% lower than nonpregnant target levels:

Premeal, bedtime, and overnight glucose 60–99 mg/dl or 3.3–5.4 mmol/L
Peak postmeal glucose 100–129 mg/dl or 5.4–7.1 mmol/L
A1c < 6.0%

Just like blood sugar levels need to be lower during pregnancy, so do blood pressure ranges. The ADA (2011a) recommends a systolic target of 110 to 129 over a diastolic of 65 to 79.

Gestational Diabetes

Gestational diabetes mellitus (GDM) is diagnosed only during the latter half of pregnancy. Blood sugars usually return to normal after delivery of the placenta. However, women who have had GDM have a 35% to 60% risk of developing diabetes in the next 10 to 20 years (CDC, 2011). The above-mentioned placental hormones cause increasing insulin resistance as the pregnancy progresses and may outpace the pancreas' ability to increase insulin production in some women. The ADA (2011a) has recently changed how gestational diabetes is diagnosed. All pregnant women between 24 to 28 weeks of gestation should receive a 2-hour, 75-g OGTT. Meeting or exceeding any *one* value is regarded as a positive test and is diagnostic of gestational diabetes.

> Fasting ≥ 92 mg/dl or 5.1 mmol/L
> 1 hour ≥ 180 mg/dl or 10.0 mmol/L
> 2 hours ≥ 153 mg/dl or 8.5 mmol/L

When an OGTT is scheduled, advise clients to fast for at least 8 hours overnight after 3 days of carbohydrate loading consisting of a daily intake of about 200 g of carbohydrates.

The ADA (2011a) recommends testing pregnant women at very high risk for GDM as soon as the pregnancy is confirmed using an A1c test. The criteria for very high risk include the following:

- Severe obesity
- Prior history of GDM
- Delivery of a large-for-gestational-age baby in the past
- Presence of glucose in the urine
- Diagnosis of PCOS
- Strong family history of type 2 diabetes

If the A1c is 6.5% or greater, type 2 diabetes is diagnosed. If it is not, then the screening test described earlier is done at 24 to 28 weeks of gestation along with all other women.

Gestational diabetes represents 90% of all pregnancies complicated by diabetes. About 135,000 cases are diagnosed each year, equaling 4% of all pregnancies in the United States (ADA, n.d.-b). With the obesity rates of women in their childbearing years (15–44) increasing and the stricter 2-hour OGTT criteria using only one abnormal value instead of two, the rate of gestational diabetes should also increase in the near future (ADA, 2011a). Three abnormalities make glucose regulation during pregnancy more difficult than normal for women diagnosed with GDM: (1) insulin resistance is common in the third trimester for all women, however, glucose metabolism of women with GDM is further hampered by impaired insulin secretion; (2) there is increased hepatic glucose production in these women, and (3) their insulin resistance is greater than in normal pregnancies during the third trimester, thus compounding the problem, resulting in hyperglycemia. The ADA (2011a) recommends that glycemic control for women with GDM include

> Preprandial ≤ 95 mg/dl or 5.3 mmol/L and either
> 1 hour postmeal ≤ 140 mg/dl or 7.8 mmol/L or
> 2 hour postmeal ≤ 120 mg/dl or 6.7 mmol/L

The good news about GDM, as stated previously, is that it goes away after delivering the placenta and its anti-insulin hormones. However, pregnant women with GDM need to continue to have blood sugars checked in the hospital to make sure they do not really have type 2 diabetes, and they will be checked again at the postpartum visit. Once a year they may be asked to have another OGTT or tested with an A1c to diagnose type 2 diabetes, if present. Weight loss and exercise are the best defenses against developing type 2 diabetes. They should be followed closely and early with each pregnancy for a return of GDM. If, however, they remain as fit and trim as possible, they may be able to avoid GDM in future pregnancies and a diagnosis of type 2 diabetes later in life.

TEACHING AND MOTIVATING PREGNANT CLIENTS

The above information gives the nurse and any healthcare professional abundant ammunition to motivate women with pregestational diabetes to control blood sugars before and during pregnancy. Following A1c levels every 3 months will evaluate the success of their efforts and indicate when attempting pregnancy is optimal. Women who are not seen regularly are more likely to become pregnant without the benefit of good glycemic control and may well develop some of the pregnancy complications discussed above. When most women plan a pregnancy, they are excited and eager to have an uncomplicated pregnancy and birth and a healthy baby. They usually are motivated to eat a healthy diet, get some exercise, and follow any medical advice given. This may be the most optimal time to teach women with diabetes good glycemic control.

Blood sugar ranges during pregnancy are the same for diabetic and nondiabetic women, a point that should make a woman with pregestational diabetes feel normal perhaps for the first time since her diagnosis. These ranges (see Table 10.1) are about 20% lower than for those who are not pregnant and are easy to achieve in nondiabetic women because their needed increase in insulin is automatic. Those who cannot overcome the pregnancy-induced insulin resistance by producing more and more insulin as the pregnancy progresses develop gestational diabetes. Because gestational diabetes increases their risk of complications during pregnancy and the risk of a large baby complicating delivery, these women should also be acutely interested in learning how to control blood sugars. The following list of topics should be covered with anyone with pregestational or gestational diabetes. It should be stressed that these are areas of concern for general diabetic care and good glycemic control and should be continued after pregnancy as well.

1. Glucose monitoring should be done at least before meals and at bedtime. Women with type 2 diabetes and gestational diabetes should periodically test 2 hours after a meal. Following 2-hour postprandial blood sugar will indicate whether or not appropriate steps are being taken to control glucose spikes because this is most strongly correlated with fetal macrosomia (Jovanovic, 2009). See Table 10.1 for normal ranges.
2. A registered dietician is often needed to review current eating habits and make appropriate recommendations for change as needed. Diets

TABLE 10.1
Normal Glucose Levels and A1c Levels During Second and Third Trimesters

GROUP	AVERAGE GLUCOSE	FASTING, PREMEAL, BEDTIME	ONE HOUR AFTER MEALS	A1c
Normal nonpregnant	97–125	70–99	123–137	5.0%–5.9%
Normal pregnancy	77.1–88.7	63.6–75	102.4–114.4	5.0%
Goals during second and third trimesters with preexisting diabetes	< 110	60–99	100–129	< 6.0%

Source: Reprinted with permission from Mertig, R. G. (2011). *What nurses know . . . Diabetes.* New York: Demos Health.

that do not accommodate a client's likes and dislikes or her financial constraints are a waste of time and effort. Individualizing a diet to meet the nutritional requirements of pregnancy is paramount. Decreasing carbohydrates to 45% of total calories may be necessary to blunt postprandial blood sugars for women with type 2 and gestational diabetes who are not administering insulin. For obese women, it might be necessary to decrease not only carbohydrate intake but also the total amount of calories as well. An average nonpregnant American woman who is not overweight has a caloric intake of 2,400 kcal per day. Pregnant women need to increase this amount by roughly 340 Kcal during the second trimester to account for the increase in maternal tissue (breast, uterus, and blood supply) and the placenta and fetus. During the third trimester calories should increase by 452 kcal per day to provide for the growth of the fetus. No extra calories are needed during the first trimester. With breastfeeding, roughly 300 more calories over a nonpregnant intake are needed to produce breast milk with the amount of fat, protein, nutrients, and increased fluid volume needed by the baby (Jovanovic, 2009). A caloric intake of 2,700 to 2,850 kcal might be a drastic reduction for those with type 2 or gestational diabetes. However, this caloric amount should achieve a weight gain of around 15 pounds for those who are obese, resulting in a normal size baby of between 7 to 8 pounds and weight loss for the woman during postpartum. A diet low in fat, moderate in animal protein, and high in whole grains and fiber with five to nine servings of fresh fruit and vegetables and four servings of low-fat dairy should meet the needs of pregnancy. See Table 10.2 for nutritional requirements during pregnancy and breastfeeding.

3. Moderate exercise is recommended for all pregnant women who do not have a medical or obstetrical contraindication. It is particularly important to help maintain glycemic control in women with diabetes.

TABLE 10.2
Nutritional Requirements for Pregnancy and Breastfeeding

WOMEN AT VARIOUS STAGES SHOULD CONSUME THE FOLLOWING NUTRIENTS
PER DAY

NUTRIENTS	ADULT WOMAN	SECOND TRIMESTER	THIRD TRIMESTER	BREAST-FEEDING
Calories	2,400	2,740	2,852	2,700
Protein	100–120 g	130–170 g	130–170 g	130–170 g
Carbs	130 g	175 g	175 g	210 g
Total fiber	25 g	28 g	28 g	29 g
Folate	400 mcg	600 mcg	600 mcg	500 mcg
Iron	8 mg	27 mg	27 mg	9 mg

The concern for anyone pregnant is to avoid exceeding a heart rate of 150 beats per minute and lasting no more than 1 hour, especially during the first trimester (Zavorsky & Longo, 2011). Prevention of dehydration and heat exhaustion is important, for these conditions affect the baby as well. Low-impact aerobic and weight-bearing exercise three times per week should greatly enhance a feeling of well being. After 20 weeks, they should avoid exercises that require lying flat on the back, which could decrease return to the heart of venous blood from the legs, thereby decreasing total blood volume to mother and fetus. Healthcare professionals can help women to schedule time for exercise. Anyone administering insulin should be cautioned to exercise after eating and to test blood sugar first to prevent hypoglycemia. If blood sugar is less than 150 mg/dl before exercise, they should be advised to eat 15 g of carbohydrate (a serving of fruit). Monitoring blood sugar 2 hours after exercise is also wise because hypoglycemia can occur several hours later, depending on the intensity and duration of the physical activity.

4. Insulin does not cross the placenta (Jovanovic, 2009) and is the drug of choice for both type 1 and type 2 clients during pregnancy. Those with type 2 diabetes on oral or injectable hypoglycemic agents may need to be switched to insulin prior to pregnancy. The long-acting insulin analog glargine (Lanthus) was compared with human NPH in a study whose conclusion indicated "There were no statistically significant differences in the occurrences of fetal outcomes" (Pollex, Moretti, Koren, & Feig, 2011). If they are taking antihypertensives, especially ACE inhibitors and ARBs, they need to know that other medications will be substituted because these drugs are particularly teratogenic. The literature supports use of older antihypertensives, such as methyldopa (Aldomet), hydralazine (Apresoline), nifedipine (Procardia),

diltiazem (Cardizem), clonodine (Catapres), labetalol (Normodyne), and prazosin (Minipress) during pregnancy (ADA, 2011a). Women with gestational diabetes may be able to control blood sugars with diet and exercise or may need medication such as glyburide, metformin, or insulin to control blood sugars once they are diagnosed (Wisconsin Diabetes Mellitus Essential Care Guidelines, 2011).

5. Breastfeeding, after delivery, is generally recommended even after a cesarean birth because it helps to stabilize blood sugars. If a client is administering insulin, requirements may be as much as 25% lower than before pregnancy. Advise all breastfeeding clients to increase fluid intake while nursing their infants and, if they are administering insulin, to add a carbohydrate snack before breastfeeding to minimize hypoglycemia, and keep glucose tablets close by to treat it if blood sugar drops. Nocturnal hypoglycemia is especially common while breastfeeding (Jovanovic, 2009). Insulin does appear in breast milk, but the infant's gastric juices destroy it so the baby does not absorb any of it. Some women with type 2 diabetes may not need any medication at all while breastfeeding as long as they continue the healthy eating and exercise habits they developed during pregnancy. Most oral diabetic medication, with the exception of glyburide, glipizide, and metformin, should not be taken while breastfeeding. Insulin and metformin have been proven safe for use during breastfeeding (Feig, Briggs, & Koren, 2007). If glyburide or glipizide are used, infants should be observed for signs of hypoglycemia, including irritability, tremors, jitteriness, lethargy, high pitched or weak cry, apnea or irregular breathing, convulsions, or localized seizures (Wisconsin Diabetes Mellitus Essential Care Guidelines, 2011). Anyone who breastfeeds for one year reduces her risk of developing type 2 diabetes by 14%. Breastfeeding also helps infants by protecting them from childhood obesity and type 2 diabetes as well as early development of type 1 diabetes if they are breastfeed for at least 6 month (Crume et al., 2011). In addition, breastfeeding decreases the incidence of respiratory infections, asthma, and hyperallergic reaction to environmental stimuli. It also decreases the future risk of hypertension for the infant (Plagemann & Harder, 2011). Because maternal diet influences the quality of human milk, this may be an added incentive for new mothers to eat healthier and decrease intake of empty calories. Breastfeeding is the healthiest thing a mother can do for herself and her baby. Most pediatricians prefer that infants drink either breast milk or formula for the first 12 months of life, so breastfeeding is also very economical.

Pregnancy, although high risk, is safe for women who have diabetes, especially if blood glucose levels are fairly well controlled (A1c of ≤7%) prior to and during the pregnancy, and advice from the healthcare team is followed.

The nurse's role in helping these women understand how diabetes affects their pregnancy, delivery, and newborn is invaluable. Listening to their real concerns and working with them will help ensure their compliance with instructions. They may be some of the most motivated clients with whom the nurse has ever worked.

CLINICAL EXAMPLE: In reviewing the learning principles used in Chapter 7 and listed in Figure 7.1, this population is usually eager to learn; willing to increase their knowledge of glycemic control; usually interested in having a healthy pregnancy, easy delivery, and healthy baby; and willing to learn or relearn how to monitor blood sugars and actively participate in the decision making that results. If the client is new to diabetes (first pregnancy with gestational diabetes), the nurse must remember to pick and choose what is taught and add to that body of knowledge later to avoid overwhelming the client. "Learning ability plateaus and time is needed to process information already learned before there is interest and motivation to learn more" (see Figure 7. 1 in Chapter 7). One last encouraging point to use with pregnant women and new mothers is the fact that they can be positive role models in families living with diabetes by serving and eating healthy foods and increasing physical activity.

GENETIC IMPLICATIONS OF DIABETES

In the beginning of this book, I discussed my guilt for bringing this disease into my family and adding to the list of hereditary diseases in my children's family medical history. After some research, I discovered that their risk of being diagnosed with type 1 diabetes was very small. You and your clients may also be interested in the genetic implications of a diagnosis of diabetes.

Diabetes is caused by genetic factors and environmental factors. Most people with type 1 diabetes have inherited risk factors from both parents. It is also more prevalent in the White race. In order for this genetic factor to become manifest, there must be an environmental trigger. Research studies to date have isolated cold weather and certain viruses as possible triggers. Breastfeeding infants and feeding solids only after 6 months of age seems to be protective. Nurses and other healthcare professionals should encourage all new mothers to breastfeed and delay solid foods, but this advice may have greater significance to women with type 1 diabetes. Breastfeeding also decreases insulin needs. Because this is an autoimmune disease, those who may get type 1 diabetes in the future usually have autoantibodies against beta cells in their blood well before they have depleted their beta cell population. Siblings of type 1 diabetics could be tested for these autoantibodies to pancreatic beta cells and, if present, could be directed to clinical studies doing research on ways to prevent beta cells destruction.

See www.ClinicalTrials.gov for a list of current trials and Chapter 1 for more on what may be on the horizon to prevent type 1 diabetes.

Type 2 diabetes has a much stronger genetic component. A family history of type 2 diabetes is a very strong risk factor for getting the disease; however, other components, such as obesity, a high-fat, low-fiber diet, and a sedentary lifestyle, may make the difference between one family member who develops the disease and another who does not. Women who are diagnosed with gestational diabetes more often than not were infants of a mother with gestational diabetes (Dabelea et al., 2005).

The ADA lists on their website www.diabetes.org/diabetes-basics/ genetics-of-diabetes.html the following genetic statistics. A child of a person with the listed characteristics has the following risk of developing the same type of diabetes:

1. Male with type 1 → child 1 in 17
2. Female with type 1 birthing the child before age 25 → child 1 in 25
3. Female with type 1 birthing the child after age 25 → child 1 in 100
4. Both parents have type 1 diabetes → child between 1 in 10 and 1 in 4
5. Male or female with type 2 diagnosed before age 50 → child 1 in 7
6. Type 2 diagnosed after age 50 → child 1 in 13
7. Mother has type 2 diabetes → child at increased risk
8. Both parents with type 2 → child 1 in 2

The prevalence of type 2 diabetes in some families is clearly genetic as well as learned behavior. Families often teach children by example, including behaviors such as poor food choices and avoidance of physical activity. Convincing a parent to turn this around for her children's sake, as well as controlling her own diabetes, could be very empowering for the client and the healthcare practitioner giving advice.

POTENTIAL IMPACT OF DIABETES IN ADULTHOOD

Adults with diabetes may face several challenges in adulthood beside pregnancy that make controlling blood sugars more difficult. This is true whether they have grown up with type 1 diabetes or are diagnosed with type 1 or type 2 diabetes as adults. Here are some of the issues that healthcare professionals need to consider as they interact with and teach these clients what they need to know to manage this disease, and motivate them to want to work at doing so.

Family Life and Conflicting Demands

Dealing with diabetes self-management takes time and energy that others of the same age and family circumstances do not need to think about. Time needs to be allocated for frequent blood sugar monitoring, injecting insulin or taking short-acting oral agents before a meal, and the care of children who depend on them. Luckily my children were school age when I was diagnosed with type 1 diabetes, but I remember on many occasions rushing in from work, sitting down to dinner, and trying to have a conversation with my husband and children when I would realize that I, not only did not do a blood sugar but also had not administered my insulin dose. I can just imagine how much more complicated this would have been if, in addition to the above scenario, I had very young children to care for.

There are many ways you can suggest for clients to stay organized with diabetes:

■ Keep everything needed to take care of diabetes in one place and make it portable like a cooler or backpack. Assign part of a shelf in the refrigerator or cupboard for healthy lunch items to grab and pack before going to work.

■ Buy a small refrigerator for the office or place a container in a work area or lunch room refrigerator with extra, unexpired insulin, and some 6 ounce cans of orange juice. This container should be labeled with the person's name and any pertinent details that might be needed.

■ Have a computer file listing all medications, over-the-counter drugs, and any herbal or vitamin supplements with dosages and when taken. Date this list and change the date when the list is updated. Carry a current copy to present to doctors, pharmacists, and diabetes educators, or for emergencies.

■ Keep a log on the computer or in a notebook to record blood sugars, insulin or other medication, food intake, and/or exercise schedule with date, time, and any emotions experienced so healthcare practitioners can help put the pieces of the puzzle together.

■ Wear or carry some kind of medical identification with name and phone number of the medical provider or diabetes educator, whoever is taking care of health issues related to diabetes. Include emergency contact information.

Men and women both may find dealing with diet and exercise intrusive in their busy work schedule and embarrassing if they need to explain to coworkers why they have to do something like monitor their blood sugar or refrain from doing what everyone else is doing. There are many ways to get around these impediments, depending on how comfortable these clients are with talking about their diabetes.

CLINICAL EXAMPLE: When going out to lunch with coworkers, suggest that they have someone else drive so a blood sugar can be done before arriving at the restaurant. When a lunch meeting is planned, suggest that they bring a low-fat dessert or a large salad to share.

Many people do not want anyone to know that they have diabetes. Nurses and healthcare professionals should discuss this with clients and find out if this is so and the rationale for feeling this way. Clients may be embarrassed, ashamed, or hate feeling different and want diabetes to remain their secret. In Chapter 5, I discuss the need for someone in their immediate environment to know in case they need help with treating hypoglycemia. This is a safety issue. Diabetes should not be viewed as a punishment for dietary indiscretions in the past but, perhaps, a wake-up call to change lifestyle, embark on a healthy eating plan, and increase physical activity. They might be encouraged to become a role model for others in the work or family environment. There are many people who are on the verge of being diagnosed with type 2 diabetes and observing a coworker or family member take charge of his or her health in a positive way may have a great influence on them. Clients can also advocate for healthier choices in the cafeteria or vending machines at work or school. Beginning in 2014, restaurants with more than 20 locations and vending machine with items that do not have nutrition labels on their packaging will have to have caloric and other nutrient values listed on menus and drive-through menus as part of the requirements of the *Patient Protection and Affordable Care Act (PPACA)* passed by Congress in December 2009 and signed into law by President Barack Obama on March 23, 2010. This may or may not help everyone make better choices in what they eat, but it should help clients with diabetes who have a vested interest in doing what they can to lose weight and stay healthy.

Family life often revolves around get-togethers, birthday parties, holidays, and other special events. These all usually include food and sometimes alcohol, which can make glycemic control more difficult. Immediate and extended family members and close friends should be supportive of a client's need to eat healthy food and manage carbohydrate intake but sometimes are not. When a person drinks too much it is even more difficult to exercise control over food intake. Ask clients about family support issues and how they handle parties and other social events. They may need help to decide how to indulge in a piece of birthday cake or other carbohydrate-rich foods without running blood glucose levels too high.

CLINICAL EXAMPLE: If a client is taking insulin at meals, it could be as simple as adding more to his dose. If clients only take long-acting insulin analogs (Lanthus or Levemir) and/or oral or injectable anti-diabetic medications (Byetta, Victosa, or Symlin), they can be advised to avoid or minimize eating other carbs at this meal so this piece of cake can be eaten. See Chapters 2 and 5 for more examples.

It is very possible that there is a "dessert pusher" in the crowd that thinks a person with diabetes can go off the "diet" just this once, which really means that this person feels sorry for the friend or relative with diabetes. There may also be a member acting as the "diabetes police" watching everything that the client eats or making intrusive remarks about weight gain or lack of loss, or asking about the latest blood sugar and giving unsolicited advice. This may undermine the client's resolve to take charge of diabetes self-management. Clients with diabetes may need some help developing responses to these individuals that will not cause a family or neighborhood feud. One very helpful place to direct them to is the Behavioral Diabetes Institute's website http://behavioraldiabetesinstitute.org and look for their *Diabetes Etiquette for People Who Don't Have Diabetes* card. It can be downloaded from http://behavioraldiabetesinstitute.org/downloads/Etiquette-Card.pdf. and sent to friends and family, which might be very appropriate for someone newly diagnosed, or simply printed and posted on the refrigerator. It uses a do's and don'ts format to help others realize what behavior is helpful and what is not (Polonski, n.d.).

Another motivating strategy to encourage someone with diabetes to take control of his or life and diabetes may be driving safety. The ADA (n.d.-a) recommends the following precautions:

- Checking blood glucose prior to getting behind the wheel should always be done. If the drive is long, monitoring blood sugars periodically may be necessary.
- Carrying a blood glucose meter and plenty of snacks—including quick-acting sources of sugar.
- Pulling over if signs of hypoglycemia occur, and checking blood glucose level.
- If it is low, eating a snack that contains a fast-acting sugar source, such a juice, non-diet soda, hard candy, or glucose tablets. They should wait at least 15 minutes and recheck blood sugar to make sure it is in target range before resuming the drive.
- A person experiencing hypoglycemia unawareness must stop driving and consult his or her healthcare provider. The person should not drive until awareness has been restored.
- Getting regular eye exams for early detection of diabetes-related vision problems is a must. If diabetic retinopathy impairs vision in both eyes, driving is not permitted.

CLINICAL EXAMPLE: Necessary visual acuity varies somewhat from state to state; however, most require 20/40 at least in one eye with or without correction and peripheral vision of at least 140 degrees to get and keep a driver's license (Wong, 2007). Peripheral vision may be diminished by the number and frequency of laser photocoagulation to prevent vitreal hemorrhage. See Chapter 6 for more on the treatment for diabetic retinopathy and other visual complications.

Discrimination in Employment

One reason that adults might want to hide the fact that they have diabetes is the fear of discrimination in the work place. People with diabetes have several federal and state laws on their side to protect them from discrimination and that also mandate reasonable accommodations to take care of their diabetes. Any client who has been discriminated against or fears that this might happen can be referred to the ADA for help with this matter. Healthcare professionals and their clients can visit www.diabetes.org/Living-with-diabetes/know-your-rights/discrimination/employment-discrimination for more information and links to other sites with specific job and accommodation mandates.

"Employers may not inquire about an individual's health status—directly or indirectly and regardless of the type of job—before making a job offer, but may require a medical examination or make a medical inquiry once an offer of employment has been extended and before the individual begins the job . . . Employers also may obtain medical information about an employee when the employee has requested an accommodation and his or her disability or need for accommodation is not obvious" (ADA, 2011b). Only those healthcare practitioners who are involved in conducting evaluations of the fitness of an employee to continue at his current employment should have access to the person's medical information. Any reports concerning the medical condition of an employee must be kept separate from the person's personnel file. The ADA recommends that all jobs, including high-risk jobs, such as law enforcement officer, fire fighter, commercial transportation worker, or airline pilot, be individualized based on established guidelines for that particular job classification and the medical evaluation by a diabetes healthcare professional who is familiar with the person with diabetes. Most employment opportunities for which the person is educationally and otherwise qualified to do should be available to all applicants who apply, regardless of their medical conditions. The potential for hypoglycemia when a person is administering insulin or taking oral sulfonylureas should not be used to discriminate against hiring or continued employment of a person with diabetes. Only if there are repeated episodes of severe hypoglycemia that cannot be explained or corrected by a change in medication or dosage or with more frequent blood sugar monitoring and frequent small meals can this be used to determine that this person may not be able to safely perform a particular job or task (ADA, 2011b).

The U.S. Equal Employment Opportunity Commission's publications can be found at www.eeoc.gov. These downloadable publications deal not only with race, gender, religious, and sexual orientation discrimination but also with disability discrimination, which includes discrimination based on medical conditions such as diabetes. It includes discrimination against a job applicant simply because he has a medical condition or firing, demoting, or otherwise discriminating against such a person when diabetes is diagnosed.

The most helpful of the EEOC publications explains the Americans with Disabilities Act of 1990 and its most recent amendment (2008). Congress, when it originally enacted this law recognized that physical and mental disabilities in no way diminish a person's right to fully participate in all aspects of society, but that people with physical or mental disabilities are frequently precluded from doing so because of prejudice, antiquated attitudes, or the failure to remove societal and institutional barriers. However, in 1999 the Supreme Court in *Sutton v. United Air Lines, Inc.*, and its companion cases had narrowed the broad scope of protection intended to be afforded by the Americans with Disabilities Act legislation, thus eliminating protection for many individuals whom Congress intended to protect. Also in *Toyota Motor Manufacturing, Kentucky, Inc. v. Williams* (2002), the court further narrowed the broad scope of protection intended to be afforded by the Americans with Disabilities Act legislation. Both of these rulings removed diabetes and many other conditions from the Americans with Disabilities Act list of clients protected from discrimination. Under the Americans with Disabilities Act Amendment Act (ADAAA) of 2008, people with diabetes and other chronic illnesses—people that Congress clearly intended to cover when it passed the original Americans with Disabilities Act in 1990—are once again within the law's umbrella of protection. This protection includes any reasonable accommodations needed.

Reasonable accommodations are defined as any modifications or adjustments to a job or work environment that enable qualified applicants or employees with disabilities to participate in the application process or to perform essential job functions. Reasonable accommodations also include adjustments to ensure that qualified individuals with disabilities have rights and privileges in employment equal to those of employees without disabilities. Examples of common reasonable accommodations for individuals with diabetes as outlined by the ADA (n.d.-c) include

- Breaks to check blood glucose levels, eat a snack, take medication, or go to the bathroom.
- A place to rest until blood sugar level normalizes.
- The ability to keep diabetes supplies and food nearby. This might include a cooler, lunch box, or small refrigerator supplied by the person affected.
- The ability to test blood glucose and inject insulin anywhere at work.
- If requested, a private area to test blood glucose or administer insulin.
- Modifications to no-fault attendance policies to ensure that someone experiencing a hypoglycemic episode is not forced to drive to work or to a meeting until it is safe to do so.
- Leave for treatment, recuperation, or training on managing diabetes (an employee may also be entitled to this under the Family and Medical Leave Act).
- The opportunity to work a modified work schedule or to work a standard shift as opposed to a rotating or swing shift. For anyone working in a hospital or other industry this may mean working an 8-hour shift

instead of a 12-hour one or being allowed to stay on the same shift instead of rotating between all shifts.

■ For individuals with diabetic neuropathy, permission to use a chair, or stool.

■ For individuals with diabetic retinopathy, large screen computer monitors, or other assistive devices.

What Is the Family Medical Leave Act (FMLA)?

FMLA is a law that protects workers who must miss work due to their own serious health condition or to care for a family member, such as a child, spouse, or parent with a serious health condition. Diabetes qualifies as a serious condition if it requires hospitalization or if it requires a person to see a medical provider at least twice a year. This fact may motivate some with diabetes to make and keep these appointments. If a person qualifies under FMLA, their employer is required to allow them to take up to 12 weeks of unpaid leave in addition to any paid vacation and sick leave. This leave can be taken all at once, for example 12 back-to-back weeks; or in smaller chunks, for example an hour at a time when needed. FMLA also allows a parent to take leave to care for a child with diabetes, for example when a child is newly diagnosed or is hospitalized, or to respond to a diabetes emergency at school. For more information on FMLA with regard to diabetes, visit the ADA's website on this topic at www.diabetes.org/Living-with-diabetes/know-your-rights/discrimination/employment-discrimination/medical-leave. If clients think they have been discriminated against because they have diabetes, healthcare professionals should direct them to the ADA's website at www.diabetes.org/Living-with-diabetes/know-your-rights/?utm_source=WWW&utm_medium=DropDownLWD&utm_content=KnowYourRights&utm_campaign=CON for help with advice and directions as to how to pursue a claim.

Health Insurance

Another important issue with diabetes is health insurance. According to the *Patient Protection and Affordable Care Act*, effective by January 1, 2014, the employer's insurance company can no longer exclude diabetes-related problems, even if it is a preexisting condition prior to employment, if this employer has 50 or more employees and offers health insurance. As stated earlier, diabetes is an expensive disease and those who are diagnosed with it need good health insurance and prescription drug coverage. If someone does not have group health insurance from his employer, it is definitely worth shopping around for one. The better glycemic control a person has, the more likely he or she can get insurance that is affordable. They probably will not get the cheapest rate, but may, with an exam and a note from their medical provider, attesting to good A1c percentages, they could qualify for a standard rate. When glycemic control is poor, the cost of private health insurance may be prohibitive. This fact may motivate clients to be more diligent in monitoring and controlling blood glucose levels and to lose weight if needed. For more information on health insurance options by state, visit: www.diabetes.org/Living-with-diabetes/treatment-and-care/health-insurance-options/health-insurance-in-your-state. If private health insurance is not an option, direct these individuals to clinics and Medicaid Services in the area where they live or work.

Self-Esteem and Sexual Concerns

Diabetes and depression are often linked. Chapters 11 and 12 discuss this more completely; however, as with any chronic illness there is a certain amount of loss of self-esteem and the view of the "perfect" self. When sexual dysfunction complicates the picture, it provides a blow to one's ego that must be dealt with. This includes men with erectile dysfunction and women experiencing diabetes-related sexual dysfunction. Diminished self-confidence and shame attached to sexual difficulties may prevent men and women from talking to medical providers and asking for help. This may be improving, at least with men, as a result of the advertisements for erectile dysfunction (ED) medication depicting men who ask for help as being very masculine and romantic. See Chapter 6 for more on autonomic neuropathy, which is the root cause of this complication. For men a referral to a medical provider for a prescription for Viagra, Cialis, or Levitra may only deal with half the problem. For many men (and women), sexual concerns may stem from low self-esteem, depression, extreme anxiety, intimacy concerns, and other psychological issues. Being unable to perform sexually or having a decreased libido may be demoralizing and increase these feelings (Stevens, 2007). A referral may be needed to a clinical psychologist or licensed clinical social worker who deals with sexual dysfunction associated with psychological issues as well as smoking cessation and drug and alcohol abuse, if these are needed. The underlying physical cause(s) of sexual dysfunction, such as hyperglycemia, hypertension, hypercholesterolemia, and obesity, need to be explored as well. These causes may be easier to treat than any psychological causes of sexual dysfunction. Nurses and other healthcare professionals may be able to use treatment of sexual dysfunction as motivation for clients to work on improving lifestyle with diet, exercise, and good blood sugar control. Listening to concerns may also help with self-esteem issues.

SENIORS AND DIABETES

The pancreas is an organ that ages along with the rest of the body. Its long-term function is related to how healthy it has always been and how old it is. I heard someone say once that in the nursing home population, 80%

of 80-year-olds have type 2 diabetes as do 90% of 90-year-olds. If this is true, then the longer one lives, the more likely one is to have a pancreatic failure resulting in insufficient insulin to remain normoglycemic. Some people in their 80s have had diabetes for decades and others have just been diagnosed. Most have type 2 diabetes but some have type 1, even if newly diagnosed. See the section on LADA in Chapter 1. What this population knows and understands about diabetes self-management runs the gamut, from outdated information and even old wives' tales to completely correct and up-to-date information. Assessment of individuals in this population's knowledge base is as crucial to successful teaching as it is with any other age group, maybe even more important. Additionally, the elderly may be experiencing comorbid conditions such as cardiovascular disease and other diabetes-related complications, arthritis, and visual and/or hearing impairment that are more common in an older population with or without diabetes. Nurses and healthcare practitioners need to adjust their teaching and expectations to accommodate any physical conditions an older person may be dealing with. Diabetes may or may not be his or her most important concern. Tight glycemic control should not be a goal if anyone already has end-stage renal disease or severe vision loss because the purpose of working at tight control is to prevent these and other long-term complications. Tight glycemic control also increases the likelihood of hypoglycemia, which can cause falls, strokes, and heart attacks in seniors. When advocating for good glycemic control to prevent complications in 10 or 20 years, life expectancy is an issue. For someone to want to control a chronic disease in order to increase healthy longevity, life has to be worth living. If a small piece of pie or cake a few times a week puts a smile on an 80-year-old's face, he or she might be convinced to give up other carbohydrates at that same meal. Bargaining with older people is a teaching strategy worth exploring.

Overall, nutrition in the older population is often not assessed. Some seniors continue to eat well-balanced meals as long as someone provides them, such as in an elder care facility, through Meals on Wheels, or by living with a son or daughter. Some seniors in such settings, however, may choose high-fat, low-fiber options or not eat enough or overeat. Making the assumption that an older person who has access to prepared meals is eating a nutritionally sound diet often leads to an inadequate assessment. Eating is a social event. When taste buds and sense of smell decrease and energy level to cook wanes, the only pleasure in eating may be the company and the conversation. The problem may not be an unwillingness to follow a healthy diet, but loneliness. Helping an older person connect with others of like mind in the community such as at a senior center or a Senior Helping Seniors organization can improve dietary intake. It is worth a call to the Agency on Aging Center for available resources in the area or suggest that the client or a family member do so. Volunteering can also improve an older person's outlook on life and willingness to work at blood sugar control to make it happen.

Exercise is also more enjoyable in a group. Older people who participate in dancing, low-impact aerobics, and other group activities, like the rest of us, do so because it is fun, not because it helps to regulate blood sugar. All someone might need is encouragement to join a dance or aerobic group for their age level with the benefit of making new friends. Most of us need incentives to move out of our comfort zone and seniors are no different. Older people who go shopping daily may live longer than their peers who do not follow this habit. "Retail Therapy" may be more appealing to an older individual because of its informality as opposed to formal exercise and the interaction with others in the retail environment. It may keep someone's mind sharp because it requires them to handle money and make decisions about what to purchase and whether or not something is a good buy. The CDC (n.d.) recommends that seniors who have no limiting health conditions spend at least 2½ hours doing aerobic activity of moderate intensity every week. This can be divided into 30 minutes, 5 days a week. Even the 30 minutes can be divided into three 10-minute sessions. Muscle-strengthening exercises should be added to this on 2 or more days per week. Physical activity for seniors can increase muscle mass and improve balance as well as help with glycemic, blood pressure, and cholesterol control and help in weight management.

Good glycemic control, meaning an A1c of less than 7%, is recommended by the ADA (2011a) for most older people who don't have comorbid diseases. Testing blood sugars regularly is one means of achieving this goal. This should be taught using a meter commensurate with a person's physical and visual abilities. Many older persons have difficulty putting a strip in the tiny slot of the meter, so one that contains the strips and produces it at the touch of a button is helpful. Lancing devices should be easy to use and produce a small prick, making it less painful and preventing blood from going everywhere. Most older people take aspirin and other NSAIDs for pain daily, which prevent clots from forming, so finger sticking can get messy. It also helps to use a strip that requires a small amount of blood. Rationale for testing blood sugar needs to be convincing for anyone to spend the money and time to do it.

CLINICAL EXAMPLE: A rationale that I use for monitoring blood sugars is that this is a means of ruling in or ruling out hypo- or hyperglycemia when patients do not feel well and helps them to determine what to do next. That is a good strategy for anyone with diabetes but is very motivating for seniors. Another is the fact that research demonstrates lowering blood glucose levels improves memory and the ability to concentrate, and increases one's enjoyment of life (Sakharova and Inzucchi, 2005). For some this might be very empowering. Just getting older people to consider their options and discuss their fears and concerns may improve the odds that they will follow through with what they have learned.

Some seniors need more time to process information but probably will resent being talked down to. Demonstrating respect for their years of survival on this earth may be as simple as listening to how they used to have to boil glass syringes and sharpen needles, or how the first-generation oral agents made them feel, or how surviving diabetes without blindness or amputations years ago was considered a miracle. Anyone who has lived more than three quarters of a century has stories to tell and wisdom to share. It takes longer to repeat instructions again and again than it does to listen to stories of the past in exchange for an attentive 10 to 20 minutes of learning about some aspect of diabetes self-management.

Hearing impairment may be very debilitating for the client who does not hear all of the words during a teaching session. One-on-one instructions often work best for seniors. Complaints by anyone that people mumble or talk too fast as well as frequent request to speak louder, inappropriate responses to questions, or the more easily recognized leaning forward posture with hand cupped over one ear are clues to the fact that this person is having a hard time hearing you. In addition, we lose the ability to hear higher pitched sounds as we age, making it more difficult to be understood if a healthcare practitioner has a very high-pitched voice. They may or may not be willing to admit to hearing loss or put on their hearing aid in your presence. The reason they may not wear a hearing aid all of the time may be that it is uncomfortable or gives them too much background noise. My father used to turn his off because it was "so peaceful." However, please do not assume that anyone over a certain age has hearing problems. Wallhagen, Pettengill, and Whiteside (2006) offer these interventions that improve communication with someone who is hearing impaired:

- Face the person directly and assess whether or not he is paying attention.
- Speak in a normal tone of voice but pronounce words distinctly and avoid dropping your voice at the end of the sentence.
- Do not cover your mouth with your hand or some object in case the client is lip reading.
- Rephrase whatever is not understood instead of repeating exactly what was previously said.
- If the client wears glasses or a hearing aid, be sure they are on. Batteries for hearing aids may need to be replaced or recharged.
- Stop periodically and ask specific questions to assess what the client has understood. Do not just ask him if he has any questions because he may take the easy way out and say no.
- Keep teaching sessions short and, with the client's permission, have a friend or family member present to help the client with recall later and to ask his or her own questions.

Visual impairment may be more difficult to deal with, depending on whether or not the client is also experiencing hearing impairment and peripheral neuropathy of the hands as well. Peripheral neuropathy may limit what feedback a person gets from feeling the medication or syringe and skin. Adequate assessment of how this client copes with visual compromise may give the nurse or pharmacist clues to what other abilities this person can use for self-care. Traditional methods of testing blood sugar or giving injections may need to be modified. There are glucose meters that give instructions and state results of blood sugars. There are visual assisting devices that help with filling syringes and insulin pens with loud clicks to let a person know how many units he or she has dialed. The ADA lists in their Consumer Guide each year the products that are available. Visit http://forecast.diabetes.org/files/images/v64n1_p56-57_Aids_For_Visual.pdf to see and read about current aids to help the visually impaired with diabetes self-care. The client may also be able to repeat instructions and follow directions perfectly, especially if the rewards for doing so are empowering.

CLINICAL EXAMPLE: My mother, with compromised eyesight from a retinal detachment, was able to fill her medication holders by feeling the containers and the shapes of the pills. She would also check each medication before taking them by feeling the shape of each pill, stating what it was, and counting them. In addition, she could give herself subcutaneous injections in her thigh and abdomen by holding the syringe like a dart, resting the base of her palm on the body part, and rocking her hand forward until she felt the tip of the needle touch her skin. She would then push the syringe into the skin and inject the medication. She needed someone to fill the syringes, but otherwise she continued to give herself injections into her mid 80s. She could have had a nurse come to her home every day, but she would have had to be homebound for Medicare to authorize and pay for this service, or she could have used her limited energy to go to the doctor's office every day in the senior center van. Instead she chose to give herself the injections so she could get out of the house and go with her friends to lunch and enjoy their company.

Medication is another area of concern for seniors with diabetes. A person does not have to have nephropathy to have decreased renal function. Aging causes loss of nephrons in all of us, so medication is not excreted as easily as it had been. Nurses and other healthcare professionals with the insights from the client's family and/or friends need to assess for symptoms of medication accumulation. During and immediately after any illness, older persons should be observed for uncharacteristic changes in mood and behavior. Somnolence, lethargy, irritability, irrational thought, hallucinations, and confusion that is atypical if reported by family members or friends need to be taken seriously because they may mean an accumulation of drug levels in the body. Recovery time from any ailment is usually prolonged, and an older person may need a referral to a home health agency for needed rehabilitation or may need supervision preparing and taking medication. Local pharmacies can fill pill containers for those having difficulty doing so and usually deliver them to the recipient's home. They may even be able to fill prescribed insulin syringes to be refrigerated and administered by the client each day.

In doing research for this chapter, I was particularly interested in the recommendation for continuing use of insulin pumps with seniors. Many older persons cannot achieve glycemic control without insulin. Herman et al. (2005) found that older type 2 diabetics with a mean disease duration of 16 years were able to achieve glycemic control of less than 7% from an average A1c of 8% or higher with either multiple insulin injections or the use of an insulin pump. Both groups experienced only a minimal number of mild (self-treated) hypoglycemic episodes and were satisfied with the treatment and the results. It is important to note that these clients neither had cognitive impairments nor had any severe impairment of cardiac, liver, or renal function. This study demonstrates what was stated in Chapter 4 concerning the progressive nature of type 2 diabetes. In order to achieve an A1c of less than 7%, most will eventually need insulin therapy. In this study group, both multiple injections of insulin and insulin delivered by pump did the job and provided client satisfaction (Herman et al., 2005).

The learning principles described in Chapter 7 are applicable to all adult clients discussed in this chapter. How they are used with each group and with individuals within each group depends on a thorough assessment of each person and the creativity of the nurse and other healthcare professionals in applying the data collected to each one of the principles. The results are certainly worth the effort.

REFERENCES

American Diabetes Association. (n.d.-a). *Driving safety.* Retrieved May 24, 2011, from www.diabetes.org/Living-with-diabetes/know-your-rights/discrimination/drivers-licenses/driving-safety.html

American Diabetes Association. (n.d.-b). *What is gestational diabetes?* Retrieved July 10, 2010, from www.diabetes.org/diabetes-basic/gestational/what-is-gestational-diabetes.html

American Diabetes Association. (n.d.-c). *Common reasonable accommodations for individuals with diabetes.* Retrieved March 24, 2011, from www.diabetes.org/Living-with-diabetes/know-your-rights/discrimination/employment-discrimination/reasonable-accommodations-in-the-workplace/common-reasonable-accommodations.html

American Diabetes Association. (2011a). Standards of medical care in diabetes—2011. *Diabetes Care, 34,* S11–S61.

American Diabetes Association. (2011b). Standards of medical care in diabetes—2011: Diabetes and employment. *Diabetes Care, 34,* S82–S86.

Centers for Disease Control and Prevention. (2011). *National diabetes fact sheet: National estimates and general information on diabetes and prediabetes in the United States, 2011.* Atlanta, GA: U.S. Department of Health and Human Services, Centers for Disease Control and Prevention.

Centers for Disease Control and Prevention. (n.d.). *How much physical activity do older adults need?* Retrieved May 25, 2011, from www.cdc.gov/physicalactivity/everyone/guidelines/olderadults.html

Clausen, T. D., Mathiesen, E., Ekbom, P., Hellmuth, E., Mandrup-Poulsen, T., & Damm, P. (2005). Poor pregnancy outcome in women with type 2 diabetes. *Diabetes Care, 28,* 323–328.

Correa, A., Gilboa, S. M., Besser, L. M., Botto, L. D., Moore, C. A., Hobbs, C. A., . . . Reece, E. A. (2008). Diabetes mellitus and birth defects. *American Journal of Obstetrics and Gynecology, 199*(3), 237.

Crume, T. L., Ogden, L., Maligie, M., Sheffield, S., Bischoff, K. J., Daniels, S., . . . Dabelea, D. (March, 2011). Long-term impact of neonatal breastfeeding on childhood adiposity and fat distribution among children exposed to diabetes in utero. *Diabetes Care, 34*(3), 641–645.

Crump, C., Winkleby, M. A., Sundquist, K., & Sundquist, J. (2011). Risk of diabetes among young adults born preterm in Sweden. *Diabetes Care, 34*(5), 1109–1113.

Dabelea, D., Snell-Bergeon, J. K., Hartsfield, C. L., Bischoff, K. J., Hamman, R. F., & McDuffie, R. S. (2005). Increasing prevalence of gestational diabetes mellitus (GDM) over time and by birth cohort. *Diabetes Care, 28,* 579–584.

Feig, D. S., Briggs, G. G., & Koren, G. (2007) Oral antidiabetic agents in pregnancy and lactation: A paradigm shift? *The Annals of Pharmacotherapy, 41*(7), 1174–1180.

Herman, W. H., Ilag, L. L., Johnson, S. L., Martin, C. L., Sinding, J., Harthi, A. A., . . . Raskin, P. (2005). A clinical trial of continuous subcutaneous insulin infusion versus multiple injections in older adults with type 2 diabetes. *Diabetes Care, 28,* 1568–1573.

Jovanovic, L. (2009). *Medical management of pregnancy complicated by diabetes, 4th ed.* Alexandria, VA: American Diabetes Association.

Mertig, R. G. (2011). *What nurses know . . . Diabetes.* New York: Demos Health.

Moore, T. R. (2007). Glyburide for the treatment of gestational diabetes: A critical appraisal. *Diabetes Care, 30,* S209–S213.

Morgan, A. R., Thompson, J., Murphy, R., Black, P. N., Lam, W.-J., Ferguson, L. R., & Mitchell, E. A. (2010). Obesity and diabetes genes are associated with being born small for gestational age: Results from the Auckland Birthweight Collaborative Study. *BioMed Central Medical Genetics, 11,* 125–134.

Plagemann, A., & Harder, T. (March, 2011). Fuel-mediated teratogenesis and breastfeeding. *Diabetes Care, 34*(3), 779–781.

Pollex, E., Morretti, M. E., Koren, G., & Feig, D. S. (2011). Safety of insulin glargine use in pregnancy. *The Annals of Pharmacotherapy, 45*(1), 1–8.

Polonski, W. (n.d.). *Diabetes etiquette for people who don't have diabetes.* Retrieved September 4, 2010, from http://behavioraldiabetesinstitute.org/downloads/Etiquette-Card.pdf

Refuerzo, J. S. (2011). Oral hypoglycemic agents in pregnancy. *Obstetrics & Gynecology Clinics of North America, 38*(2), 227–234.

Sakharova, O., & Inzucchi, S. (2005). Treatment of diabetes in the elderly: Addressing its complexities in this high-risk group. *Postgraduate Medicine, 119*, 19–29.

Stevens, S. (2007, July 12). *Viagra research says that self esteem not boosted*. Retrieved May 25, 2011, from www.ukmedix.com/viagra-self-esteem.cfm

Wallhagen, M. I., Pettengill, E., & Whiteside, M. (October 2006). Sensory impairment in older adults: Part 1: Hearing loss. *American Journal of Nursing, 106*(10), 40–48.

Wisconsin Diabetes Mellitus Essential Care Guidelines. (2011). *Section 12: Preconception, pregnancy, and postpartum care*. Retrieved May 23, 2011, from www .dhs.wisconsin.gov/health/diabetes/PDFs/GL12.pdf

Wong, R. V. (2009, December 7). *You only need good vision in one eye to keep driving!* Retrieved June 1, 2011, from www.retinaeyedoctor.com/2009/12/ states-require-one-eye-for-drivers-license

Zavorsky, G. S., & Longo, L. D. (2011). Exercise guidelines in pregnancy: New perspectives. *Sports Medicine, 41*(5), 345–360.

ELEVEN

Diabetes and Mental Illness

Mental illness is nothing to be ashamed of, but stigma and bias shame us all.
—Bill Clinton

The National Institute of Mental Health (NIMH) estimates that over 26% of adult Americans experience a psychiatric disorder in any given year (Kessler, Chiu, Demler, Merikangas, & Walters, 2005). Of these, approximately 6% suffer from a serious and disabling mental illness, and nearly half meet diagnostic criteria for two or more disorders. According to the World Health Organization (2011), major depressive disorder is the leading cause of disability in the United States for people aged between 15 and 44.

With the prevalence of these psychiatric disorders, it is inevitable that some of the estimated 25.8 million Americans with diabetes (National Diabetes Information Clearinghouse, 2011) will suffer from at least one mental illness at some point in their lives, potentially worsening these individuals' overall prognoses and increasing their healthcare costs. Compounding the problem, there is evidence that the emotional burden of diabetes, as well as its metabolic effects, may negatively impact mental health. There are also increasing concerns that certain medications commonly used in the treatment of psychiatric disorders can contribute to the development of diabetes or complicate disease management.

Severe mental illnesses, such as major depression, bipolar disorder, and schizophrenia, adversely affect individuals' cognition, functioning, communication, and motivation, sometimes making it more difficult for these clients to seek and receive adequate care, either for their psychological or physiological symptoms. The fragmentation and specialization within the healthcare system often create a barrier to comprehensive care. Other barriers can be internal, related to clients' knowledge and perceptions about their situations.

Sometimes when people recognize emotional problems and seek help, financial constraints can interfere with the ability to receive timely and appropriate care. Despite all the popular rhetoric about the mind–body connection and the publicized information about the detrimental impact of stress on physiological functioning and the immune system, mental health treatment is undervalued for its adjunctive potential in the management of chronic health conditions. Many insurance plans have special caveats and limitations regarding mental disorders compared with other illnesses, with lifetime capitations, higher deductibles, and limited treatment options.

Though the concurrent management of mental disorders and diabetes clearly presents a challenge, the challenge can be met with knowledge, initiative, effective communication among providers, and careful health monitoring. A holistic approach that results in effective diagnosis and management of both psychological and physiological conditions can help prevent complications of each and improve the client's general well-being. In this chapter, we will examine the implications of two of the most problematic psychiatric symptoms—depression and psychosis—in terms of the management of diabetes and how healthcare providers may best impact the care of individuals who suffer from co-occurring physical and psychiatric conditions.

DIABETES AND DEPRESSION

The presence of any chronic or severe illness, including diabetes, increases an individual's risk for development of a depressive disorder. Conversely, depression may have a negative impact on physiological disease outcomes by lowering immunity and interfering with individuals' ability and motivation to engage in healthy self-care practices and manage treatment regimens. Independent of the psychological effects of disease, there is growing evidence that the neuroendocrine changes involved in depression are themselves risk factors for the development of physiological illnesses, such as cardiovascular disease and diabetes.

Research has indicated that people with diabetes are up to twice as likely as those without to suffer from depression (Anderson, Freedland, Clouse, & Lustman, 2001). This risk is greatest among individuals who have other chronic conditions or suffer cardiovascular or neurological complications of diabetes (O'Connor, Crain, Rush, Hanson, Fischer, & Kluznik, 2009). Depression is associated with poor glycemic control and problems with adherence to self-care regimens related to medications, exercise, smoking cessation, and diet (Gonzalez et al., 2007), which contributes to long-term complications of diabetes. The complications, in turn, create stressors that increase susceptibility to depression. Individuals with type 1 diabetes, whose self-care behaviors are more vulnerable to the effects of depression, are more likely to experience poor outcomes (Aikens, Perkins, Piette, & Lipton, 2008). There is compelling evidence that co-occurring depression and diabetes results in a significantly higher all-cause mortality risk than diabetes alone (Katon, 2010).

The Chicken or the Egg?

Although the association between diabetes and depression is well established, the nature of the relationship is not well understood. It was long assumed that depression, related to the ongoing situational stress of managing a chronic illness, followed diabetes. However, the relationship might be bidirectional for some individuals, especially those with type 2 diabetes. Depression can lead to altered biochemical activities in the brain that decrease insulin sensitivity. Furthermore, depression is associated with hypothalamic-pituitary-adrenal axis (HPA) dysregulation, increased cortisol levels, changes in autonomic nervous system homeostasis, and higher levels of inflammatory factors, all of which affect outcomes in diabetes (Katon, 2010).

Regardless of which occurs first—diabetes or depression—several circumstances can contribute to individual risk. Among these are the psychosocial adjustment to a diagnosis of depression, stress resulting from disease management, discomfort associated with symptoms and complications, the metabolic effects of the disease itself on the brain, factors such as age or the presence of other chronic illnesses, and even genetics. Genes have been identified that predispose individuals to both depression and obesity, the leading risk factor for type 2 diabetes. Healthcare providers can play a critical role in interrupting the diabetes–depression cycle. It is necessary to integrate treatment of both disorders in the client's plan of care in order to have a positive effect on diabetes management and disease progression, as well as the client's quality of life.

Challenges in the Management of Co-Occurring Depression and Diabetes

Depression presents significant health risks, especially for people who also have diabetes. The symptoms of depression often include fatigue, inactivity, appetite disturbance, forgetfulness, loss of concentration, and apathy, all of which can have serious implications in the management of diabetes. Not surprisingly, the focus on management of the physiological consequences of the disease process frequently overshadows concerns about the client's mental health. By the time a serious problem with depression is recognized, the client's overall health has suffered. Even low levels of depression can have a negative impact on self-care practices and medication adherence. Therefore, the recognition that depression is present is the first challenge in the management of diabetes and depression.

Diagnosis

Like it or not, the majority of individuals with problems such as depression and anxiety are going to present to their primary care provider, not a mental health professional. This could represent a reluctance by some people to admit to experiencing emotional problems or a lack of recognition of the problem as psychological in origin. Mental illness still carries with it a stigma. Clients, especially those who are older, of lower socioeconomic status, or of ethnic and racial minorities, are relatively unlikely to seek care for psychological issues until a situation becomes unbearable. Clients may even believe that emotional distress simply "comes with the territory" of coping with a chronic illness such as diabetes and may not bring up the topic unless the provider asks specific assessment questions. Unfortunately, providers who share this assumption may tend to minimize or overlook signs of depression or anxiety. Although to some extent it is true that a degree of distress associated with coping with diabetes might be expected (information that is covered well in earlier chapters), when distress becomes persistent and interferes with functioning, more aggressive intervention may be necessary.

What You Can Do

First, assess, assess, assess! Allow me a moment atop my soapbox: The lifetime prevalence of depression in the general population is so high that ALL patients should be routinely assessed for depression, but it is particularly important to include this type of assessment in the care of individuals with diabetes. Remember that you may be picking up on a condition that preexisted the diabetes or one that has been exacerbated or triggered by the presence of diabetes. According to the National Institute of Mental Health (2010), about 17% of individuals will experience depression at some point during their lives, with women being 70% more likely than men to suffer depression. All clients should be asked about a personal and family history of depression, because the disorder is highly recurrent and there may be a genetic predisposition to the development of depression within families (Burcuso & Iacono, 2007). This information can alert you to clients who may benefit from close monitoring. Consider depression when clients present with issues without a clear physiological etiology.

CLINICAL EXAMPLE: Many people with depression complain of fatigue, insomnia, or physical symptoms, such as backache, headache, diarrhea, constipation, itching, or blurred vision. Such broad and overlapping symptoms can make accurate diagnosis more difficult, and providers may or may not be attuned to the potential for these types of symptoms to be warning signs of depression.

Of course, a thorough assessment should include an evaluation of whether the depressive symptoms could be caused by medications or an interaction of medications that the client might be taking. This could be particularly important for clients with multiple conditions. Many medications, including antihypertensives, steroids, and hormones, can contribute to depression for some clients. One listing of such medications can be obtained online at www.medicinenet.com/script/main/art.asp?articlekey=55169.

There are numerous brief tools that can be used to screen for depression (Valence & Saunders, 2005). These can be self-administered and may even be presented to patients with routine check-in paperwork. One easy tool—the Patient Health Questionnaire (PHQ-9)—was designed to be used in a primary care setting and has been successfully used to screen individuals with diabetes (Acee, 2010). The PHQ-9 is free and can be accessed online at www.depression-primarycare.org/clinicians/toolkits/materials/forms/phq9/.

CLINICAL EXAMPLE: Asking two questions assessing whether the client has experienced either of the two critical features of depression ("Over the past 2 weeks, have you felt down, depressed, or hopeless?" and "Over the past 2 weeks, have you felt little interest or pleasure in doing things?") can alert the provider to serious symptoms that require further investigation. These questions can easily be incorporated into the routine intake information, and are a good starting point for your assessment. (Keep in mind that negative answers to the questions do not automatically rule out depression, as more subtle symptoms of depression or subclinical symptoms can still affect motivation and behavior.) If you suspect that your client is depressed, it is critical that your assessment include questions concerning thoughts of death or suicide. Sometimes people respond to passive suicidal thoughts by neglecting their own care or taking health risks and to active suicidal thoughts by overdosing on potentially lethal medications. The risks of such a scenario involving a person with diabetes are apparent.

Next, be sure that your clients with diabetes, and their families, recognize the signs of depression and the importance of seeking help promptly if depression is suspected. This type of education can be included in diabetes teaching and reinforced throughout the ongoing care process. Do not be afraid that bringing up the subject will somehow trigger depression in vulnerable or suggestible clients. Instead, with this knowledge, you are providing clients with one more tool to optimize their own well-being. If you sense that your client is hesitant to admit to experiencing emotional problems, emphasizing the prevalence of depression and focusing on its biological origin can sometimes help increase his or her comfort level.

Treating Depression: Antidepressant Medications

Healthcare providers can work together to ensure that clients receive appropriate treatment. Assessment for and detection of a problem are pointless unless it is addressed. Treatment should be individualized to the client's circumstances, symptoms, and preferences. Typical interventions include antidepressant medications, stress-management modalities, and psychotherapy. Often, individuals can be effectively treated for depression in the primary care setting, but a referral to a mental health professional may be warranted, especially in cases of severe depression or in the presence of suicidal thoughts. Nonpharmacological treatments have been used successfully to treat depression in individuals with co-occurring depression and diabetes (Wang, Tsai, Chou, & Chin, 2008). Clients who have diabetes can safely take antidepressants, but should be followed carefully because of the potential side effects of the medications. Selective serotonin reuptake inhibitors (SSRIs) can increase risks of hypoglycemia, whereas tricyclic antidepressants (TCAs) are associated with hyperglycemia. Monoamine oxidase inhibitors (MAOIs), another class of antidepressants, can contribute to hypoglycemia and also require dietary restrictions that would be an additional burden to a client who is already coping with managing a healthy diet. Recently, pharmaceutical companies have been aggressively marketing medications such as quetiapine (Seroquel), typically used to treat psychoses, as adjunctive treatments for depression. These medications should be used with caution because of metabolic effects discussed below.

An adverse effect of antidepressant use that is of particular concern for clients with diabetes is weight gain, so weight should be monitored and weight control measures, such as diet and exercise, might require adjustment. Although TCAs and MAOIs are the worst culprits, SSRIs can also have this effect. Bupropion (Wellbutrin) is a unique category of antidepressant that is less well-researched, but has been effectively and safely used to treat depression in people with type 2 diabetes (Lustman, Williams, Sayuk, Nix, & Clouse, 2007). A benefit of bupropion is that it does not cause weight gain and may even lead to weight loss. Bupropion is also useful as a smoking cessation aid, which could be a bonus when this serious risk factor for complications of diabetes is present.

Finally, it should also be noted that antidepressant therapy can decrease the symptoms of diabetic neuropathy for some clients (Bril et al., 2011). Some of the same neurotransmitters, such as serotonin and dopamine, responsible for regulating mood also have a role in the transmission of pain signals in the brain. It is important to emphasize to clients that these medications do not treat or inhibit the progression of neuropathy, so maintenance of their prescribed diabetes management regimen is imperative.

DIABETES AND CHRONIC, SEVERE MENTAL ILLNESSES

Certainly depression can be both chronic and severe, but mental illnesses that involve psychotic symptoms and more pronounced interference with cognition, motivation, and thought processes can be even more challenging, both for clients to cope with and for providers to treat. Fortunately, these disorders are less prevalent than depression. Approximately 1% of the world's population suffers from schizophrenia, and the estimates for the prevalence of bipolar disorder are around 3% (Kessler, Chiu, Demler, Merikangas, & Walters, 2005). These psychiatric disorders are not typically managed solely by the primary care provider, because care often involves complex medication regimens and clients are less likely to be independent in following up with their own care. The care of such clients is traditionally fragmented. Attention to the more overt symptoms exhibited by clients with chronic mental illnesses means that physical symptoms do not take priority in the treatment plan, and lack of coordination of care often results in inadequate treatment for the physical health needs of these clients.

In terms of healthcare and community services, people with chronic mental illnesses are truly marginalized. The symptoms of their disorders often prevent them from following through with their own routine healthcare. Many live in adult group homes, or are homeless, with little psychosocial support. They receive their healthcare in clinics and agencies that accept Medicaid compensation or provide free services, which are generally limited in human and material resources. Deinstitutionalization and the closing of many long-term psychiatric beds has contributed to a large population of mentally ill individuals who are poor and whose multiple psychiatric and physical illnesses lead to deficits in functioning and self-care. So, access, financial constraints, and the disease processes are major barriers to adequate management of diabetes and other illnesses for those with chronic, severe mental illnesses.

Studies have shown that the chronic mentally ill population experiences higher rates of most diseases, but cerebrovascular, cardiovascular, endocrine, and pulmonary disorders are the major physiological contributors to the excess mortality rate (about double the general population) of individuals with chronic and severe mental illnesses (Kennedy, Salsberry, Nickel, Hunt, & Chipps, 2005). Clients with severe mental illnesses are two to three times more likely than those in the general population to have diabetes, and much *less* likely to be appropriately diagnosed and treated. When working and teaching in inpatient psychiatric settings, I have been struck by the number of clients with hypertension and diabetes, often not well controlled.

Numerous factors contribute to higher morbidity and mortality. As with depression, psychosis can contribute to an imbalance of corticosteroids, affecting glucose utilization in the body. Detrimental lifestyle habits, such as poor diet, sedentary activities, and smoking, are associated with chronic and severe mental illnesses and are—as we know—risk factors for type 2 diabetes. Obesity is common, which is a problem in itself, and increases people's risk for other illnesses. Inadequate self-care, poor adherence, and a lack of regular healthcare contribute to complications of diabetes, such as vision loss and amputation, resulting in further functional impairment.

Most people with chronic severe mental illnesses require medications to enhance their ability to function in their daily lives. Unfortunately, medications used to treat psychiatric disorders are notorious for contributing to weight gain. This is particularly an issue for clients controlling their symptoms with mood stabilizers, such as lithium and the valproates (e.g., Depakote), and antipsychotic medications. The weight gain is a common reason that clients cite for lack of adherence to their prescribed psychotropic medication regimens—the most frequent cause of relapse. Weight loss programs are not routinely available in mental health settings. The medications also tend to cause dry mouth and increase thirst, leading to an excessive intake of sugar-laden beverages. Certain antipsychotic medications have additional metabolic effects that are of particular concern for individuals with diabetes as discussed later.

Antipsychotic Medications and Hyperglycemia

In addition to weight gain, antipsychotic medications have numerous troublesome side effects. The advent of atypical (newer) antipsychotics was welcomed by clinicians and clients alike because they seemed to have a lower risk of extrapyramidal side effects (movement disorders), were less sedating, and treated a wider range of symptoms than the conventional antipsychotic medications, such as haloperidol (Haldol). Although some are quite expensive, these medications are widely used, and new ones are introduced to the market regularly. Unfortunately, several of the newer generation of antipsychotics are known to impair glucose metabolism, exacerbate existing diabetes, and contribute to new-onset type 2 diabetes by inducing metabolic changes via a mechanism that is not well understood. Like many other medications, they cause weight gain, but the gain is often rapid, centered in the midsection, and can occur even without a change in intake or exercise levels. This weight gain, theorized to be related to insulin resistance, can lead to *metabolic syndrome*—hypertension, increased cholesterol, hyperlipidemia, and increased blood glucose, which in combination sharply increase an individual's cardiovascular and endocrine risks (Meyer, 2007).

There is increasing evidence that cardiovascular and metabolic effects can occur even in the absence of significant weight gain, with the medication acting physiologically to elevate triglyceride levels and increase insulin resistance (Stahl, Mignon, & Meyer, 2009). Furthermore, the metabolic abnormalities may persist even with medication changes, probably because the antipsychotic medications are only one piece of the equation. In rare cases, atypical antipsychotic medications have been associated with sudden diabetic ketoacidosis and hyperglycemic hyperosmolar syndrome, both life-threatening conditions. Although the degree of cardiometabolic risk differs among atypical antipsychotic medications, the concern is sufficiently serious that the FDA now requires pharmaceutical companies to include a warning about a possible link with diabetes on the product labels of all medications in this category, and to provide information about metabolic syndrome in their packaging (Bender, 2010).

Does this mean that atypical antipsychotic medications should be avoided for clients with diabetes? Not necessarily. Using conventional antipsychotic medications is not always the easy solution because of their problematic side effect profiles. Certain atypical antipsychotic medications carry lower cardiometabolic risks, so it is preferable to use those when possible (Stahl, Mignon, & Meyer, 2009). Limited data exist about the newest atypical antipsychotics; however, six medications have a substantial research base. Clozapine (Clozaril) and olanzapine (Zyprexa) are associated with the greatest amount of weight gain, as well as diabetes and metabolic risks. Risperidone (Risperdol) and quetiapine (Seroquel) are also associated with weight gain, although the information about metabolic risks is less definitive. Ziprasidone (Geodon) and aripiprazole (Abilify) appear less likely to cause weight gain, and have not been associated with diabetes or metabolic syndrome. In 2004, the ADA, along with the American Psychiatric Association, the American Association of Clinical Endocrinologists, and the North American Association for the Study of Obesity, published a consensus statement recommending baseline and ongoing assessment of fasting serum glucose and lipid profiles for everyone receiving antipsychotic medications. These guidelines are especially critical for anyone with risk factors for diabetes or diagnosed diabetes, with regular monitoring and attention to changes in glucose levels during administration of the medications. Clients should also be monitored for symptoms of hypoglycemia, indicating a possible need to adjust their diabetes medications or inappropriate self-administration of medication. Symptoms such as confusion, fatigue, loss of concentration, and depressed mood can be misinterpreted as medication side effects or psychiatric symptoms but may actually be hypo- or hyperglycemia. (See Chapter 5 for more on glycemic control.) Clients certainly should not have to choose between controlling their diabetes or their psychotic symptoms, but the coexistence of both problems translates into a need for knowledgeable coordination of care to manage both conditions.

CLINICAL EXAMPLE: A 48-year-old male client with chronic schizophrenia was seen in a mental health clinic for a medication check. Four weeks earlier, the client's medications had been changed to olanzapine (Zyprexa) after he experienced symptoms of a movement disorder while on his previous medication. The client was noted to have gained 12 pounds, stating an increase in appetite and thirst. He was advised to walk daily and to drink water instead of soda. Six weeks later, the client had gained another 18 pounds, bringing his BMI into the overweight range. He complained of fatigue and said he was not able to tolerate daily walks. Lab results indicated an elevated serum glucose level. His medication was changed once again, this time to aripiprazole (Abilify), and he was referred to the endocrinology clinical for follow-up. His case manager also arranged for him to receive transportation to a community center for individuals with chronic mental illnesses 3 days per week, where he would be able to participate in activities and consult weekly with the nurse, who would be available to assist him with monitoring his nutrition, weight, exercise, and glucose levels.

What You Can Do

All healthcare providers can take an active role in monitoring lab work, maintaining awareness of medication effects and side effects, noting symptoms that clients may exhibit and promoting early intervention. Perhaps in no population is your role as client advocate more critical. As a client advocate, you can communicate with other providers, document findings thoroughly, and do your best to ensure that clients' symptoms are adequately evaluated and that clients receive appropriate treatment. The importance of close monitoring of both physiological and psychological status has been previously stressed, but for clients who are mentally ill, this is harder to achieve. You may work with case managers to ensure that clients follow-up with appointments and have assistance with transportation and other needs if necessary. Self-care and medication adherence for anyone is challenging—clients with chronic mental illnesses are likely to be overwhelmed without support. If they live alone, they may need help connecting with resources and with obtaining medications, equipment, and food to effectively manage healthy diets. It is important to include mental health professionals as part of the diabetes healthcare team for all clients who are known to have mental illnesses or who are at particularly high risk. Providers skilled in the assessment and treatment of mental illnesses should also be available as resources to collaborate when referrals are necessary. If you are unsure whether a mental health problem exists, are uncertain about the appropriate treatment, or if the symptoms of mental illness worsen or do not improve, it is always prudent to refer your client to a mental health professional. Even in the absence of a clinically diagnosable mental illness, counseling can be helpful for clients who are feeling overwhelmed by any aspect of their disease or its management. Unless you are a licensed therapist, your involvement in direct intervention for the client's psychiatric illness may be minimal, but understanding this aspect of the client's care will better equip you to approach the client as a whole person rather than as a group of serious diagnoses. Keeping your knowledge current about psychiatric illnesses and their implications, including the use of psychotropic medications for clients with diabetes, can give you a baseline upon which you can individualize care based upon each client's needs. A quick note: if you are going to be working with clients with severe and chronic mental illnesses, take stock of your own beliefs and opinions, fears, and concerns about interacting with them, so that your own anxiety does not hinder your effectiveness.

TEACHING AND MOTIVATING CLIENTS WITH MENTAL ILLNESSES

If your client is profoundly depressed, acutely psychotic, or severely anxious, you will have to wait until these symptoms are controlled before any teaching interventions will be effective. A strong therapeutic alliance is a powerful tool in facilitating learning, adherence, and motivation in clients with severe mental illnesses. Approach clients with patience and a nonjudgmental attitude, so that they will feel safe in honestly sharing their perceptions. Really listen to them, acknowledge their feelings, whether or not you believe they are realistic, and let them know that their concerns have been heard. Avoid arguing, trying to convince them that they should feel differently, or minimizing their feelings—this invalidates them. Avoid false reassurances: "You'll feel a lot better once you learn how to work this glucometer." (The likelihood is that YOU are the one who will feel better.)

Try to elicit their beliefs about mental illness and about diabetes. This allows you to approach the situation from their perspective and to offer information that can dispel misconceptions. Clients with mental illnesses often have low self-esteem, leading them to feel helpless and ineffectual. They may not feel competent to perform required self-care. You can help to counteract this tendency to focus on limitations by pointing out what they are doing well. Provide ongoing encouragement and let them know that you believe they can be capable collaborators in their own healthcare.

Loss of concentration, difficulty making decisions, and slowed thought processes are other common symptoms. Present your information in short spurts. Clients will not be able to take in a lot of complex information at once. Understand that more repetition and time than usual may be necessary to ensure that they comprehend the information. If they are not readily able to demonstrate their understanding to you, it does not mean they were being inattentive. Allow time for what you are saying to sink in and for questions to be formulated and asked. If you are working with a client who has a chronic and severe mental illness, you have to be prepared for ongoing teaching. Because of problems with memory and cognition related to their illnesses, such clients generally need frequent reinforcement of information. Education provided in an individual or family context, rather than in a group setting, is often more effective for clients who have cognitive deficits, because it is less stimulating and anxiety-producing. Written logs to help clients keep track of glucose checks, nutrition, activity, energy levels, and stress levels may be helpful. Examples of logs, as well as other helpful tools to assist with assessment and ongoing care of individuals with co-occurring severe mental illnesses and diabetes, were created by a group of advanced practice nurses at the University of Illinois. Practice guidelines and tools are available at www.uic.edu/nursing/pma/services/diabetes/research/index.htm

Realize that low motivation, apathy, and low energy levels are prominent symptoms of many mental illnesses. If your client also has impairment in cognition and concentration, it is imperative to be sure that the client will have frequent follow-up and support in his or her self-care efforts. Successful control of symptoms is much more likely with the involvement of supportive family members or others. Goals for glycemic control should be realistic and tailored to each client, given the competing time and resources needed to manage the mental illness. McDevitt and colleagues (2003) note that setting a conservative goal, at least initially, can help avoid complications of hypo- or hyperglycemia while the healthcare team collaborates with the client to determine a holistic plan of care that is based on the individual's abilities, resources, and overall circumstances.

You are already aware of the importance of teaching clients with diabetes about diet and exercise to help promote glycemic control. You can point out to clients that healthy diets and exercise also have the benefit of improving mood and decreasing fatigue. Strenuous exercise programs are not likely to be met with much success, but short intervals of exercise, walking, and noncompetitive activities can be helpful. It is important to remember that even minimal weight loss and exercise can have a beneficial effect. If you are able to help the client persist in healthier lifestyle behaviors long enough to exact a sense of improved well-being, the likelihood of maintaining the behaviors is improved. Engaging significant others in this effort or facilitating the involvement in interactive leisure activities in the community can help decrease isolation and encourage health-promoting habits.

Factors such as the amount of social and family support people receive, their previous coping skills, and their beliefs about diabetes and their own ability to manage their self-care can impact people's adjustment to a diagnosis of diabetes and the long-term management of diabetes. Conditions such as depression and anxiety can be short-lived or chronic. The potential stigma of mental illness should be acknowledged, and clients can be approached from the perspective of addressing overall well-being. Although many people are able to overcome debilitating psychological distress without professional intervention, we can do our best to ensure that they don't have to! Continued assessment is useful to minimize the impact of the distress and prevent the situation from worsening. Regular screening and prompt psychological interventions as needed should be incorporated into standard care. Healthcare providers can facilitate this by using brief standardized instruments, asking questions that elicit information about support, beliefs, and psychological distress associated with diabetes, and determining the degree to which distress impairs personal functioning. For individuals with known severe psychiatric disorders, it is critical to ensure that the disorders are adequately treated and resources for ongoing care are in place. Ideally, case managers are available to assist with the coordination of the care necessary to address the complex needs presented by both diabetes and severe, chronic mental illnesses. Effective care requires ongoing assessment of physical, psychological, cognitive, and psychosocial status, with frequent communication among providers on the client's healthcare team. In this way, clients receive the information, support, and treatment they need to increase their physiological and psychological stability and maximize their individual potential for self-care.

REFERENCES

Acee, A. M. (2010). Detecting and managing depression in patients with type II diabetes: PHQ-9 is the answer! *Med-Surg Nursing, 19*(1), 32–38.

Aikens, J. E., Perkins, D. W., Piette, J. D., & Lipton, B. (2008). Association between depression and concurrent type 2 diabetes outcomes varies by diabetes regimen. *Diabetic Medicine, 25*, 1324–1329.

American Diabetes Association, American Psychiatric Association, American Association of Clinical Endocrinologists, North American Association for the Study of Obesity. (2004). Consensus development conference on antipsychotic drugs and obesity and diabetes. *Diabetes Care, 27*, 596–601.

Anderson, R. J., Freedland, K. E., Clouse, R. E., & Lustman, P. J. (2001). The prevalence of depression in adults with diabetes: A meta-analysis. *Diabetes Care, 24*, 1069–1078.

Bender, K. J. (2010). Are FDA warnings on antipsychotics heeded? *Psychiatric Times, 27*(4). Retrieved May 5, 2011, from http://www.psychiatrictimes.com/display/article/10168/1550442

Bril, V., England, J., Franklin, G. M., Backonja, M., Cohen, J., Del Toro, D., et al. (2011). Evidence-based guideline: Treatment of painful diabetic neuropathy. *Neurology.* Retrieved April 28, 2011, from http://www.neurology.org/content/early/2011/04/08/WNL.0b013 e3182166ebe

Burcuso, S. L., & Iacono, W. G. (2007). Risk for recurrence in depression. *Clinical Psychology Review, 27*(8), 969–985.

Gonzalez, J. S., Safren, S. A., Cagliero, E., Wexler, D. J., Delahanty, L., Wittenberg, E., et al. (2007). Depression, self-care, and medication adherence in type 2 diabetes: Relationships across the full range of symptom severity. *Diabetes Care, 30*, 2222–2227.

Katon, W. (2010). Depression and diabetes: Unhealthy bedfellows. *Depression and Anxiety, 27*, 323–326.

Kennedy, C., Salsberry, P., Nickel, J., Hunt, C., & Chipps, E. (2005). The burden of disease in those with serious mental and physical illnesses. *Journal of the American Psychiatric Nurses Association, 11*, 45–51.

Kessler, R. C., Chiu, W. T., Demler, O., Merikangas, K. R., & Walters, E. E. (2005). Prevalence, severity, and comorbidity of twelve-month DSM-IV disorders in the National Comorbidity Survey Replication (NCS-R). *Archives of General Psychiatry, 62*(6), 617–627.

Lustman, P. J., Williams, M. M., Sayuk, G. S., Nix, B. D., & Clouse, R. E. (2007). Factors influencing glycemic control in type 2 diabetes during acute- and maintenance-phase treatment of major depressive disorder with bupropion. *Diabetes Care, 30*(3), 459–466.

McDevitt, J., Snyder, M., Breitmayer, B., Paun, O., & Wojciechowksi, E. (2003). *Diabetes management in the context of serious and persistent mental illness: Clinical practice recommendations. Evidence-based guidelines for integrated care.* Chicago: The Nursing Institute, College of Nursing, University of Illinois. Retrieved May 11, 2011, from http://www.uic.edu/nursing/pma/services/diabetes/research/index.htm

Meyer, J. (2007). The metabolic syndrome and schizophrenia: Clinical research update. *Psychiatric Times, 23*(2). Retrieved May 5, 2011, from http://www.psychiatrictimes.com/display/article/10168/46441

National Diabetes Information Clearinghouse. (2011). Fast facts on diabetes. *National diabetes statistics, 2011.* Retrieved April 26, 2011, from http://diabetes.niddk.nih.gov/dm/pubs/statistics/index.htm#fast

National Institute of Mental Health. (2010). *Major depressive disorder among adults.* Retrieved May 30, 2011, from http://www.nimh.nih.gov/statistics/1MDD_ADULT.shtml

O'Connor, P. J., Crain, A. L., Rush, W. A., Hanson, A. M., Fischer, L. C., & Kluznik, J. C. (2009). Does diabetes double the risk of depression? *Annals of Family Medicine, 7*, 328–335.

Stahl, S. M., Mignon, L., & Meyer, J. M. (2009). Which comes first: Atypical antipsychotic treatment or cardiometabolic risk? *Acta Psychiatrica Scandinavica, 119*, 171–179.

Valence, S. M., & Saunders, J. (2005). Screening for depression and suicide: Self-report instruments that work. *Journal of Psychosocial Nursing, 43*, 22–31.

Wang, M., Tsai, P., Chou, K., & Chin, C. (2008). A systematic review of the efficacy of non-pharmacological treatments for depression on glycaemic control in type 2 diabetes. *Journal of Clinical Nursing, 17*, 2524–2530.

World Health Organization. (2011). *Mental health: Depression.* Retrieved April 28, 2011, from http://www.who.int/mental_health/management/depression/definition/en/

TWELVE

Client Noncompliance (Nonadherence)

Nothing is a waste of time if you use the experience wisely.
  —Rodin

No book about teaching clients with a chronic illness would be complete without a chapter on noncompliance or nonadherence. What is it and what can those of us in the healthcare field do about it? I wrote the first edition of this book for the many former nursing students who saw me in the hospital setting, where they worked as I oriented new nursing students. They were constantly telling me about their noncompliant patients and how the patients were not listening to what they were trying to teach them. I started asking these former students if they had diabetes, would they comply with this advice and, if so, how hard would it be for them to do so. By the blank looks in their faces, I guessed they had never thought about it in that way before. Life has to be worth living as defined by the person living it.

DEFINITIONS

Noncompliance means different things to different healthcare practitioners. The online medical dictionary at www.medterms.com/script/main/art.asp?articlekey=10159 defines *noncompliance* as "the failure or refusal to comply: the failure or refusal to conform and adapt one's actions to a rule or to necessity. The term 'noncompliance' is used in medicine particularly in regard to a patient not taking a prescribed medication or following a prescribed course of therapy."

Nonadherence is defined as "Patient or client refusal of or resistance to medical, psychological, or psychiatric treatment" (APA, Thesaurus of Psychological Index Terms, 8th ed.) found online at http://medconditions.net/patient-non-adherence.html. Neither of the above definitions helps a healthcare professional understand why this is happening or what to do about it.

I was asked to speak to a group of nurses doing chronic disease management for a major insurance company as part of their in-service education. Out of a list of topics concerning diabetes, they chose "the noncompliant patient," as I thought they might. There is nothing more frustrating to a healthcare professional than to be rebuffed by a client after trying so hard to convince him or her to do what the professional knows he or she ought to do to stay healthy. I had spoken to this group previously, and they knew that I had type 1 diabetes. Their list of behaviors that constituted noncompliance was very enlightening for me, as I fit many of them. They included the following:

- Not following physicians' orders
- Not following the diabetic diet
- Not taking medications as ordered
- Not losing weight
- Not testing blood sugars as often as requested
- Not exercising as prescribed

On the other hand, my definition of *noncompliance* is "a knowledgeable and conscious decision by a person to reject all help and a total refusal to try in any way to do anything that might be helpful in preserving his or her life and preventing complications, both acute and chronic—in other words, a decision by the client to cause his or her own eventual death." No one can be helped as long as he or she feels this way. All you can do is let this person know that you are available to help if and when the person changes his or her mind.

Berne (1964/1992), in *Games People Play*, discusses how many adults use various "games" to manage and manipulate their world. Some of these strategies were learned and/or developed in childhood and continue to be practiced today for some psychological gain perhaps not known or understood by the person doing it. Some of these "games" played by clients that get in the way of learning and effective diabetes self-management include

- *Kick Me:* The client states he does not want or is fearful of developing diabetes complications but seems to do nothing to control blood sugars. With an unconscious expectation that there is nothing he can do about the inevitable, he is relieved from any responsibility for self-care. He is also playing the "poor me" game.
- *See What You Made Me Do:* These clients may blame others for their plight in life. If blood sugar or A1c is high, it must be because Aunt Sallie brought her six-cup-of-sugar pound cake to the family reunion.
- *Ain't It Awful:* This is another blame game where clients look at others' behaviors and discuss why they are fat, or have a complication, or are experiencing this or that physical or emotional problem. Secretly they are glad it is happening to someone else. This, however, does not seem to motivate them to prevent similar occurrences in their own life.
- *Why Don't You . . . Yes But:* This is played often in healthcare. The professional teaches, advises, or demonstrates something the client needs to know, understand, or practice. The client indicates she appreciates

or accepts the concept but states, "It will never work because . . . ." For example: "I can't cook that way or serve that food because my family won't eat it." "I can't exercise because I don't have time." "I can't check my blood sugar because the strips are so expensive." There is always a plausible reason to excuse their nonadherence.

By acknowledging in a nonthreatening manner that the client is giving himself an excuse to avoid taking charge of his diabetes, the healthcare practitioner may be able to help him get past the games and move on to better control.

Although, since 1993, the Joint Commission on Accreditation of Healthcare Organizations (JCAHO), now called The Joint Commission (TJC), has required all healthcare agencies to document that patients and families are taught what they need to know to participate in decision making concerning their health, there is little accountability on the patient to demonstrate behavior change based on this teaching (Rankin, Stallings, & London, 2005). Maybe that is what frustrates nurses so much. They do their part by teaching and yet some clients don't seem to want to take part in their own care. Some of the reasons why noncompliance or nonadherence occurs can be summed up under the two categories of "can't" and "won't."

THE "CAN'T" CATEGORY

Under the "can't" category, there are many valid reasons why clients do not comply with instructions given.

Financial Considerations

Diabetes is a very expensive disease. Blood glucose strips cost a dollar or more each, which may limit the number of times a client is able to test his or her blood sugar. Clients are also frustrated when they "waste" a strip, if they get an error message instead of a glucose number and, if their meter requires periodic calibrations, may be reluctant or refuse to use strips to do glucose controls. Human insulin costs $50 or more a vial, and the cost can be as high as $100 per vial for the newer human insulin analogs, such as Humalog, Novolog, Apidra, Lanthus, and Levemir. Even with a prescription drug card and 90-day supplies, co-pays can be substantial. This may influence the number of injections and amount of insulin taken. The same applies to newer oral agents prescribed to control diabetes. It may be embarrassing for some to admit they cannot afford to comply with medical orders or that they need help seeing or taking medications. This is especially true of older clients or anyone on a fixed income. Nurses and other healthcare professionals can help them to troubleshoot these difficulties by asking open-ended questions about how they manage their health in a concerned and respectful manner. Many drug companies will provide medication with a physician's prescription to those who qualify for such assistance. Clients and/or family members can be directed to the website www.pparx.org for the Partnership for Prescription Assistance. (See Chapter 4 for other helpful websites.) Also know that many clients reuse syringes and lancets without apparent adverse effects. Good health insurance can be found by checking www.diabetes.org/living-with-diabetes/treatment-and-care/health-insurance-options/health-insurance-in-your-state as discussed in Chapter 10.

Physical Limitations

Clients may also not have the manual dexterity or visual acuity to use the meter they have or may not accurately draw up the correct dose of insulin, especially if two insulins are mixed, which often leads to uncontrolled blood sugars. Observing the client using his or her meter or drawing up insulin will provide the nurse or pharmacist with valuable insights as to what difficulties exist for this person in his or her self-care. The client and/or family can be directed to the American Diabetes Association resource information guide at http://forecast.diabetes.org/magazine/features/consumer-guide-2011.jsp for more appropriate meters that require less manual dexterity and have larger readouts. Pharmacies sell magnifiers that slide over syringes, and there are 30-unit syringes with more space between the lines, which increases the accuracy for small doses of insulin. A premixed insulin in a pen form may be another appropriate option. If clients are covered by Medicare, a referral to home health agencies can be made by the physician. A home health nurse can prepare a week's supply of insulin in syringes that are then refrigerated and/or prepare a week's supply of medication in pill containers for this purpose. Pharmacies also provide these services and usually deliver the medication to the patient free of charge.

Deficient Knowledge

The most common reason for lack of compliance under the "can't" category is lack of understanding. Too often, nurses and others make the assumption that a client with long-standing diabetes has learned what he or she needs to know. With short hospital stays or no hospitalization at all, the initial instruction after the diagnosis of diabetes may have been overwhelming to the client and family and most of it may have been either not comprehended at that time or forgotten in the intervening years. Moreover, many things have changed in diabetes treatment over the past several years and most clients need periodic updates as new research broadens the understanding of how diabetes affects the body. Clients do not need healthcare practitioners to repeat what was not understood the first time. They need it explained in a different manner or they may need more current information. Nurses should ask about how the client deals with their diet, medication, exercise, and glucose monitoring to assess what is understood and what needs clarification and amplification. To get useful feedback from clients, avoid yes or no questions.

Literacy

Another reason for client ignorance concerning diabetes self-management is literacy. A client with a low literacy level cannot comprehend most printed educational materials and may not understand the terminology used in educational videos. Assumptions are made that adults have a high school education, and teaching is done at that level using vocabulary and pamphlets that may not be appropriate. When clients fail to ask questions, or have a flat affect, or avoid participating in discussions about their diabetes management, do not assume they are disinterested or consciously plan to disregard advice given. DeYoung (2003, p. 99) gives other behavioral examples of low literacy to watch for

- Not reading or even looking at printed material given
- Stating that printed material will be shared with family members later
- Claiming the need for eyeglasses that are broken or left at home
- Stating they have a headache or are too tired to read over printed material
- Mouthing words as they attempt to read anything written

CLINICAL EXAMPLE: My own mother, who dropped out of high school at the beginning of her junior year, hated to read and threw out printed instructions that did not have corresponding pictures. This did not diminish her intelligence but did significantly alter how she learned best. I was with her when she was admitted to the hospital once and watched as she convinced the nurse to fill out her medical history for her. After stating her birth date correctly, she then proceeded to add her age, 86, to that year to answer the question about today's date. The nurse misunderstood and said it was not 1986. I interrupted and told the nurse to wait until my mother finished her calculations. She got the year correct and knew it was close to Christmas. Not bad for someone who had been homebound for 2 years and never read the newspaper.

It takes a great deal of assertiveness and self-esteem to interrupt a nurse or physician and ask that the discussion proceed in a simpler format. This is often too much to expect of older adults, immigrants with minimal English language skills, or those with less education. Even when asked if they understand what has been said, they are really not "verbalizing understanding" when they simply nod their heads or say "yes." Why not request that they demonstrate understanding by asking them some "what if" questions? "What if you started to sweat and shake and were confused about what was happening to you? What would you do?" This encourages interaction, helps evaluate their vocabulary usage and problem-solving ability, as well as notes their understanding of the teaching on hypoglycemia. This must be done in a respectful manner so the client does not feel that the nurse is talking down to him or her. It is much more difficult to teach or interact with someone "not like us," including differences in age, education, culture, and experiences. These differences between healthcare professionals and our clients truly put our ability to be understood by others to the test, a challenge we must accept if we are to reach others and have a meaningful impact on their lives.

Culture

Cultural differences can potentially be enormous obstacles to compliance with diabetes management. Culturally sensitive questions must be asked, using an interpreter if needed, to gather the data necessary to understand any barriers to compliance. "Cultural awareness is the process whereby the nurse becomes respectful, appreciative, and sensitive to the values, beliefs, and problem-solving strategies of a client's culture" (DeYoung, 2003, p. 79). We need to examine and recognize our own prejudices concerning other cultures and work at discarding them or, at least, blocking them from interfering with the care we give to others. Until nurses and all healthcare practitioners understand that they have those biases, they will not see how these biases interfere with the appropriateness of how they deal with members of another culture. By asking questions and gathering data through reading, workshops, or the Internet, nurses can begin to understand what cultural values and beliefs might interfere with client compliance. This openness to learning about a client's culture will help to break down barriers to meaningful communication. This open communication may need to start with the interpreter who may not translate everything that we say because he or she may be offended by or misinterpret instruction due to his or her own cultural bias. Speaking fluent English does not negate cultural upbringing.

CLINICAL EXAMPLE: My father immigrated to the United States from Quebec, Canada, when he was 16, learned to speak English, and formed his own construction company. Despite this, his cultural beliefs concerning the need for preventative medicine and routine visits to doctors and dentists remained as it had been growing up on a farm in Canada. Doctors were called when someone was dying. By the time he saw a dentist for the first time in his 30s, he had no back teeth (all pulled out the old-fashioned way with a string tied to a door knob). I have my wise, though less educated, mother to thank for insisting that my brother and I receive routine medical and dental care. When my father was diagnosed with lung cancer, resulting in a lobectomy and then radiation therapy, he asked no questions of the doctor. After talking to him, I discovered he had no understanding of how ill he was or how radiation could affect him. His oncologist told me that patients only ask when they are ready for the information. With my father's cultural background, he believed that the doctor would tell him what he needed to know. There was a huge disconnect between them. On my insistence, his physician agreed to see my father again to explain in nonmedical terms what my father's situation was. However, he never asked him to repeat his understanding of it. On the way home, I did that using open-ended questions. That is the only way to evaluate another person's understanding, especially if he or she comes from a different cultural background.

In order to obtain culturally sensitive healthcare information from clients, DeYoung (2003) suggests variations of the following questions be incorporated in the interview:

- How do you explain the problem you have?
- What do you think caused this problem? (This is a question that should be asked of everyone.)
- When did it start?
- How does it make you feel?
- How bad is it?
- What are you afraid of most about this illness?
- What difficulties has it caused you at home, at work?
- How do you think it should be treated?
- What are the most important results you hope for from this treatment?

All of these questions may not be necessary in order to evaluate differences in cultural beliefs that could pose a communication problem between a healthcare practitioner and a client. One answer may lead to other more pertinent questions, but whatever is asked must be done in the spirit of acquiring the necessary information that will make teaching, learning, and disease management more likely.

Religious Constraints

If the client's religious beliefs prevent him or her from following through with prescriptive measures to control blood sugars, the client may not be compliant. Again, open-ended questions concerning if, and, or how religious beliefs impact treatment of diabetes might yield useful information. A client may believe this diagnosis is a punishment from God(s) for past sins. This may lead to a lack of adherence with the treatment regimen because the belief may be that he or she must suffer and that attempts to control the disease are defying God's will. Prevention of complications may be a totally unholy pursuit. In high school, I actually had a nun preach about sinful touching of breasts and looking at oneself naked in the mirror. I didn't know much about breast self-exams at the time, but I have often wondered about the rate of breast cancer in the members of that order at that time. Other religious beliefs might influence a client to pray more or give service to others rather than work at something as "self-centered" as diabetes self-management.

Some religions are distrustful of modern medical practices and believe in the power of spiritual healers and their remedies. Also women in many religions and cultures are treated as second-class citizens and may not be deemed worthy of the time and expense that control of diabetes entails. They may need the express permission of a male relative (husband, father, brother, son) to access the healthcare options that will keep them well. Those of us in healthcare professions need to ask good questions to obtain this information and understand the constraints that may prevent compliance. There may be subtle ways to work around these religious constraints and free the client to make better self-management choices. Just because a nurse does not agree with something that is not the norm, he or she must still deal with its reality in the client's life.

Support System

Whether or not a client with any chronic disease can cope mentally and/or physically with the regimen to treat that illness depends a great deal on his or her support network. Negative interactions with family members and friends can make or break the greatest resolve to do what is needed to live a fulfilling life despite diabetes. In " 'They care but don't understand': Family Support of African American Women with Type 2 Diabetes," the authors interviewed several women who perceived a lack of understanding of their needs by members of their social network (Carter-Edwards, Skelly, Cagle, & Appel, 2004).

CLINICAL EXAMPLE: I experienced this after my own diagnosis with diabetes. Family and friends may want to help but do not understand the disease or know what the client needs from them. Nurses can help explain the disease process and treatment options, but they need to empower clients to ask for what they specifically need from each of their support persons (Rubin, n.d.). Sometimes it may be to back off or to treat them as they had prior to the diagnosis. It may also include avoiding tempting foods or drink that the client needs to minimize. No one wants to be treated as fragile or different, but pretending one does not have special needs after being diagnosed with diabetes is not an option. Helping clients to verbalize what irritates them and plan how to dialogue with significant others is useful. Asking, "How would you like your family/friends to treat you?" is a start. Then, "What can you do to make that happen?" would be the next step. Trial and error is a reality, and the more options nurses can help the client realize, the closer he or she might come to getting the support he needs. A good website to explore for some of these options is the Behavioral Diabetes Institute mentioned in Chapter 10. Their card with do's and don'ts of *diabetes etiquette for those who do not have diabetes* can be downloaded or printed from http://behavioral-diabetesinstitute.org/downloads/Etiquette-Card.pdf.

THE "WON'T" CATEGORY

When a client refuses to follow prescribed advice and you have ruled out all of the areas covered under the "can't" category, the following issues should be explored. Some of these reactions to a diagnosis are part of the grief stages described by the late Dr. Elisabeth Kübler-Ross in *On Death and Dying* and discussed in the introduction to this book using personal examples. Some of the following may be based on a client's personality and life experiences and some may need medication and/or psychological intervention.

Denial

Denial is an unconscious defense mechanism that protects us from a threat to self. In order to deal with the perceived loss of health that a diagnosis of diabetes brings, most people react with shock and denial. By refusing to accept this diagnosis, getting a second opinion, or remaining in a dazed state, the mind bides its time and allows for reality to sink in slowly. When we are ready to begin coping with this new entity, we can then listen to instructions and learn what we need to do. This is normal coping strategy and needs to be indulged by healthcare professionals, at least for a while. During this time clients and/or family members can be taught what is needed to improve the immediate health problem or threat to life, the "survival skills." They can learn to test blood sugar, give insulin, or take oral medication. What they may not be able to grasp is that diabetes is a chronic illness and that lifestyle changes and medication are for life. Denial becomes pathological only when it persists beyond this initial stage and interferes with the process of acceptance so necessary in achieving good glycemic control. Healthcare providers may contribute to this by stating that type 2 diabetes is the "mild" form, nothing to worry about. Clients may comment that they have "a touch of sugar" or that they do not really need to worry about what they eat or about losing weight.

Taking oral agents to control diabetes is like taking a vitamin pill. It is "no big deal." This attitude increases resistance to using insulin because "going on the needle" works against their denial.

CLINICAL EXAMPLE: I have spoken to several clients with type 2 diabetes on oral antidiabetic agents or experiencing neuropathy and cardiovascular complication indicating years of hyperglycemia, who state they have never been diagnosed with diabetes. Denial is very powerful and difficult to break through. Nurses and healthcare professionals can talk about good healthcare practices for everyone and focus on improving whatever clients are willing to deal with, like the numbness and tingling of feet or the decrease in circulation. Whatever lifestyle changes clients are willing to make will improve blood sugar control or at least prevent further deterioration of their current condition. Giving client handouts concerning diet, exercise, medications, and weight loss that mention diabetes may be a nudge in the right direction. Listening to their thoughts about diabetes may uncover personal fears that they will become like a neighbor or relative who suffered and died of diabetic complications. Knowing what is behind this prolonged and counterproductive denial may give the nurse insight and information with which to formulate "an offer the client can't refuse." If a client wants to do something specific with his or her life, like a career, family, sports, or longevity, he or she may fear that acceptance of this diagnosis will make it impossible. Knowing that gives you a tool to motivate the client to work at control in order to improve the odds that his or her dreams will be realized. Most people need to work at one thing at a time. Help the client choose which area he or she is willing to deal with first. It may be quitting smoking (diabetes and smoking are a deadly combination). This might lead to brisk walking because he or she has more energy and lung capacity, which usually results in weight loss and improved blood glucose control.

Anger and Frustration

Anger is ever-present in most people diagnosed with a chronic illness. "Why me?" is always under the surface and can spring up even after years of good control. A client may state or act as if he or she just does not want to deal with "it" anymore or needs a break from doing blood sugars, counting carbs, and/or taking medication or insulin. Because people with type 1 diabetes will get very ill quickly if they stop taking insulin, their choice may be to eat whatever they want and stop testing their blood sugar for a few days or longer. It will quickly become apparent that this plan is making them sick and less able to enjoy life. Nurses can use this realization to reinforce the importance of glycemic control while understanding the client's need to take a vacation from the tedious regimen. Those with type 2 diabetes can last much longer avoiding control before feeling bad. However, clients usually can talk about life changes that have happened over this noncompliant time, which they may relate to the aging process; changes discussed include decreased energy level, disinterest or lack of enjoyment in things that once held their attention, like sports or grandchildren, and falling asleep after eating. Once you know what they miss doing, you can use this to motivate them to return to good control. Some people use anger at diabetes to lash out at others, which causes problems with family and work relationships. Focusing on the cause of anger can help to vent feelings of frustration at having diabetes and being forced to change lifestyle. Anger can also help people assert and protect themselves. Teach them to learn to use their anger to work for better diabetes care (ADA, n.d.-a). When I experience anger at diabetes, I always remember what a wise physician once said in the early days of my diabetic career: "Diabetics have to do what everyone else ought to do." Now instead of being angry, I feel challenged to lead a healthy lifestyle, to be an example to my family and peers, and to be a leader. How empowering!

Nurses need to be good listeners and encourage clients to get their feelings out. Once the issues bothering someone are on the table, the client can recognize them for what they are and begin to deal with them. As long as they remain inside, these issues simply cause agitation, anger, and frustration.

CLINICAL EXAMPLE: To get a discussion going, ask, "What is it like to live with diabetes?" or "How does having diabetes make you feel?" If the client is experiencing anger, be prepared for him or her to let you really know in no uncertain terms. You may have opened up the floodgates bottled up for years. Always remember that the client's anger is not directed at you but at the disease. Once the flood of words has subsided, you can ask, "So what would you like to do about it?" You may have given him or her the first opportunity to come to grips with this new life change no matter how long it has been since diagnosis. Please remember that a client's anger can be a powerful force leading to new learning and growth in self-care. Listening and allowing the client to dump all of his or her pent-up emotions can be the catalyst for this change.

Depression

In the process of accepting the loss of good health, the loss of being "normal," whatever that means to an individual, or the diagnosis of a chronic illness, some sadness or depression is typical and necessary.

Without it people remain in the stages of denial and anger. As the reality of how life has been altered forever by a diagnosis of diabetes sets in, a client may withdraw from loved ones or display signs of hopelessness and helplessness even while doing some of the activities necessitated by the diagnosis. The client may check his or her blood sugar and give insulin or take oral medication but be unable to problem solve when blood sugars are not what they should be. Lack of energy may make physical activity impossible. Other signs of depression include loss of pleasure at doing things a person loves to do, changes in sleep patterns (too much or too little), changes in appetite (eating too much or too little), and perhaps even suicidal thoughts (ADA, n.d.-b).

CLINICAL EXAMPLE: A meta-analysis to examine the relationship between depression and treatment nonadherence in patients with type 1 and type 2 diabetes was done by Gonzalez et al. (2008), which determined that a significant association between depression and treatment nonadherence in patients with diabetes existed. Destructive behaviors such as imbibing in alcoholic beverages, smoking, or relying on mind-altering drugs (prescribed, over the counter, or illegal), may take over. Thoughts of suicide, the ultimate escape, may take center stage. Nurses need to evaluate whether the sadness and depressed mood exhibited by the client is part of the coming to terms that is a normal and expected phase to acceptance or a true situational depression necessitating psychiatric intervention. When in doubt, get an order for a psychiatric evaluation. Depression is covered in more depth in Chapter 11.

Stress and Excessive Fear

Stress hormones are released in response to either physical or mental difficulties. Stress hormones, such as cortisol and adrenaline, cause an increase in blood pressure, pulse, and breathing rate as well as an increase in the release of stored glucose by the liver. This is very important in the fight-or-flight response but not useful when a person really does not need to fight or flee. Stress moves the focus away from taking care of one's health and diabetes. Long-term stress can also damage the cardiovascular system and cause stomach ulcers. This is true whether or not a person has diabetes.

All stress is not bad; whether it is good or bad depends on the level of stress someone is experiencing. Mild stress levels are needed motivators of behavior. If we were not hungry, we might not get out of bed in the morning. Moderate concern over health issues may cause a person to make or keep an appointment with a medical provider, work on a healthier diet, increase their exercise level, or monitor blood sugar and blood pressure. However, high anxiety levels can be incapacitating. We have difficulty seeing the big picture because the stressors are so overwhelming. It makes conscious, logical thought very difficult and figuring out what to do about a situation next to impossible. Stress is also produced by happy events, as anyone getting married, having a baby, changing jobs, or making any other positively anticipated change in one's life can attest.

If someone has extremely high anxiety or is overly fearful about something, it is important to assess for this and ascertain the cause. Because stress hormones increase blood glucose levels, it may make clients look as if they are not working at diabetes control when they may be doing all they can at any given moment. To complicate this situation even further, stress blocks the release of insulin in type 2 diabetes, and some of these people may also be even more sensitive to some of the stress hormones than the norm (ADA, n.d.-c).

A healthcare provider may or may not be able to help clients solve whatever problems are causing the stress, but at least listening to them talk about it should help them feel better about themselves. When everyone else believes clients are noncompliant, thus increasing their stress and perhaps their anger, at least you are giving them a chance to express what is going on in their lives that might explain the higher than normal blood sugars. By allowing them to talk, you may also be helping them to hear themselves verbalize the anxieties that may only have been vague notions in their minds. This verbalization may help them to see the problems for what they are and formulate their own solutions.

Fatalism

"Traditional educational interventions are designed to give the same information to everyone and to teach new coping skills without first addressing the well-established beliefs that drive the selection of coping strategies" (Redman, 2004, p. 24). If there is a family history of diabetes with negative consequences, this diagnosis can either help a client do what relatives did not do to improve survival or lead the client to believe that there is nothing he or she can do that will make his or her fate any different than that of others with diabetes complications. I have heard a variation of both themes from people diagnosed with diabetes.

CLINICAL EXAMPLE: If a person concludes that his or her grandmother died of diabetic complication because she did nothing to control blood sugar, I know that person is open to learning how to prevent the same consequences from happening to him or her. If, however, he or she believes in the inevitability of similar consequences happening to him or her, I know I have my work cut out for me. People in the latter category have no incentive to make lifestyle changes or monitor their blood sugars because they believe it will not make any difference in the long run. About 10 years ago, a family practice physician told me informally that he would rather die than take insulin injections. I answered that I felt sorry for his patients. According to the literature, this attitude is not uncommon and leads to more preventable long-term complications when type 2 diabetics are not switched to insulin if glycemic control is not achieved (Peyrot et al., 2005). This attitude on the physician's part may contribute to the fatalism that some with type 2 diabetes feel.

Diabetes Burnout

Diabetes care is a 24/7 proposition. Everyday there are hundreds of things that someone with diabetes, especially type 1 diabetes, must think about and make decisions about. There are meals: what to eat, when to eat, depends on blood sugar; exercise: whether to do it or not, when, what kind, depends on blood sugar; medication: when to take it in relation to meals and exercise and how much to take, depends on blood sugar. Is it safe to get behind the wheel of a car? It depends on the blood sugar. How long can I do something before I will need to eat? It depends on blood sugar. After many years of doing their best day after day, many people with diabetes just want to take a break, a diabetes vacation, and stop obsessing over all the rules, just do what everyone else does, be normal for a while. Because clients may have been labeled noncompliant, no matter what they say about needing a break, they may feel guilty even thinking about it. Women may be especially prone to burnout because they often put their needs last after the needs of their families. Folz-Gray (2010) with LifeScript gives some ideas for healthcare professionals to help clients who are tempted to quit their diabetes self-management. We can pass these tips on to clients when they get down about all that diabetes self-management entails, including

- Making sure these behaviors are not masking depression.
- Giving in to frustration and venting once in a while.
- Gaining perspective and focusing on what is going right in life.
- Cutting calories not the enjoyment of food. A new cookbook or restaurant might help.
- Taking a short, well-planned diabetes vacation (but not from meds) and making it restorative. They could sleep late or go out with friends or skip exercise for a week.
- Consulting a diabetes educator for new ideas to make life easier and increase motivation.
- Finding a diabetes support group or a diabetes buddy to talk to. Visit www.diabetessister.org for forums, blogs, and online programs for women with diabetes.
- Getting rid of the need to do herculean exercise routines or drop 5 dress sizes. Making goals realistic can be motivating.
- Putting it on paper or on the computer—food intake, any physical activity, feelings, goals, blood sugars—so they can be appreciated. Reward accomplishments and avoid getting down about what still needs improvement. Today is the first day of the rest of one's life.

healthcare practitioners must avoid making discouraged clients feel worse about an A1c that is too high and focus on how to make it better. Clients usually know why it happened and may need to vent their frustration at life with diabetes. They certainly don't need to be scolded.

Self-Determination

Many people with chronic illnesses develop strategies of self-management that differ from the prescribed regimens. They may use alternative therapies or alter when they take medications or do blood sugars. Some self-management strategies are stricter or more difficult than what is prescribed. All of these patients may be labeled noncompliant by their healthcare practitioner. In diabetes as in all other experiences in life, one size never fits all. Clients who want to manage their diabetes "my way" need to be in a collaborative relationship with their healthcare team. No one knows a person's history, beliefs, likes, and dislikes, and how his or her body deals with glycemic control better than the client. What clients need from nurses and other healthcare practitioners are tools to make good choices and cope with life and the ups and downs of blood sugars.

CLINICAL EXAMPLE: When anyone asks me how often I check blood sugars, my answer is "as often as I need the information." That might mean 4 times a day or up to 10 times. I might need the information in the middle of the night or before I go for a walk. Clients need to be encouraged to test after meals, not just before meals. The real proof of control is whether a 2-hour postprandial blood sugar stays under 140 mg/dl.

VALUES CLARIFICATION

Help the client who are having difficulty with diabetes control do values clarification concerning health to get him or her to develop realistic goals that he or she is willing to work toward. Here are the steps and how you might word them:

1. "What do you see are your choices of actions now that you have diabetes?" The client might need help with this. One choice may be to do nothing.
2. "What might the consequences of each of these choices be?" Again help may be needed.
3. "How would you feel about each of these consequences?"
4. "Which of these choices would you like to pursue **at this time?**"
5. "Who should know about this choice you are making and how do you plan to explain this choice to them?" This is especially important if he chooses to do nothing.

6. "How can I help you to deal with this choice?" (It must remain the client's problem and thus his or her choice).

7. MAKE THEM AN OFFER THEY CAN'T REFUSE!

   a. "You say you will do anything as long as you don't have to be on insulin (type 2). Here are some options that might improve the odds that you will not have to take insulin (lose 15 to 20 pounds and/or exercise)."

   b. "Your stated goal is to minimize low blood sugars. The best way to do that is to test blood sugars often and count carbohydrates. Here is how to do that . . . . . "

   c. "You want to be able to eat anything you want, so why don't you test your blood sugar before and after you eat to see what effect a particular food has? If it elevates your blood sugar, then we can work on how to prevent that (by decreasing other carbs in the same meal or by increasing insulin or changing oral agents.)" Then communicate with the prescriber.

   d. "Because it sounds like you have decided not to participate in your care, how are you going to protect your loved ones from bearing the consequences of your decision?" (Financially and emotionally—they may hate you for not taking care of yourself, for in fact killing yourself.) Sometimes you have to be blunt to help clients understand what they are really saying and doing.

Use of the Internet

There is so much written about diabetes today that healthcare practitioners need to realize they are not the only voice a client hears. Nurses need to know what their clients are reading and who they are listening to. Some of the recent offers I have received in the mail include titles from the American Diabetes Association, titles from the Mayo Clinic, *Johns Hopkins White Papers*, and publications such as *Diabetes Self-Management* as well as some of dubious value touting weight loss without dieting and exercise or the sugar cure for diabetes. The Web is also a source of well-researched and useful information, as well as personal opinions, products pushing "cures," and other unsubstantiated guides. We need to help clients evaluate these resources by asking them to note the author or organization contributing the information and the date when it was posted. Outdated information is not useful. Other questions to ask include the following: "Is the article selling something?" "Does it include studies proving the points made?" and "Does it make sense?" If an article states what a client wants to hear, it may indeed be too good to be true.

The proof of any self-management strategy is in the hemoglobin A1c. There are clients that are compliant and have A1cs above 7%. That may mean they are "cheating" or, more likely, the current medication regimen is inadequate. There are also clients who are considered noncompliant with A1c levels consistently below 7%. Nurses should conclude that these clients must be doing something right. In a recent article on patient compliance in *Family Practice Management,* the author states, "The physician has to recognize the opportunity for intervention, reframe it in a way that makes it meaningful to the patient and generate a sufficient sense of urgency to compel the patient to take action. At the same time, the physician has to maintain a partnership with the patient, based on trust and understanding" (Pawar, 2005, p. 44). I could easily substitute "the nurse" for the physician in this quote. In other words, nurses need to encourage discourse, listen carefully, use what the client says to "make an offer he or she cannot refuse." In order to convince the client to change, the nurse must "sell" good glycemic control in a way that the client can understand and that makes sense to him or her. Tips given by Pawar (2005) to improve patient satisfaction and compliance include the following:

1. Establish a trusting and caring relationship. Clients must believe we value them as people not just as work-related charges.
2. Uncover patients' actual needs and concerns. Ask follow-up questions to get at the real issues that trouble the client.
3. Use dialogue, not monologue. Encourage participation and really listen to what clients say.
4. Don't force or threaten; little steps are better than nothing. Keep the client in charge of his or her own care. Ask "Are you willing to do blood sugars before each meal for 1 week?" Incremental steps are often needed.
5. Follow-up is paramount. This may be by phone if you see the client in an office or other outpatient setting or it may be as simple as checking in on an inpatient client each day you are working, even if he or she is not part of your assignment.
6. Call often to get a progress report and give PRAISE and encouragement about being honest with you. Ask how the client feels about this report. Remind the client and self that perfection is not part of the human condition.
7. Be understanding when the report is not what you'd like. Ask the client what he/she thinks happened. Then work with that.
8. Never assume you know the answer. There may be an unavoidable reason that was not under the client's control.
9. Don't judge the client's lapse as "noncompliance" or "nonadherence." Whose life is it anyway?
10. Be a client advocate. Troubleshoot between the client and the physician, pharmacist, insurance company, family. Or suggest ways that the client and/or the family could improve the situation between the physician, pharmacist, insurance company, family.
11. Seize the TEACHABLE MOMENTS! This is your window of opportunity to convince the client to change his or her ways!
    - Any hospitalization or illness
    - Family vacation
    - Holidays
    - Participation in sports

- Birth, birthday, anniversary
- Another's death, diagnosis of chronic complication (other's or the client's)
- Whenever the client calls for any reason indicates that the client is reaching out to you; grab the opportunity!

Avoid burnout—yours and the client's by doing some of the following:

- Give it a rest.
- Try a new approach.
- Refer the client to a colleague.
- Pat yourself and the client on the back for whatever success is attained.
- Look back at how far the client and you have come.
- A client may not be ready for your teaching now, but when ready, the client knows he or she will get a straight talker, who cares and who will listen.

Attitude Is Everything (Yours and Theirs)

Share the following words of wisdom with clients:

"Control will set you free!"
"Today is the first day of the rest of your life!"
"Be all that you can be!"
"A diabetic *has to* do what everyone else *ought to* do!"
"When life hands you a lemon, make lemonade!"
"Master the possibilities!"
"*You* control your diabetes. Don't let *it* control you!"

Ask the client to make a commitment to good health. All decisions have consequences. Choosing to do nothing in self-care is a decision but with perhaps devastating consequences.

If healthcare practitioners were to use the above selling strategies and respect the right of clients to refuse or to modify diabetes management strategies, they would look at their jobs with a greater sense of fulfillment and would experience less burnout themselves. Hopefully, we, as nurses and healthcare professionals, will stop the ineffectual labeling of patients as noncompliant or nonadherent and realize that there is a reason, maybe even several, why a client cannot or will not comply with the medical regimen prescribed. Until we know and understand what these reasons are, we cannot help the client in his or her struggle to improve diabetes self-management. Each time we work with clients who might be considered noncompliant, we cannot write them off. Trying some of the strategies listed in this book and any others that we can think of will help us learn from these challenges and work at perfecting our approach to such clients. We as nurses may never see the results of our efforts, but we know that we have given the client something to think about when no one else may have bothered to do so.

REFERENCES

American Diabetes Association. (n.d.-a). *Anger*. Retrieved September 20, 2010, from www.diabetes.org/living-with-diabetes/complications/mental-health/anger.html

American Diabetes Association. (n.d.-b). *Depression*. Retrieved September 21, 2010, from www.diabetes.org/living-with-diabetes/complications/mental-health/depression.html

American Diabetes Association. (n.d.-c). *Stress*. Retrieved September 17, 2010, from www.diabetes.org/living-with-diabetes/complications/stress.html

Berne, E. (1964, renewed 1992). *Games people play*. New York, NY: Ballantine Books.

Carter-Edwards, L., Skelly, A. H., Cagle, C. S., & Appel, N. J. (2004). "They care but don't understand": Family support of African American women with type 2 diabetes. *Diabetes Education, 30*(3), 493–501.

DeYoung, S. (2003). *Teaching strategies for nurse educators*. Upper Saddle River, NJ: Prentice Hall.

Folz-Gray, D. (2010, November 24). *13 tips for fighting diabetes burnout*. Retrieved June 7, 2011, from www .lifescript.com/Health/Conditions/Diabetes/13_Tips_for_Fighting_Diabetes_Burnout.asp

Gonzalez, J. S., Peyrot, M., McCarl, L. A., Collins, E. M., Serpa, L., Mimiaga, M. J., & Safren, S. A. (2008). Depression and diabetes treatment nonadherence: A meta-analysis. *Diabetes Care, 31*(12), 2398–2403.

Pawar, M. (2005). Five tips for generating patient satisfaction and compliance. *Family Practice Management, 12*(6), 44–46.

Peyrot, M., Rubin, R. R., Lauritzen, T., Skovlund, S. E., Snoek, F. J., Matthews, D. R., et al. (2005). Resistance to insulin therapy among patients and providers. *Diabetes Care, 28*, 2673–2679.

Rankin, S. H., Stallings. K. D., & London, F. (2005). *Patient education in health and illness* (5th ed.). Philadelphia, PA: Lippincott Williams & Wilkins.

Redman, B. K. (2004). *Advances in patient education*. New York, NY: Springer Publishing.

Rubin, R. R. (n.d.). *Tips for really helping a person who has diabetes*. Retrieved May 16, 2011, from www.diabetes.org/living-with-diabetes/connect-with-others/support

Glossary

Acanthosis nigricans—condition characterized by discolored patches in the skin folds of the armpits, neck, or groin, ranging from tan to dark brown. Acanthosis nigricans is associated with hyperinsulinemia (a higher than normal level of insulin in the blood), which results from obesity-related insulin resistance.

ACE inhibitor—angiotensin-converting enzyme inhibitor, an antihypertensive that prevents an enzyme from causing the conversion of angiotensinogen to angiotensin-constricting blood vessels and thus raising blood pressure.

Adhesion—band of scar-like tissue that forms between two surfaces inside the body and causes them to stick together. The causes include surgery, trauma, and inflammation. This can happen anywhere in the body, such as in joints and inside the abdomen or pelvis.

Aerobic exercise—any physical exercise that requires additional effort by the heart and lungs to meet increased demand by the skeletal muscles for oxygen resulting in increased heart and lung efficiency.

Alpha cells—cells in the islets of Langerhans of the pancreas that produce glucagon, which causes the liver to release stored glucose in the form of glycogen.

Alpha-glucosidase inhibitors—work in the small intestine to delay and/or block the digestion of carbohydrates (starches and sucrose) and decrease the peak postprandial glucose levels, allowing insulin production to better match glucose absorption. Examples include Precose and Glyset.

Amsler Grid—series of vertical and horizontal lines with a dot in the middle. You may use the Amsler Grid on a daily basis, testing each eye separately. In this way, someone with macular degeneration will become familiar with his or her own pattern of distortion. Any new waviness should be reported to the doctor. This may be a sign of active "wet" macular degeneration.

Amylin—hormone produced by the beta cells of the pancreas, as is insulin. It is secreted in response to eating and helps to reduce postprandial glucagon levels, thus lowering blood glucose. Symlin is a synthetic amylin analog.

Anaerobic exercise—exertion of muscles without the need to take in more oxygen.

Antihyperlipidemics—drugs that lower cholesterol.

Antihypertensives—drugs that lower blood pressure.

ARB—angiotensin receptor blocker, a type of antihypertensive that prevents blood pressure from going up by blocking the receptors for angiotensin, a powerful substance that makes the blood vessels contract, causing blood pressure to rise.

Arrhythmia—any deviation from the normal pattern of the heartbeat, or an irregular beat.

Atherosclerosis—occurs when fatty deposits stick to the inner layers of the walls of large and medium arteries.

Autonomic neuropathy—inflammation or degeneration of nerves in the autonomic nervous system caused by hyperglycemia. Neurogenic bladder, gastroparesis, and erectile dysfunction are examples.

Basal metabolic rate—amount of energy used by a fasting, resting person to maintain vital functions.

Beta blockers—antihypertensives that block beta receptors on blood vessels so stress hormones cannot cause them to constrict. They also prevent an increase in heart rate.

Beta cells—part of the islets of Langerhans that produce insulin in response to a rise in blood glucose.

Biguanides—antidiabetic drugs that act primarily to decrease the liver's inappropriate release of glycogen into the blood, thus increasing blood sugar. It also improves tissue insulin sensitivity, both problems in type 2 diabetes. Glucophage, Glumetza, and Fortamet are examples.

Body mass index—calculation of body fatness based on the relationship between a person's height and weight. It is calculated by using body weight in kilograms divided by height in meters squared.

Calcium channel blockers—slow the movement of calcium into the cells of the heart and blood vessel walls, which makes it easier for the heart to pump and widens blood vessels.

Carb counting—method of keeping track of the number of grams of carbohydrates for weight loss and blood sugar control. Foods high in dietary carbohydrates include sugar; starchy foods, such as potatoes and pasta; and grain-based foods, such as breads and cereals. Carbohydrates can also be found in dairy products and fruits and starchy vegetables, as well as many beverages.

Cardiovascular disease—conditions or diseases of the heart and blood vessels in general, including coronary artery disease, angina, congestive heart failure, high blood pressure, and stroke.

Carotid artery—main artery that carries oxygenated blood from the heart to the brain. There is one on each side of the neck.

Carotid endarterectomy—surgical procedure used to prevent stroke, by correcting the stenosis (narrowing) in the common carotid artery. Endarterectomy is the removal of material on the inside (end-) of an artery.

Carotinoids—precursors to vitamin A found in yellow and orange vegetables.

Carpal tunnel syndrome—median nerve entrapment, often caused by repetitive motion, such typing or painting, that irritates the tendons around the median nerve at the wrist. This causes swelling, which makes the bony tunnel space narrower and compresses the nerve.

Cerebral arteries—arteries in the brain that carry oxygenated blood to the cells of the brain.

Charcot's joint—neuropathic osteoarthropathy, also known as Charcot arthropathy (often "Charcot foot"), refers to progressive degeneration of a weight-bearing joint, a process marked by bony destruction, bone resorption, and eventual deformity.

Cholesterol—sterol lipid (fat) synthesized by the liver and transported in the bloodstream to the membranes of all animal cells; it plays a central role in many biochemical processes and, as a lipoprotein that coats the walls of blood vessels, is associated with cardiovascular disease. Cholesterol can also be found in many animal food sources.

Congenital anomalies—birth defects.

Congestive heart failure—condition caused by the inadequacy of the heart so that as a pump it fails to maintain the circulation of blood by pumping it forward, with the result that congestion and edema develop in the tissues, first in the lungs and then in the rest of the body.

Continuous glucose monitoring system—device that tests blood glucose levels every 5 minutes or so, depending on the system. This continues for 72 hours or more before the site must be changed. It wirelessly transmits the information to a receiver (cell phone size) or an insulin pump that displays the results.

Coronary artery disease—narrowing or blockage of the arteries and vessels that provide oxygen and nutrients to the heart muscle.

Crohn's disease—chronic inflammatory disease, primarily involving the small and large intestine but that can affect other parts of the digestive system as well.

CT scan—computed tomography scan (also known as a CAT scan), a computerized X-ray procedure. A CT scan produces cross-sectional images of the body. The images are far more detailed than X-ray films and can reveal disease or abnormalities in tissue and bone. The procedure is usually noninvasive and brief.

DASH diet—Dietary Alternative to Stop Hypertension; includes fresh fruit, vegetables, and whole-grain products. It is a diet high in potassium and low in sodium.

Dermopathy—also called *shin spots*, is a skin condition that develops as a result of changes to the blood vessels that supply the skin as a result of hyperglycemia. Dermopathy appears as a shiny round or oval lesion of thin skin over the front lower parts of the lower legs. The patches do not hurt, although rarely they can be itchy or cause burning. Medical treatment generally is not necessary.

Diabetes self-management—proactive way to look at client-controlled management of a complex disease. It involves the client's willingness to learn how to control the disease, take the steps to actively participate in the treatment, seek help when needed, and self-tailor this treatment on the basis of knowledge of his or her own body.

Diabetic ketoacidosis—condition that occurs when the body cannot burn glucose for energy because there is insufficient insulin to move it into cells. The body then burns fat, and the by-product of this burning creates fatty acids and ketones.

Dietary Guidelines for Americans—jointly issued and updated every 5 years by the U.S. Department of Agriculture and the U.S. Department of Health and Human Services. They provide authoritative advice for people 2 years and older about how good dietary habits can promote health and reduce risk of major chronic diseases.

Diuretics—make kidneys excrete more water in the urine, thus lowering blood pressure.

DPP-4 inhibitor—class of medications (like Januvia and Onglyxa) that help the body lower too-high blood glucose levels in people with type 2 diabetes by increased incretin levels (GLP-1 and GIP), which inhibit glucagon release, the effect of which, in turn, decreases blood glucose but, more significantly, increases insulin secretion and slows gastric emptying.

Endocrinologist—physician who specializes in the diagnosis and treatment of conditions affecting the endocrine system, including the thyroid and the pancreas.

Fat-soluble vitamins—vitamins that dissolve in dietary and body fat (vitamins A, D, E, and K). They are metabolized and absorbed only in the presence of dietary fat. Because excess fat-soluble vitamins may be stored in the body fat, several weeks' supply may be consumed in a single dose or meal.

Fetal demise—death of the fetus during pregnancy.

Fetal surveillance—indirect way to measure fetal well-being and the adequacy of fetal oxygenation, includes periodic ultrasound, fetal monitoring, fetal movement assessment, periodic fetal heart rate, continuous electronic fetal heart rate monitoring, fetal amniotic fluid analysis, and more.

Frozen shoulder—or adhesive capsulitis is a painful restriction of shoulder movement.

Gestation—another word for pregnancy.

Gestational age—how many weeks old a fetus is.

Gestational diabetes mellitus—diabetes that occurs only during pregnancy.

Gingivitis—inflammation of gums in the mouth. Gums become red, swollen, and often bleed.

Glomerulus—capillary tuft in the kidney that performs the first step in filtering blood to form urine.

Glucose—simple sugar. Cells use it as a source of energy. Glucose is one of the main products of photosynthesis. Starch and cellulose are polymers derived from the dehydration of glucose.

Glucose challenge test—measures the amount of glucose (sugar) in the bloodstream after the woman is "challenged" with a 50-g glucose solution. It determines whether she can produce enough insulin in 1 hour to keep blood sugar levels from rising. This test is given between 24 and 28 weeks of pregnancy to screen for gestational diabetes.

Glucose tolerance test—administration of a premeasured amount of glucose drink (usually 75–100 g) to determine how quickly it is cleared from the blood and homeostasis is maintained. The test is usually used to test for diabetes, insulin resistance, and sometimes reactive hypoglycemia.

Glycogen—glucose that is stored in the liver and skeletal muscles for later use.

Glycosuria or glucosuria—condition that exists when glucose is found in urine.

Heart failure—condition in which a problem with the structure or function of the heart impairs its ability to supply sufficient blood flow to meet the body's needs.

Hemodialysis—method for removing waste products, such as creatinine and urea, as well as free water from the blood when the kidneys are in renal failure.

Hemoglobin A1c (HbA1c)—blood test that measures the average percentage of blood glucose over a 2- to 3-month period. It can be used to diagnose diabetes.

High-density lipoprotein—type of lipoprotein that consists of about 50% protein and 19% cholesterol. It protects against cardiovascular disease by removing cholesterol deposits from arteries or preventing their formation. It is also known as good cholesterol.

Human leukocyte antigen markers—associated with specific autoimmune diseases. Some human leukocyte antigens offer protection against certain autoimmune diseases. We get these genetic markers from our biological parents.

Hydrogenated fat—unsaturated fat to which hydrogen has been added to make it more stable and solid at room temperature. Partially or completely hydrogenated oils both contain *trans*-fat.

Hypercholesterolemia—another name for high cholesterol levels in the blood.

Hyperglycemia—another word for high blood sugar, usually defined as 180 mg/dl or higher, but symptoms may not start to become noticeable until blood glucose is over 250 mg/dl.

Hyperinsulinemia—higher than normal level of insulin in the blood. This is common in overweight and obese individuals who are insulin resistant. They may or may not develop diabetes.

Hyperosmolar hyperglycemic nonketotic syndrome—serious condition most frequently seen in older persons with type 2 diabetes caused by an illness or infection. Blood sugar levels are usually over 600 mg/dl and there is severe dehydration from the kidneys' attempt to get rid of the glucose. There is enough insulin produced to use some of the sugar, so fat is not burned for energy (nonketosis). Severe dehydration may lead to seizures, coma, and eventually death.

Hyperthyroidism—autoimmune disease caused by overactive tissue within the thyroid gland, resulting in overproduction and thus an excess of circulating free thyroid hormones: thyroxin (T_4), triiodothyronine (T_3), or both. Symptoms include nervousness, irritability, increased perspiration, a racing heart, hand tremors, anxiety, difficulty sleeping, thinning of the skin, fine, brittle hair, and muscular weakness, especially in the upper arms and thighs. Weight loss, sometimes significant, despite a good appetite may occur, as well as vomiting, and, for women, menstrual flow may lighten and menstrual periods may occur less often. Treatment includes medically obliterating the thyroid gland or surgically removing it.

Hypoglycemia—another word for low blood sugar, usually defined as lower than 70 mg/dl. Glucose levels of 40 and below constitute severe hypoglycemia, a life-threatening emergency.

Hypothyroidism—autoimmune disease caused by decreased activity of the thyroid gland. Symptoms may include weight gain, sluggishness, dry skin, intolerance to cold, and slowing of bodily processes. Treatment includes prescribing oral dosages of the thyroid hormone.

Incretin mimetics—synthetic version of the human incretin hormone GLP-1 (glucagon-like peptide-1) that is secreted in the small intestines, but it lasts longer. This drug classification includes Byetta (exenatide) and Victoza (liraglutide).

Insulin analogs—man-made substances resembling insulin in which the molecular structure has been altered for a more desirable effect. Some insulin analogs are rapid acting (Humalog, NovoLog, Apidra) or long acting (Lantus, Levemir).

Insulin-to-carbohydrate ratios—ratio between 1 unit of insulin and the specific number of grams of carbohydrates it will take care of, such as 1 unit to 10 g of carbs.

Intermittent claudication—pain in one or both legs that a person experiences when walking or exercising due to insufficient blood flow to bring enough oxygen to the active muscle. The pain is intermittent and goes away when the person rests.

Interstitial fluid—fluid between the cells of the body.

Islets of Langerhans—irregular clusters of endocrine cells scattered throughout the tissue of the pancreas that secrete insulin and glucagon. They are named after Paul Langerhans, the German scientist who discovered them in 1869.

Ketonemia—occurs when fat is burned for energy and the by-product, ketones, build up in the blood.

Ketonuria—condition in which ketones from fat metabolism are present in the urine.

Lactation—another word for the process of breastfeeding.

Large for gestational age—means that a newborn is larger than the range of normal weight at that gestational age or greater than the 90th percentile for that gestational age. For example, a baby born at 40 weeks' gestation should weigh between 6.6 and 8.8 pounds.

Laser photocoagulation—coagulation (clotting) of tissue using a laser that produces light in the visible green wavelength that is selectively absorbed by hemoglobin, the pigment in red blood cells. It is used to seal off bleeding blood vessels in the back of the eye.

Low-density lipoprotein—type of lipoprotein that transports cholesterol and triglycerides from the liver to peripheral tissues and blood vessels. Because higher levels of low-density lipoprotein particles promote health problems and cardiovascular disease, they are often called "bad cholesterol."

Macrosomia—leads to a large-for-gestational-age baby whose birth weight lies above the 90th percentile for that gestational age.

Macular degeneration—medical condition that usually affects older adults that results in a loss of vision in the center of the visual field (the macula) because of damage to the retina. It occurs in dry and wet forms. It is a major cause of visual impairment in older adults (over 50 years of age). Macular degeneration can make it difficult or impossible to read or recognize faces, although enough peripheral vision remains to allow other activities of daily life.

Macula edema—most common cause of vision loss in people with diabetes. *Macula edema* develops in nonproliferative retinopathy and threatens central vision unless treatment begins soon. The *macula* is the site on the retina that focuses on central vision needed to see straight ahead for reading, driving, and doing any close work, such as knitting or needlepoint.

Magnetic resonance imaging—use of nuclear magnetic resonance of protons to produce proton density images.

Meglitinide—classification of drugs that make the pancreas produce more insulin in response to glucose. It works much faster than sulfonylureas and does not last as long. Prandin is the only example to date; it should be taken right before a meal.

Metabolic syndrome—condition that includes obesity, insulin resistance, diabetes or prediabetes, hypertension, and high lipids.

Microalbuminuria—small amounts of protein found in the urine. It is a highly sensitive indicator of glomerular disease and a sign that kidneys are not functioning properly.

Monounsaturated fat—kind of fat in which one or more pairs of electrons in the atom making up the fat molecule form a bond with a pair of electrons from another atom (a double bond). Monounsaturated fats contain one double bond and are found in peanuts, peanut butter, olives, and avocados. They are heart-healthy fats.

Necrobiosis lipoidica diabeticorum—condition thought to be caused by changes in the collagen and fat content underneath the skin. The overlaying skin area becomes thinned and reddened. Most lesions are found on the lower parts of the legs and can ulcerate if subjected to trauma. Sometimes the condition is itchy and painful.

Nephrons—working units of the kidney that remove waste and extra fluids from the blood. Each kidney is made of approximately 1 million nephrons.

Nephropathy—serious kidney disease that can occur in people who have had diabetes for a long time, particularly if their diabetes has been poorly controlled.

Neuropathy—any disease or injury affecting nerves or nerve cells.

Noncompliance—failure or refusal of a knowledgeable and financially able person to cooperate and carry out those activities that have been communicated to this person by healthcare practitioners as being appropriate to control the disease and therefore exerts his or her own control knowing that by doing so he or she is purposely shortening life expectancy.

Nonproliferative retinopathy—initial stage in diabetic retinopathy. High levels of blood glucose cause damage to the blood vessels in the retina. The blood vessels leak fluid, which can collect and cause the retina to swell. This stage usually does not cause decrease in vision unless the edema is in the macula.

Normoglycemic—having a normal amount of glucose in the blood. Normal fasting blood sugar is 70 to 99 mg/dl.

Olestra or Olean—fat substitute that adds no fat, calories, or cholesterol to products. It has been used in the preparation of traditionally high-fat foods, such as potato chips, thereby lowering or eliminating their fat content.

Ophthalmologist—medical doctor who diagnoses and treats all diseases and disorders of the eye, including surgical treatment. Ophthalmologists can also prescribe glasses and contact lenses.

Optometrist—doctor of optometry, a primary healthcare professional for the eye. Optometrists examine, diagnose, treat, and manage diseases, injuries, and disorders of the eye. They prescribe glasses, contact lenses, and low-vision aids. Optometrists cannot perform surgery.

Pancreatitis—inflammation of the pancreas. It can be acute or chronic and can be caused by alcoholism, trauma, infection, and some drugs. It can be extremely painful and may require treatment with pancreatic digestive hormones as well as insulin as it heals.

Pedometer—device worn on the belt, usually on one side. It counts steps and can calculate miles walked, and some may calculate pounds lost, heart rate, and other information based on parameters preprogrammed into it by user.

Periodontal disease—set of inflammatory diseases affecting the tissues that surround and support the teeth. Periodontitis involves progressive loss of the alveolar bone around the teeth and, if left untreated, can lead to the loosening and subsequent loss of teeth.

Peripheral artery disease—includes all diseases caused by the obstruction of large arteries in the arms and legs.

Peripheral neuropathy—condition of the nervous system that usually begins in the hands and/or feet with symptoms of numbness, tingling, burning and/or weakness. It can be caused by certain anticancer drugs and by hyperglycemia.

Peristalsis—is the rippling motion of muscles in the digestive tract. In the stomach, this motion mixes food with gastric juices, turning it into a thin liquid. In the intestines, this motion moves the contents along until it exits at the anus.

Peritoneal dialysis—treatment for persons with severe chronic kidney failure. The process uses the peritoneum in the abdomen as a membrane across which fluids and dissolved substances (electrolytes, urea, glucose, albumin, and other small molecules) are exchanged from the blood. Fluid is introduced through a permanent tube in the abdomen and flushed out either every night while the person sleeps (automatic peritoneal dialysis) or via regular exchanges throughout the day (continuous ambulatory peritoneal dialysis).

Peritonitis—infection of the gut wall or peritoneum. It can be a complication of peritoneal dialysis or caused by a ruptured appendix or other sources of abdominal infection.

Pilates—exercise system that is focused on building strength without bulk, improving flexibility and agility, and helping to prevent injury.

Placebo—inert compound or treatment that should have no effect.

Placebo effect—when the client expects something to happen and it does, even though the client was not given the *real* medication or treatment.

Podiatrist—doctor of podiatric medicine, also known as a podiatric physician or surgeon, who is qualified by his or her education and training to diagnose and treat conditions affecting the foot, ankle, and related structures of the leg.

Polyunsaturated fat—kind of fat in which one or more pairs of electrons in the atom making up the fat molecule form a bond with a pair of electrons from another atom (a double bond). Polyunsaturated fats contain two or more double bonds and are found in oils such as corn, sunflower, and soybean. They are heart-healthy fats.

Postprandial—after meals.

Preconception—prior to pregnancy, usually refers to prepregnancy health evaluation and care.

Prediabetes—occurs when there is impaired fasting glucose, impaired glucose tolerance, a fasting glucose of 100 to 125 mg/dl or an A1c between 5.7% and 6.4%. Individuals with prediabetes have an increased risk of developing diabetes in the near future if weight loss and lifestyle changes are not instituted.

PreDx Diabetes Risk Score Test—simple blood test that Tethys Bioscience says can identify persons with a high risk of developing type 2 diabetes within 5 years.

Pregestational—before pregnancy.

Pregnancy-induced hypertension—hypertension after 20 weeks of pregnancy that is accompanied by proteinuria and edema above the waist. It is a dangerous condition of pregnancy that can develop over a number of weeks, or it can have a sudden onset and end in convulsions. Older terms are *preeclampsia* (before a seizure) and *eclampsia* (seizure).

Prematurity—in regard to gestation, before 37 completed weeks or the first day of the 38th week.

Preprandial—before meals.

Proliferative retinopathy—fourth stage of diabetic retinopathy, in which signals sent by the retina for nourishment trigger the growth of new blood vessels, which are abnormal and fragile. They grow along the retina and the surface of the clear vitreous gel that fills the inside of the eye. They can bleed into the vitreous gel and cause blurred vision or blindness if bleeding is extensive.

Proteinuria—condition in which an excessive amount of protein is found in the urine.

Renal tubules—microscopic chemical factories in the kidneys that manufacture urine from filtered blood, at the same time conserving essential nutrients and other substances required by the body, such as protein.

Retina—light-sensitive lining of the back of the eyeball that transmits signals to the optic nerve, which sends them to the brain for interpretation.

Retinopathy—complication of diabetes that is caused by changes in the blood vessels of the retina. When blood vessels in the retina are damaged, they may leak blood and grow fragile, brush-like branches and scar tissue. This can blur or distort the vision images that the retina sends to the brain.

Rheumatoid arthritis—chronic autoimmune disease with inflammation of the joints and marked deformities; something (possibly a virus) triggers an attack on the joint by the immune system, which releases cytokines that stimulate an inflammatory reaction that can lead to the destruction of all components of the joint.

Saturated fat—type of fat that has been shown to increase the risk of heart disease. Found in animal foods such as butter, full-fat dairy foods, and fatty meats, as well as many processed and take-out foods.

Scleroderma diabeticorum—skin problem that affects people with type 2 diabetes, causing a thickening of the skin on the back of the neck and upper back.

Secretagogue medications—drugs that make the pancreas increase its production of insulin.

SGLT2 inhibitors—work by inhibiting the SGLT2 molecules (sodium-glucose co-transporter) in the kidney tubules that cause reabsorption of sugar and sodium that otherwise would be excreted in the urine. The result is that more sugar and sodium are excreted, resulting in lower blood sugar, weight loss, and lower blood pressure. Dapgliflozin and canagliflozin are examples, but no drugs in this class are yet on the market.

Standard of care—treatment that another prudent healthcare professional, of similar background and training, would give to the same client. It is usually the recommended treatment option for this person for this problem.

Stent—man-made tube inserted into a natural passage/conduit in the body to prevent, or counteract, a disease-induced localized flow constriction. It is used as part of an angioplasty procedure to correct a blockage in a coronary or peripheral artery, such as in the leg.

Sugar alcohols—food additives that are used as sweeteners and texturizing agents in foods. The limited absorption and metabolism of sugar alcohols are important factors in their use in dietetic foods. The list includes mannitol, sorbitol, xylitol, maltitol, and other *-itol* sweeteners. They do contribute to blood sugar but are slowly absorbed. They also stimulate the bowels, and even a listed serving size may cause cramps and diarrhea in some people.

Sulfonylureas—group of hypoglycemic drugs that act on the beta cells of the pancreas to increase the secretion of insulin.

Systemic lupus erythematosus—chronic autoimmune connective tissue disease that can affect any part of the body. As occurs in other autoimmune diseases, the immune system attacks the body's cells and tissue, resulting in inflammation and tissue damage.

Tai Chi—Chinese system of slow meditative physical exercise designed for relaxation, balance, and health.

Thiazolidinediones—class of drugs (such as pioglitazone and rosiglitazone) that are thiazolidine derivatives used to reduce insulin resistance in the treatment of type 2 diabetes.

trans-fat—type of unsaturated fat with *trans*-isomer fatty acid(s), usually made by food manufacturers by partially hydrogenating mono- or polyunsaturated oils so that foods last longer on shelves or in cans. Eating *trans*-fats increases the risk of some illnesses, such as heart disease.

Transient ischemic attack—risk factor for stroke. Transient ischemic attacks are caused by temporary interruptions to the blood supply of the brain. Their symptoms are similar to stroke symptoms but disappear within a few minutes.

Trigger finger—also called *trigger thumb*, or *trigger digit*, is a common disorder of later adulthood characterized by catching, snapping, or locking of the involved finger flexor tendon, associated with dysfunction and pain. It can be corrected with outpatient surgery or eased with massage and stretching exercises.

Triglycerides—common blood fats that trigger the liver to create more cholesterol. If blood glucose is high, triglycerides are usually high. Elevated triglycerides can also be due to overweight/obesity, physical inactivity, cigarette smoking, excess alcohol consumption, and a diet very high in carbohydrates (60% of total calories or more).

Type 1 diabetes mellitus—form of diabetes mellitus that results from autoimmune destruction of insulin-producing beta cells of the pancreas. The subsequent lack of insulin leads to increased blood and urine glucose.

Type 2 diabetes mellitus—disorder that is characterized by high blood glucose in the context of insulin resistance and relative insulin deficiency.

Valsalva maneuver—performed by forcible exhalation against a closed airway, usually done by closing one's mouth as when pushing down to have a stool.

Vitrectomy—surgical procedure that removes the vitreous gel from the back of the eye and replaces it with saline solution. It is usually an outpatient procedure done under local anesthesia.

Water-soluble vitamins—are not stored in the body and must be replenished on a daily basis. Water-soluble vitamins include the B complex of vitamins (thiamin, riboflavin, niacin, pyridoxine, biotin, folic acid, B_6, and B_{12}) and vitamin C.

Xerostomia—dry mouth.

Yoga—healing system of theory and practice. It is a combination of breathing exercises, physical postures, and meditation that has been practiced for more than 5,000 years.

Resources

The following is a list of diabetes organizations and diabetes professional organizations:

American Academy of Physical Medicine and Rehabilitation
330 Wabash Ave., Suite 2500
Chicago, IL 60611
Phone: 312-464-9700
www.aapmr.org

American Association of Diabetes Educators
100 West Monroe, 4th Floor
Chicago, IL 60603-1901
Phone: 800-338-3633 for names of diabetes educators
312-424-2426 to order publications
www.aadenet.org

American Association of Kidney Patients
3505 East Frontage Rd., Suite 315
Tampa, FL 33607
Phone: 800-749-2257
E-mail: info@aakp.org
www.aakp.org

American College of Sports Medicine
P.O. Box 1440
Indianapolis, IN 46206
Phone: 317-637-9200
www.acsm.org

American Council on Exercise
4851 Paramount Drive
San Diego, CA 92123
Phone: 888-825-3636 (toll free)
www.acefitness.org

American Diabetes Association
1701 North Beauregard St.
Alexandria, VA 22311
Phone: 703-549-1500
800-ADA-ORDER to order publications toll free
800-DIABETES (800-342-2383) for diabetes information
www.diabetes.org
www.diabetes.org/for-parents-and-kids/for-teens.jsp

American Dietetic Association
National Center for Nutrition and Dietetics
216 West Jackson Blvd., Suite 800
Chicago, IL 60606-6995
Phone: 800-366-1655 Consumer Nutrition Hotline
(Spanish speaker available)
800-745-0775
www.eatright.org

American Heart Association National Center
7272 Greenville Ave.
Dallas, TX 75231
Phone: 214-373-6300
www.heart.org/HEARTORG

American Kidney Fund
6110 Executive Blvd., Suite 1010
Rockville, MD 20852
Phone: 800-638-8299 or 301-881-3052
E-mail: helpline@kidneyfund.org
www.kidneyfund.org

American Pain Foundation
201 North Charles St., Suite 710
Bethesda, MD 21201-4111
Phone: 888-615-7246 or 410-385-1832
www.painfoundation.org

American Podiatric Medical Association
9312 Old Georgetown Rd.
Bethesda, MD 20814-1621
Phone: 800-FOOTCARE (366-8227) or 301-581-9200
www.apma.org

American Psychological Association
750 First St., NE
Washington, DC 20002-4242
Phone: 800-374-2723
www.apa.org
http://locator.apa.org

To find a therapist versed in cognitive behavior therapy in your state, go to *www.psychologyinfo.com/directory/state-links.html*

American Urological Association Foundation
1000 Corporate Blvd.
Linthicum, MD 21090
Phone: 866-746-4282 or 410-689-3700
www.auafoundation.org
www.urologyhealth.org

Arthritis Foundation
P.O. Box 7669
Atlanta, GA 30357
Phone: 800-283-7800
www.arthritis.org

Children with Diabetes
8216 Princeton-Glendale Road, PMB 200
West Chester, OH 45069-1675
www.childrenwithdiabetes.com

Diabetes Education and Camping Association
PO Box 385
Huntsville, AL 35804
www.diabetescamps.org

Diabetes Exercise and Sports Association
310 West Liberty, Suite 604
Louisville, KY 40202
Phone: 800-898-4322
Fax: 502-581-0206
www.diabetes-exercise.org

Juvenile Diabetes Research Foundation International
26 Broadway
New York, NY 10004
Phone: 800-533-CURE (800-533-2873)
Fax: 212-785-9595
www.jdrf.org

Life Options Rehabilitation Program
c/o Medical Education Institute, Inc.
414 D'Onofrio Dr., Suite 200
Madison, WI 53719
Phone: 800-468-7777 or 608-232-2333
E-mail: lifeoptions@meiresearch.org
www.lifeoptions.org
www.kidneyschool.org

Lower Extremity Amputation Prevention Program
Health Resources and Services Administration
5600 Fishers Ln.
Rockville, MD 20857
Phone: 888-ASK-HRSA (888-275-4772)
www.hrsa.gov/leap

National Diabetes Information Clearinghouse
1 Information Way
Bethesda, MD 20892-3560
Phone: 301-654-3327 or 800-860-8747
www.diabetes.niddk.nih.gov

National Institute on Aging
Building 31, Room 5C27
31 Center Drive, MSC 2292
Bethesda, MD 20892
Phone: 800-222-2225
www.nih.gov/nia

National Kidney Foundation, Inc.
30 East 33rd St.
New York, NY 10016
Phone: 800-622-9010 or 212-889-2210
www.kidney.org

National Kidney and Urologic Diseases Information Clearinghouse
3 Information Way
Bethesda, MD 20892-3580
Phone: 1-866-569-1162
www.kidney.niddk.nih.gov

The Neuropathy Associations, Inc.
60 E. 42nd St., Suite 942
New York, NY 10165-0999
Phone: 800-247-6968
www.neuropathy.org

The President's Council on Physical Fitness and Sports
200 Independence Ave., SW, Room 738-H
Washington, DC 20201
Phone: 202-690-9000
www.fitness.gov
www.presidentschallenge.org

Weight-control Information Network
1 Win Way
Bethesda, MD 20892
Phone: 877-946-4627
http://win.niddk.nih.gov

Periodicals

The following journals and magazines deal with diabetes and self-care management:

Diabetes Forecast, http://forecast.diabetes.org
Diabetes Self-Management, www.diabetesselfmanagement.com
Diabetic Living, www.diabeticlivingonline.com
Diabetic Cooking, www.diabeticcooking.com
Diabetes Health, www.diabeteshealth.com
Eating Well, www.eatingwell.com
Insulin, www.insulinjournal.com

Organizations that have information about diabetes and other health issues:

Federal Government Organizations

Centers for Disease Control and Prevention
1600 Clifton Rd.
Atlanta, GA 30333
800-CDC-INFO (800-232-4636) or 770-488-5000
www.cdc.gov/diabetes

Health Resources and Services Administration
5600 Fishers Ln.
Rockville, MD 20857
www.hrsa.gov

Indian Health Service
Diabetes Program
5300 Homestead Rd., NE
Albuquerque, NM 87110
505-248-4182
www.ihs.gov/medicalprograms/diabetes/index.asp

National Diabetes Education Program
One Diabetes Way
Bethesda, MD 20814-9692
Phone: 800-438-5383
http://ndep.nih.gov/teens/index.aspx?redirect=true

National Institute of Diabetes and Digestive and Kidney Diseases
1 Information Way
Bethesda, MD 20892-3560
Phone: 800-GET LEVEL (800-438-5383) or 301-654-3327
www.niddk.nih.gov

National Diabetes Information Clearinghouse
1 Information Way
Bethesda, MD 20892-3560

Phone: 301-654-3327
Fax: 301-907-8906
http://diabetes.niddk.nih.gov/index.htm
http://diabetes.niddk.nih.gov/dm/pubs/financialhelp/index.htm

National Eye Institute
Building 31, Room 6A32
31 Center Dr., MSC 2510
Bethesda, MD 20892-2510
Phone: 301-496-5248 or 800-869-2020 (to order materials)
Fax: 301-402-1065
www.nei.nih.gov

Office of Minority Health Resource Center
U.S. Department of Health and Human Services
P.O. Box 37337
Washington, DC 20013-7337
Phone: 800-444-MHRC (800-444-6472)
www.omhrc.gov

U.S. Department of Veterans Affairs
810 Vermont Ave., NW
Washington, DC 20420
www.va.gov/diabetes

Nonfederal Government Organizations

American Optometric Association
1505 Prince St.
Alexandria, VA 22314
Phone: 800-262-3947 or 703-739-9200
www.aoanet.org

American Podiatric Medical Association
9312 Old Georgetown Rd.
Bethesda, MD 20814
Phone: 301-571-9200 or 800-ASK-APMA
(800-275-2762)
Fax: 301-530-2752
www.apma.org

**Medical Eye Care for the Nation's Disadvantaged
Senior Citizens**
The Foundation of the American Academy of Ophthalmology
P.O. Box 429098
San Francisco, CA 94142-9098
Phone: 800-222-EYES (800-222-3937)
www.faao.org

Information on living wills and advance directives for each state:

National Hospices and Palliative Care Organization
Caring Connections
http://caringinfo.org

Equipment companies for current and future meters and other paraphernalia:

Meter Companies

Abbott Diabetes Care (formerly Therasense)
Phone: 888-522-5226, 800-527-3339
www.abbottdiabetescare.com
Meters: FreeStyle Lite, FreeStyle Freedom Lite, Precision Xtra

Accu-Chek
Phone: 800-858-8072
www.accu-chek.com/us
Meters: Aviva, Compact Plus, Active, Advantage

AgaMatrix, Inc.
Phone: 603-328-6000, 866-906-4197
www.wavesense.info
Meters: WaveSense Jazz, Jazz Wireless, WaveSense KeyNote, WaveSense KeyNote Pro,WaveSense Presto, WaveSense Presto Pro

Arkray USA (formerly Hypoguard)
Phone: 800-818-8877
www.arkrayusa.com
Meters: Assure Platinum, Assure Pro, Assure 4
www.glucocardusa.com
Meters: Glucocard 01, Glucocard 01-Mini, Glucocard X-Meter, Glucocard Vital

Bayer
Phone: 800-348-8100
www.bayerdiabetes.com
www.simplewins.com
Meters: Breeze2, Contour, Contour TS A1C Now

Bionime USA
Phone: 888-481-8485
www.bionimeusa.com
Meters: Rightest GM100, Rightest GM300

Diabetic Supply of Suncoast
Phone: 866-373-2824
www.pharmasupply.com
Meters: Advocate, Advocate Duo, Advocate Redi-Code

Diagnostic Devices
Phone: 800-243-2636
www.prodigymeter.com
Meters: Prodigy Autocode, Prodigy Pocket, Prodigy Voice

Fora Care
Phone: 866-469-2632
www.foracare.com/usa
Meters: Fora G20, Fora G90, Fora V10, Fora V12,
Fora V20, Fora V22

Home Diagnostics
Phone: 800-342-7226, Ext. 3300
www.homediagnostics.com
Meters: Sidekick, True2Go, Trueresult, Truetrack

Infopia
Phone: 888-446-3246
www.infopiausa.com
Meters: Eclipse, Element, Envision, Evolution, GlucoLab

LifeScan
Phone: 800-227-8862
www.lifescan.com
Meters: One Touch UltraSmart, UltraMini, UltraMini2, UltraLink,
Ulta2

Nova Biomedical
Phone: 800-681-7390
www.novacares.com
Meters: Nova Max, Nova Max Link

U.S. Diagnostics
Phone: 866-216-5308
www.usdiagnostics.net
Meters: Acura, EasyGluco, Infinity, Maxima

WalMart
Phone: 800-631-0076
www.relion.com/diabetes
Meters: ReliOn Micro, ReliOn Ultima

Insulin Pump Companies

Animas
Phone: 877-937-7867
www.animascorp.com
Maker of the OneTouch Ping and 2020, IRI250, IR 1000
www.animas.com/Request-ping-pump-info

Insulet
Phone: 781-457-5000
www.myomnipod.com/about-omnipod/omnipod-CGM
Makers of the Omnipod Insulin pump

Metronic/MiniMed
Phone: 800-646-4633
www.minimed.com
Makers of the Paradigm 522/722 and Revel insulin pumps

Roche Diabetes Care
Phone: 317-521-3966
www.roche.com
Makers of the Accu-Chek Spirit insulin pump

Sooil Development Co. Ltd.
Phone: 858-404-0659
http://sooil.en.ec21.com/index.jsp
Makers of the Dana Diabecare II insulin pump

Tandem Diabetes Care
Phone: 858-366-6900
www.tandemdiabetes.com
Maker of t:slim insulin pump. Not available in the United States as of September 2010.

Continuous Glucose Monitor Companies

Abbott Diabetes
Phone: 866-597-5520
www.freestylenavigator.com
Makers of the Freestyle Navigator

Dexcom
Phone: 877-339-2664
www.dexcom.com
Maker of the Seven Plus System

Metronic/Minimed
Phone: 866-948-6633
www.minimed.com
Makers of the Paradigm Real Time System and Revel integrated system

Drug Companies

Amylin Pharmaceuticals Inc.
Phone: 858-552-2200
Makers of Noninsulin injections

Symlin (pramlintide)
www.symlin.com
SymlinPen
www.symlin.com/132-using-the-symline-pen.aspx
Byetta (exenatide)
www.byetta.com/Pages/index.aspx

Bayer Pharmaceuticals Corp.
Makers of Precose (acarbose)
www.rxlist.com/precose-drug-patient.htm

Bristol-Myers Squibb Company
Makers of:
Glucophage (metformin) and Glucophage XR
(metformin ER)
www.bms.com/ourcompany/Pages/uswebsites.aspx
Glucovance (metformin and glyburide)
www.rxlist.com/glucovance-drug-patient.htm
Metaglip (metformin and glipizide)
www.rxlist.com/metaglip-drug-patient.htm
Onglyza (saxagliptin)
www.onglyza.com/about/managing.aspx

DepoMed Inc.
Makers of Glumetza (metformin extended release)
www.depomedinc.com/view.cfm/1286/ourproducts

Eli Lilly & Company
Phone: 317-276-9624
Makers of:
Glucagon, Humulin R, N, Humulin 70/30, Humulin 50/50 vials
Humulin R, N, and 70/30 disposable, prefilled pens
www.lillydiabetes.com/index.jsp
Humalog, Humalog 75/25
www.lillydiabetes.com/product/humalog.jsp?reNavId=5.1
Humalog KwikPen and Humalog 75/25 Prefilled Pen
www.insidehumalog.com/hcp/humalog_insulin_hcp.jsp

GlaxoSmithKline
Phone: 888-825-5249
Makers of:
Avandia (rosiglitazone)
www.avandia.com
Avandamet (metformin and rosiglitazone)
www.avandia.com/about_avandamet/avandmet.html
Avandaryl (rosiglitazone and glimepiride)
www.rxlist.com/avandaryl-drug-patient.htm

MannKind Corporation
Phone: (661) 775-5300
Maker of Afrezza inhaled insulin
www.mannkindcorp.com/product-pipeline-diabetes-afrezza.htm

Merck & Co. Inc.
Makers of:
Januvia (sitagliptin)
www.januvia.com/sitagliptin/januvia/consumer/index.jsp
Janumet (metformin and sitagliptin)
www.janumet.com/sitagliptin_ metformin_HCl/janumet/consumer/
medication_guide/index.jsp

Novartis Pharmaceuticals USA
Phone: 888-669-6682
Makers of Starlix (netaglinide)
www.pharma.us.novartis.com/products/name/starlix.jsp

Novo Nordisk
800-727-6500
Makers of:
Prandin (repaglinide)
www.prandin.com
PrandiMet (metformin and repaglinide)
www.rxlist.com/prandiment-drug-patient.htm
Novolin R, N vials and Novolin R, N and 70/30 Penfill
www.insulindevice.com/novopen/faq.asp
NovoLog and NovoLog 70/30
www.novolog.com, *www.novologmix70-30.com*
NovoLog Flexpen
www.novolog.com/devices-flexpen.asp?s=ds&h=60
Levemir and Levemir Flexpen
www.levemir-us.com
Victoza (liraglutide)
www.victoza.com
Glucagon

Pfizer Inc.
Phone: 212-733-2323
www.pfizer.com/products
Makers of Diabinese, Glucotrol (glipizide) and Glucotrol XL (glipizide ER), Glynase Pres tabs (micronized glyburide), Glyset (miglitol), Micronase (glyburide)
www.rxlist.com/glyset-drug-patient.htm

Ranboxy Pharmaceuticals
Makers of Riomet (metformin oral solution)
www.riomet.com

Shionogi Pharma, Inc.
Makers of Fortamet (metformin extended release)
www.rxlist.com/fortamet-drug-patient.htm

Sanofi-Aventis US
Phone: 800-633-1610
Makers of:
Diabeta (glyburide)
www.sanofi-aventis.us/live/us/en/index.jsp
Amaryl (glimepiride)
www.sanofi-aventis.us/live/en/index.jsp
Apidra (glulisine insulin)
www.apidra.com
Apidra SoloSTAR Pen Lantus (glargine insulin) and Lantus SoloSTAR
Pen
www.lantus.com

Takeda Pharmaceuticals
Makers of:
Actos (pioglitazone)
www.rxlist.com/actos-drug-patient.htm
Actoplus Met (metformin and pioglitazone)
www.rxlist.com/actoplus-met-drug-patient.htm
Duetact (pioglitazone and glimepiride)
www.actos.com/duetact/home.aspx

Nutrition

The following information relates to some of the Web sites listed in
Chapter 2.

Sugar-Free Syrups and Flavorings

Atkins Nutritionals, Inc.
Hauppauge, NY 11788
Phone: 800-6-ATKINS (800-628-5467)
www.lowcarb.ca/store/sauce.html

R. Torre & Co (maker of Torani Syrups)
So. San Francisco, CA 94080
www.torani.com

DaVinci Gourmet, Ltd.
Seattle, WA 98108
Phone: 800-640-6779
www.davincigourmet.com

Baja Bob's Sugar Free Cocktail Mixers
1465 Encinitas Blvd.
Encinitas, CA 92024
Phone: 888-569-2272, 760-634-5316
www.BajaBob.com

Low-Carb Pasta

Dakota Growers Pasta Company
One Past Ave.
Carrington, ND 58421
Phone: 800-250-1917
www.dreamfieldsfoods.com

Strumba Media LLC
8605 Santa Monica Blvd., Suite 6920
West Hollywood, CA 90065
Phone: 800-948-4205
www.miraclenoodle.com

Salt Substitutes

Mrs. Dash blend of herb and spices and marinades
Phone: 800-622-DASH
www.mrsdash.com

Morton's Lite Salt
Morton International, Inc.
Chicago, IL 60606-1743
www.mortonsalt.com/products/foodsalts/lite_salt.htm

DASH Diet (Dietary Approach to Stop Hypertension)
http://dashdiet.org

Index

A1c. *See* Hemoglobin A1c
Abilify (aripiprazole), 239
Abuse. *See* Substance use/abuse
Acanthosis nigricans, 150
Acarbose (Precose), 67, 70
Accupril (quinapril), 124
ACE inhibitors, 124
Acebutolol (Prent, Sectral), 125
Acesulfame K (Sunett and Sweet One), 25
Actoplus Met (metformin/ pioglitazone), 67, 68
Actos (pioglitazone), 14, 64, 66, 68
Actos and Avandia (TZDs), 64
ADA. *See* American Diabetes Association (ADA)
Adalat (nifedipine), 125
Adhesion, 147
Adhesive capsulitis. *See* Frozen shoulder
Adolescence and their parents
    addressing nonadherence, 197–199
    adherence to, 195–197
    balancing parental involvement, 194–195
    depression, 199
    eating disorders, 199–200
    insulin omission, 199–200
    substance use/abuse, 200–202
    teaching and motivating, 191–192
    transition to self-care, 192–193
Adrenaline, stress hormones, 53, 100, 256
Adults
    pregnancy, diabetes and, 215–218
    discrimination in employment, 219–221
        Family Medical Leave Act (FMLA), 221

genetic implications of, 214–215
    gestational diabetes, 208–210
    health insurance, 221–222
    pregestational diabetes, 205–210
    self-esteem, 222
    seniors and, 222–227
    sexual concerns, 222
    pregnant clients, 210–214
    teaching and motivating, 205
Advicor (lovastatin + niacin), 122
Aerobic exercise, 46
    children and teens, 47
    defined, 47
    Diabetes Prevention Program (DPP), 48
    weight-bearing exercises, 47
Aerobic monitors, 59
Afrezza, 89
Albumin, 134
Alcohol, 200
    hypoglycemia, 41
    Johns Hopkins White Papers: Nutrition and Weight Control, 40
Alcoholic beverages, 121
Aldomet (methyldopa), 212
Alfuzosin (Uroxatral), 125
Alpha-blockers, 125
Alpha cells, 4–5
Alpha-glucosidase inhibitors, 63, 64, 67, 69, 70
Altace (ramipril), 124
Alveair, 89
Amaryl (glimepiride), 63, 64, 65, 130
American Cancer Society, 26, 37
American Diabetes Association (ADA), 54, 155, 156, 159, 215
American Heart Association, 26, 37
Americans with Disabilities Act Amendment Act (ADAAA) of 2008, 220